Marsh and Martin's Oral Microbiology

Dedications

To: Jane, Katherine, Thomas, Jonathan,
Heather, Christopher and Andrew
Mike, Ben and Sam
Lorna, Daniel, Ailish, Calum and Sioned
Andrew, Coren, Arran and Elinor

For Elsevier

Content Strategist: Alison Taylor
Content Development Specialist: Veronika Watkins
Project Manager: Andrew Riley
Designer/Design Direction: Christian Bilbow
Illustration Manager: Karen Giacomucci/Amy Naylor
Illustrator: MacPS

6th Edition

Marsh and Martin's Oral Microbiology

Professor Philip D. Marsh BSc, PhD
Chief Scientific Leader, Public Health England, Salisbury, UK; Professor
of Oral Microbiology, School of Dentistry, University of Leeds, UK

Professor Michael A. O. Lewis PhD, BDS, FDSRCPS, FDSRCS (Ed and Eng), FRCPath, FHEA, FFGDP(UK)
Professor of Oral Medicine and Dean, School of Dentistry, College of
Biomedical and Life Sciences, Cardiff University, Heath Park, Cardiff, UK

Dr Helen Rogers, MB ChB BDS BSc MFDS FDS (OMed) RCS Eng
Consultant and Honorary Senior Lecturer in Oral Medicine, University of Bristol Dental
Hospital, Bristol, UK

Professor David W. Williams BSc (Hons), PhD
Professor of Oral Microbiology, School of Dentistry, College of Biomedical and Life
Sciences, Cardiff University, Heath Park, Cardiff, UK

Dr Melanie Wilson BSc (Hons), BDS, PhD, FDSRCS, FRCPath
Senior Lecturer and Honorary Consultant in Oral Microbiology, School of Dentistry,
College of Biomedical and Life Sciences, Cardiff University, Heath Park, Cardiff, UK

Illustrations by MacPS

ELSEVIER

Edinburgh   London   New York   Oxford   Philadelphia   St Louis   Sydney   Toronto   2016

ELSEVIER

First Edition 1980
Second Edition 1984
Third Edition 1992
Fourth Edition 1999
Fifth Edition 2009
Sixth Edition 2016

ISBN 978-0-7020-6106-6

British Library Cataloguing in Publication Data
A catalogue record for this book is available from the British Library

Library of Congress Cataloging in Publication Data
A catalog record for this book is available from the Library of Congress

ELSEVIER your source for books, journals and multimedia in the health sciences

www.elsevierhealth.com

  Working together to grow libraries in developing countries

www.elsevier.com • www.bookaid.org

The publisher's policy is to use paper manufactured from sustainable forests

Contents

Preface

The aim of the latest edition of this successful textbook continues to be to describe the complex relationship between the resident oral microbiota and the host in health and disease. The Sixth Edition has been completely rewritten and updated, but retains its philosophy of explaining this relationship in ecological terms. This approach is of benefit to the reader by providing a clear set of principles to explain the underlying issues that determine whether or not the microbiota will have a beneficial or an adverse relationship with the host at a particular site. This information provides a foundation that can be exploited by research workers or health professionals to understand, prevent or control disease.

This new edition reflects the impact that the genomic era has had on the subject area. The application of molecular biology techniques has revolutionised our knowledge of the richness and diversity of the microorganisms that can be found in the mouth and highlighted that, even with the most sophisticated of techniques, only around 50% to 70% of the microbiota can be cultured in the laboratory. These molecular approaches have also implicated the involvement of complex consortia of microorganisms in the aetiology of oral diseases. This edition includes new sections on the benefits of the resident oral microbiota to the host, and on current concepts of factors driving dysbiosis in periodontal disease. There is a new chapter on the emerging role of oral microorganisms in systemic diseases, while contemporary views on therapeutic and prophylactic antibiotic use, and on infection control, have been expanded.

This new edition builds on the success of previous ones, and provides an even more comprehensive coverage of the field of oral microbiology. The layout of the book has been revamped, with Key Points highlighted throughout for ease of learning, and each Chapter now has a set of Multiple Choice Questions to assist with self-learning. The book will be suitable for undergraduate and postgraduate students, research workers and a wide range of clinical dental professionals.

Phil Marsh
Mike Lewis
Helen Rogers
David Williams
Melanie Wilson

Acknowledgements

We would like to thank the many colleagues who gave permission to reproduce figures used in previous editions, and to Mike Curtis, Deirdre Devine, Thuy Do, Josephine Meade, Wendy Rowe, Kirsty Sands, Owain Dafydd Thomas, Adam Jones, and William Wade who provided new information or images for the Sixth Edition. The authors would also like to acknowledge the legacy contributions from previous editions by Dr Mike Martin. Particular thanks also go to our families who have supported us throughout the preparation of this edition, and the publishers for their helpful contributions.

Introduction

Oral health is inextricably linked to general health, and vice versa. Evidence continues to accumulate that demonstrates that the microorganisms that inhabit the mouth have a crucial function in the normal development of the physiology of the oral cavity, and play a wider role in maintaining the well-being of the host.

The mouth is the gateway of the body to the external world and represents one of the most biologically complex sites in the body. This is where the first stages of the digestive process take place and consequently, the mouth is richly endowed with sensory functions (taste, smell, temperature and texture). It also plays a critical role in communication, whether by speech or facial expressions, and makes a significant contribution to our appearance. Maintaining a healthy mouth is therefore of vital importance for a person's self-esteem and general health.

The mouth is an easily accessible part of the body and so can provide healthcare workers with a 'window' into a person's oral and general health. Disease that is localised elsewhere in the body can be reflected in the mouth and as a result, saliva is becoming increasingly recognised as a key diagnostic fluid. For example, oral candidosis (Chapter 8) in previously healthy young adults can be the first sign of human immunodeficiency virus (HIV) infection, while antibodies against a range of viruses can be detected in saliva. Risk factors for general health, such as tobacco habits, alcohol abuse and an inadequate diet, can also have a deleterious effect on oral health whereas, in an analogous manner, oral disease can also impact on the overall health of the individual. Recent studies suggest that severe periodontal disease in some populations might be a risk factor for premature or low birth weight babies, heart disease, pulmonary disease, rheumatoid arthritis, some forms of cancer and diabetes mellitus (see later, and Chapter 11).

The mouth is one of the key interfaces between the body and the external environment and can act as a site of entry for some microbial pathogens, especially from the air or via ingestion when eating. Therefore, it is equipped with a comprehensive array of defence strategies that includes elements of both the innate and adaptive immune system (see Chapter 2). Indeed, the ability of the host to recognise and respond to invading pathogens while simultaneously tolerating a diverse resident microbiota (see Chapter 3) remains one of the most remarkable feats of evolution, and the precise mechanisms that permit this level of discrimination are still not fully understood.

HUMAN MICROBIOTA

It has been estimated that the human body is made up of over 10^{14} cells of which only around 10% are mammalian. The remainder are the microorganisms that comprise the resident human microbiota. The **microbiota** is the term used to define the full complement of microorganisms at a particular location. Another term is the **microbiome**, which describes the microbiota and its collective genetic material at a site on the human body, or elsewhere.

The resident human microbiota does not have merely a passive relationship with its host, but contributes directly and indirectly to the normal development of the physiology, nutrition and defence systems of the organism. In general, the human microbiota exists in harmony with the host and both parties benefit from the association (**symbiosis**). Loss or perturbation of the resident microbiota can lead to colonisation by exogenous (and often pathogenic) microorganisms, thereby predisposing sites to disease, and have a deleterious impact on aspects of the physiology of the host (see later, and Chapter 4).

The human genome is made up of approximately 23 000 genes, but collectively the human microbiome has more than 1 million genes. At present, only about 50–70% of the human microbiota can be cultured in the laboratory. Molecular (culture-independent) studies have shown that although the composition of the microbiota varies at specific body sites in healthy individuals, the metabolic functions of each microbiota are similar. Once formed, the composition of each microbiota in a person at a particular site is relatively

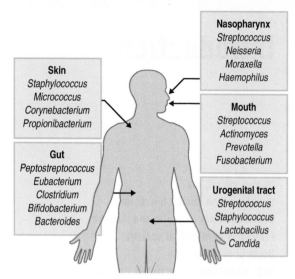

FIGURE 1.1 Distribution of the resident human microbiota. The predominant groups of microorganism at some distinct anatomical sites are listed.

stable over time, and the variation within a person over time at each site is less than subject-to-subject variation at equivalent sites.

The microbial colonisation of all environmentally accessible surfaces of the body (both external and internal) begins at birth. Such surfaces are exposed to a wide range of microorganisms originating from the environment and from other persons. However, because of differences in physical and biological properties, each surface is suitable for colonisation by only a proportion of these microbes. This results in the acquisition, selection and natural development of a diverse but characteristic microbiota at distinct sites (Fig. 1.1). For example, staphylococci and micrococci predominate on the skin surface, but rarely become established in significant numbers in the mouth of a healthy person. Similarly, less than 30 out of over 700+ types of microorganisms that can be found in the mouth are able to colonise the gastrointestinal tract, despite the continual passage (by the swallowing of saliva) of these microbes to the gut. Furthermore, the predominant species of bacteria can differ markedly at distinct surfaces in the mouth despite these organisms having equal opportunities to colonise each site, and this is again because of subtle variations in

KEY POINTS

> Humans are made up of ten times more microbial cells than mammalian cells. These microorganisms form the 'human microbiota' and confer essential benefits to the host. The composition of the microbiota varies at distinct surfaces in the body and is characteristic of that site. This demonstrates that the microbiota is directly influenced by the local environment that prevails at each site and surface, and is responsive to change.

key parameters than influence microbial growth and competitiveness (see Chapter 4).

BENEFITS OF THE HUMAN MICROBIOTA

Contemporary microbiological studies continue to identify mechanisms by which our natural human microbiota is contributing actively to the well-being and normal development of the host. Most information has been obtained from studies of the gut microbiota. These microbial consortia have been shown to:

- aid the digestion of otherwise indigestible dietary compounds;
- synthesise beneficial compounds, such as B vitamins (folic acid, biotin) and vitamin K;
- metabolise potentially harmful compounds such as bile acids, cholesterol, nitrosamines, etc.;
- generate short chain fatty acids from the metabolism of dietary polysaccharides which act as key energy sources for the human colonic mucosa;
- prevent colonisation by exogenous microorganisms (colonisation resistance); and
- promote the development of a competent immune system, and modulate proinflammatory pathways.

Bacterially-generated short chain fatty acids contribute up to 10% of the daily calorific needs of the host; in particular, colonocytes derive 60% to 70% of their energy needs from butyrate, which is a common end product of bacterial metabolism in the gut, and which may also be anticarcinogenic. These interactions are important for gut mucosal renewal and gut motility, and they also promote the development of villi and capillary networks in the villi.

Humans exist in a state of natural balance (homeostasis) with their microbiota, but a shift in this balance can lead to a deleterious relationship developing; this process is termed **dysbiosis**. In the gut, this can result in inflammatory bowel diseases (e.g., ulcerative colitis and Crohn's disease), and colorectal cancer. Changes to the composition and metabolism of the gut microbiota are also linked to obesity and insulin resistance. Thus the resident human microbiotas are not mere passengers on our mucosal surfaces, but are an integral and intimate part of our make-up; they play an essential role in promoting general health and in ensuring our normal physiological development.

ORAL MICROBIOTA IN HEALTH AND DISEASE

The mouth is similar to other sites in the body in having a natural microbiota with a characteristic composition and existing for the most part in a harmonious and positive relationship with the host, where it provides numerous benefits (see Chapter 4) in an analogous manner to that outlined previously for the gut microbiota. The oral microbiota is described in detail in Chapter 3 and its intraoral distribution is presented in Chapter 4. However, and perhaps more commonly than elsewhere in the body, this relationship can break down in the mouth (dysbiosis) and disease can occur. This is usually associated with:

- major changes to the biology of the mouth from exogenous sources (examples include: antibiotic treatment or the frequent intake of fermentable carbohydrates in the diet) or from endogenous changes such as alterations in the integrity of host defences following drug therapy, which perturb the natural stability of the microbiota;
- failure of oral hygiene practices to maintain the oral microbiota at levels compatible with health; or
- the colonisation of sites not normally accessible to oral microorganisms; for example, when oral bacteria enter the bloodstream following tooth extraction or other traumas and are disseminated to distant organs, where they can cause abscesses or endocarditis (Chapter 7), or more serious systemic conditions (Chapter 11).

Microorganisms with the potential to cause disease in this way are termed **opportunistic pathogens**, and many oral microorganisms have the capacity to behave in this manner. Indeed, most individuals suffer at some time in their life from localised episodes of disease in the mouth caused by imbalances (dysbiosis) in the composition of their resident oral microbiota. The commonest clinical manifestations of such imbalances are dental caries and periodontal diseases (see Chapter 6), both of which are highly prevalent in industrialised societies and are now on the increase in developing countries. Other acute and chronic infections occur but less frequently (see Chapter 7). Dental caries is the dissolution of enamel or root surfaces (demineralisation) by acid produced primarily from the metabolism of fermentable carbohydrates in the diet by bacteria colonising the tooth surface (dental plaque). Dental plaque is also associated with the aetiology of periodontal diseases in which the host mounts an inappropriate inflammatory response to an increased microbial load (caused by plaque accumulation) around the gingivae, resulting in damage to the supporting tissues of the teeth.

Caries and periodontal diseases pose distinct challenges when it comes to determining their microbial aetiology. These diseases occur at sites with a preexisting diverse, natural resident microbiota, although even more complex but distinct consortia of microorganisms are implicated with pathology. It is necessary, therefore, to determine which microbial species are implicated directly in active disease, which are present as a result of disease and which are merely innocent bystanders. Numerous studies have shown that these common diseases are caused by shifts in the balance of the resident microbiota, in which some minor components of dental plaque become predominant because of a change in local environmental conditions. These shifts in dental plaque composition in caries and periodontal disease are described in detail in Chapter 6.

PRINCIPLES OF MICROBIAL ECOLOGY

There is an intimate and dynamic relationship between the human microbiota and the host. The microbial composition of the microbiota varies on distinct surfaces (skin, mouth, gastrointestinal tract, etc.) because of the prevailing environmental conditions, but is reasonably stable over time on each of these surfaces. However, this stability (termed **microbial homeostasis**) can be perturbed if environmental conditions alter. Early studies showed that the occlusion of the forearm

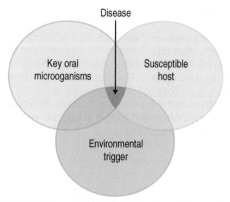

FIGURE 1.2 The interrelationships that lead to oral disease. Environmental triggers include a high sugar diet and antibiotic therapy, although host susceptibility might increase because of reduced saliva flow or immunosuppression.

(to increase local moisture levels and humidity) resulted in the skin microbiota increasing in number by several orders of magnitude, with a shift from a staphylococcal-dominated microbiota to one with high proportions of cutaneous corynebacteria. Thus the microbiome is responsive to changes in local environmental conditions, and follows ecological principles.

Dental diseases (including caries and periodontal diseases) result from a complex interaction of the environment (for example, the nature and frequency of the diet, and lifestyle factors such as smoking), the resident microbiota, and the host (Fig. 1.2). To determine the aetiology and biological mechanisms behind these diseases it is necessary to understand the factors that influence these interactions. This can be achieved by the application of the principles of microbial ecology. In this book, the relationships among oral microorganisms, and between these microorganisms and the host, will be explored. The general composition of the oral microbiota is well characterised, and more is now emerging regarding how the properties of the mouth influence the composition and metabolism of the resident microbiota in health and disease. The oral microbiota is in dynamic equilibrium with the host, and a change in a key parameter that influences microbial growth can perturb this equilibrium and determine whether the oral microbiota will have a symbiotic or dysbiotic relationship with the host.

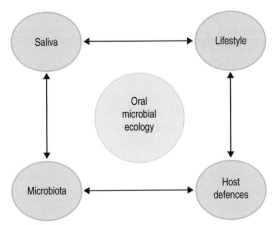

FIGURE 1.3 The interrelationships that influence the microbial ecology of the mouth in health and disease. The predominant microorganisms in the mouth might alter because of changes in saliva flow, lifestyle (e.g., tobacco habit, diet) or to changes in the integrity of the host defences. These changes may predispose sites to disease.

The philosophy of this textbook is that the key to a more complete understanding of the role of microorganisms in oral disease depends on a paradigm shift away from concepts that have been derived from studies of diseases with a simple and specific (perhaps single species) aetiology to an appreciation of ecological principles. Most diseases of the mouth have a polymicrobial (multiple species) aetiology. The ability of consortia of bacteria to cause disease depends on the outcome of various interactions both among the microbes themselves, and between these microorganisms and the host. It may be necessary, therefore, to take a more holistic approach when relating the oral microbiota to disease. The activity and behaviour of these microbes is intimately linked to other biological systems in the mouth (see Fig. 1.2 and Fig. 1.3). Thus, the composition and metabolism of bacteria at a site will be influenced by the flow rate and properties of saliva, the lifestyle of an individual (in particular, the presence of a tobacco habit, the nature of the diet and exposure to medication), and the integrity of the host defences. For example, the risk of caries may increase not only because of the frequent intake of fermentable carbohydrates in the diet, but also as a consequence of long-term medication for an unrelated medical complaint because a side effect of such treatment can be a reduced saliva flow. Similarly, smoking tobacco can impair the functioning of the host defences,

leading to a failure to control the growth of potentially pathogenic microorganisms. Oral fungal infections arise following the wearing of dentures, suppression of the host defences or antibiotic therapy that removes competing resident bacteria. Acceptance of such ecological principles can more readily explain the transition of the oral microbiota from a commensal to a pathogenic relationship with the host (dysbiosis), and also open up new opportunities for prevention, treatment and control.

Much of the terminology used in this book to describe events in microbial ecology will be as defined by Alexander (1971). The site where microorganisms grow is the **habitat**. A number of terms have been used to describe the characteristic mixtures of microorganisms associated with a site. These include the normal, indigenous or commensal microbiota, but some difficulties in nomenclature arise if any of the organisms are associated with disease on occasions. Alexander (1971) proposed that species found characteristically in a particular habitat should be termed **autochthonous** microorganisms. These multiply and persist at a site (with no distinction made regarding disease potential), and can be contrasted with **allochthonous** organisms which originate from elsewhere and are generally unable to colonise successfully unless the ecosystem is severely perturbed. Alternatively, a simpler approach has been to use the term **resident microbiota** to include the complete collection of microorganisms that are regularly isolated from a site; again, no distinction concerning disease potential is made.

The microbial species that comprise the local microbiota interact with one another and function as a **microbial community** (or **microbial consortium**) made up of populations of individual species or less well-defined groups (taxa); the properties of these communities is more than the sum of the component species. These microbial communities grow on oral surfaces in an organised manner to form complex structures termed biofilms (see Chapter 5). The significance of a biofilm lifestyle is that such microorganisms are more tolerant of antimicrobial agents and are less susceptible or accessible to the host defences. The microbiota in a specific habitat together with the biotic and abiotic surroundings with which these organisms are associated is known as the **ecosystem**. The **niche** is defined here as the function of an organism in a particular habitat. Thus, the niche is not the physical location of an organism, but is its role within the microbiota. This role is dictated by the biological properties of each microbial population. Species with identical functions in a particular habitat will compete for the same niche, although the coexistence of many species in a habitat is because of each population having a different role (niche) and thus avoiding competition.

Microorganisms that have the potential to cause disease are termed **pathogens**. As stated earlier, those that cause disease only under exceptional circumstances are described as **opportunistic pathogens**, and can be distinguished from **true** or **overt pathogens** which are consistently associated with a particular disease.

SCALE OF ORAL DISEASES

Although rarely life-threatening, oral diseases are a major problem for health service providers in developed countries because of their high prevalence within the general population and the huge costs associated with their treatment. These costs are increased still further by the treatment of a range of acute infections (predominantly dentoalveolar abscesses) and chronic conditions such as actinomycosis and fungal infections; these are described in Chapters 7 and 8, respectively. For example, the National Health Service (NHS) in the United Kingdom spent over £3 billion per annum on dental treatment between 2010 and 2011, and this figure increases to nearly £6 billion when the burgeoning private sector costs are included. Despite this investment, in a national survey of about 14000 children in England, Wales and Northern Ireland in 2013, 34% of 12-year-olds and 46% of 15-year-olds had dental caries in their permanent teeth, while nearly a third of 5-year-olds and nearly half of 8-year-olds had decay in their primary teeth. Rates of tooth decay were highest among children from deprived families. The commonest reason for primary-school aged children being admitted to hospital is to have multiple teeth extracted. Similar trends occur in other countries. Americans make about 500 million visits to dentists each year, and in 2010 an estimated $108 billion was spent on dental services, and yet dental caries still affects more than 25% of children aged 2- to 5-years-old, and 50% of those aged 12- to 15-years-old. Advanced periodontal diseases affect 4% to 12% of adults in America, whereas 25% of adults aged over 65 have no natural teeth. Untreated dental caries in permanent teeth was reported to be the most prevalent condition worldwide, with 2.4 billion people affected, whereas untreated caries in deciduous teeth was the tenth most prevalent condition, affecting 621 million children.

In general, dental health in developing countries is improving because of better oral hygiene, the use of more effective oral care products, and a greater awareness of dental disease among the general population. As a result, the incidence of dental caries has been falling in children over the past few decades. The World Health Organization (WHO) goal for 50% of 5-year-old children to have no caries has already been achieved by many countries. This has been accompanied by an increase in the number of people who retain their teeth into later life.

These trends should not induce a feeling of complacency; the increase in the number of teeth being kept means that susceptible sites and surfaces are at risk of dental disease (including caries) throughout the life of an individual. In Europe, 80% of older adults now have some natural teeth, and the average number of teeth retained by these individuals has also risen. Children who at present are enjoying low levels of decay will need to develop a lifestyle that embraces good oral hygiene, an appropriate diet and regular visits to dental professionals if they are to avoid problems later in life because of periodontal diseases or root surface caries.

Profound disparities in oral health exist within a population because of differences in socio-economic status and race or ethnicity; surveys show that around 80% of childhood caries is found in <20% of children in Europe, and similar trends exist elsewhere. There is evidence of a gradual increase in dental caries in urban areas of developing countries, probably as a result of changing dietary habits. Three-quarters of adults in some parts of the developing world have been found to suffer from periodontal disease. Few individuals in these communities take remedial action because of a general lack of awareness of the presence or consequence of such diseases. Advances in prevention

KEY POINTS

> Dental diseases are highly prevalent and are a huge economic burden to healthcare providers. Untreated caries in permanent teeth has been reported as being the most prevalent condition worldwide, affecting 2.4 billion people.
>
> Diseases such as caries and periodontal diseases are a consequence of imbalances in the normal oral microbiota (dysbiosis). Therefore understanding the dynamic relationships that exist between the host, the local environment, lifestyle and the oral microbiota (oral microbial ecology) is fundamental to educating patients and preventing disease, and can identify the risk factors that drive these deleterious changes in the microbiota.

could lead to a major reduction in the prevalence of these diseases, with the potential for massive savings in healthcare budgets.

ORAL MICROBIOTA AND SYSTEMIC DISEASE

The oral microbiota is generally considered only in the context of health and disease in the mouth, but evidence is accumulating that suggests that these microorganisms have an impact on the general health of an individual. In periodontal diseases for example, large numbers of Gram-negative bacteria accumulate around the roots of the teeth and produce virulence factors such as lipopolysaccharide (LPS), cytotoxic metabolites, and immunoreactive molecules. The host mounts an inflammatory response to the microbial insult, and prostaglandins and proinflammatory cytokines are produced. These bacterial and host factors can enter the bloodstream because of the high vascularity of the periodontium and can affect distant sites in the body.

Recent human epidemiological studies and animal experiments have demonstrated that periodontal diseases represent a previously unrecognised and potentially clinically significant risk factor for preterm low birth weight babies, either as a direct consequence of preterm labour or to premature rupture of membranes, although this has not been confirmed in all population groups. Furthermore, inflammatory changes associated with periodontal microorganisms can predispose to diabetes or affect glycaemic control. Additionally, oral microorganisms, including periodontal pathogens, can enter the bloodstream during transient bacteraemia, where they may play a role in the development and progression of atherosclerosis, thereby increasing the risk for coronary heart disease. Studies have also reported associations between oral bacteria and rheumatoid arthritis, inhalational pneumonia and colorectal cancer. The role of oral bacteria in systemic disease will be discussed in greater detail in Chapter 11.

The mouth may also affect general health by acting as a reservoir for opportunistic pathogens. Oral hygiene is poor among patients in intensive care, and dental plaque from these patients contains large numbers of potential respiratory pathogens. Aspiration of these pathogens (and bacteria implicated in periodontal disease; Chapter 6) into the lower respiratory tract can increase the likelihood of serious lung infection, especially in immunocompromised or elderly people. *Helicobacter pylori* is also detected in dental plaque on occasions, and this organism is strongly associated with chronic gastritis and peptic ulcers, and is a risk factor for gastric cancer. *H. pylori* is not a normal bacterial inhabitant of the mouth, and its presence may be associated with gastrooesophageal reflux. Its intermittent persistence in the mouth is linked with the presence of deep periodontal pockets, and this carriage may aid its transmission from person to person. Cystic fibrosis (CF) is often accompanied by lung infection caused by opportunistic pathogens such as *Pseudomonas aeruginosa, Haemophilus influenzae, Burkholderia cepacia* and staphylococci. Studies have shown that a number of oral sites in patients with CF can be colonised by *P. aeruginosa*, suggesting that the mouth could act as reservoir for this organism. Evidence of transfer of these bacteria to dental equipment has been reported, which highlights the need for effective cross-infection control strategies (Chapter 12).

The properties of the mouth that influence its function as a microbial habitat together with the major groups of microorganisms that reside there will be described in the next two chapters. Subsequent chapters will describe the acquisition and development of the oral microbiota (Chapter 4), especially dental plaque (Chapter 5). The remainder of the book will consider the role of the oral microbiota in disease, including infections in the mouth caused by exogenous microbes, and the role of the oral microbiota in systemic diseases (Chapter 11), and will describe strategies for infection control in the dental surgery (Chapter 12).

KEY POINTS

> Oral microorganisms can have an impact on the general health of an individual. Periodontal pathogens, together with the host's inflammatory response to subgingival bacteria, may be risk factors for cardiovascular disease, preterm or low birth weight babies, rheumatoid arthritis or diabetes. Oral bacteria can act as opportunistic pathogens at distant sites in the body, e.g., following entry to the bloodstream (bacteraemia) or aspiration into the lungs. Oral bacteria may be linked to some forms of cancer. The mouth may also act as a reservoir for pathogenic bacteria such as *Pseudomonas aeruginosa* and *Helicobacter pylori*, emphasising the need for effective infection control strategies in the dental surgery.

CHAPTER SUMMARY

The human body has ten times more microbial cells than human cells. These microorganisms make up the human microbiota; each body surface has a microbiota with a characteristic composition. The human microbiota is natural and beneficial and is essential for the normal development of the physiology and defence systems of the host. The mouth is similar to other surfaces of the body in having a resident microbiota with a characteristic composition that exists, for the most part, in harmony with the host, and which also delivers key benefits.

Components of the microbiota can act as opportunistic pathogens when the habitat is disturbed or when microorganisms are found at sites not normally accessible to them. Dental diseases are caused by imbalances in the resident microbiota (dysbiosis) and are highly prevalent and extremely costly to treat. Dental diseases may also act as risk factors for more serious medical conditions, such as heart and pulmonary disease, diabetes, poor birth outcomes and rheumatoid arthritis; the mouth can also act as a reservoir for exogenous pathogens such as *H. pylori* and *P. aeruginosa*, emphasising the need for effective infection control strategies.

Oral health has a strong influence on the quality of life of an individual and is more than merely preserving the integrity of the teeth and their supporting tissues. An understanding of the relationship between the oral microbiota and the host, and how this relationship can be perturbed by exogenous and endogenous factors (oral microbial ecology), is critical to understanding oral diseases and in developing new preventative strategies.

FURTHER READING

Alexander M. *Microbial ecology.* New York: John Wiley; 1971.

Bengmark S. Gut microbiota, immune development and function. *Pharmacol Res.* 2013;69:87-113.

Cho I, Blaser MJ. The human microbiome: At the interface of health and disease. *Nat Rev Genet.* 2012;13:260-270.

Dowsett SA, Kowolik MJ. Oral *Helicobacter pylori:* Can we stomach it? *Crit Rev Oral Biol Med.* 2003;14:226-233.

Hooper LV, Littman DR, Macpherson AJ. Interactions between the microbiota and the immune system. *Science.* 2012;336(6086): 1268-1273.

Kassebaum NJ, Bernabé E, Dahiya M, et al. Global burden of untreated caries: A systematic review and metaregression. *J Dent Res.* 2015;94:650-658.

Maddi A, Scannapieco FA. Oral biofilms, oral and periodontal infections, and systemic disease. *Am J Dent.* 2013;26:249-254.

Marsh PD. Are dental diseases examples of ecological catastrophes? *Microbiol.* 2003;149:279-294.

Olsen I. From the acta prize lecture 2014: The periodontal-systemic connection seen from a microbiological standpoint. *Acta Odontol Scand.* 2015;73:563-568.

Relman DA. The human microbiome: Ecosystem resilience and health. *Nutr Rev.* 2012;70(suppl 1):S2-S9.

Ruby J, Goldner M. Nature of symbiosis in oral disease. *J Dent Res.* 2007;86:8-11.

Wade WG. The oral microbiome in health and disease. *Pharmacol Res.* 2013;69:137-143.

Walker AW, Lawley TD. Therapeutic modulation of intestinal dysbiosis. *Pharmacol Res.* 2013;69:75-86.

Wilson M. *Microbial inhabitants of humans. Their ecology and role in health and disease.* Cambridge: Cambridge University Press; 2005.

Wilson M. *Bacteriology of humans: An ecological perspective.* Oxford: Blackwell; 2008.

Wade WG. New aspects and new concepts of maintaining 'microbiological' health. *J Dent.* 2010;(suppl 1):S21-S25.

Useful Links

National Dental Epidemiology Programme for England: Oral health survey of five-year-old children 2012.

A report on the prevalence and severity of dental decay. <www.nwph.net/dentalhealth/survey-results5.aspx?id=1>.

CDC. Oral health. Preventing cavities, gum disease, and oral cancers.

<www.cdc.gov/chronicdisease/resources/publications/aag/doh.htm>.

MULTIPLE CHOICE QUESTIONS

Answers on p. 249

1 *Which of the following statements is true about the resident microbiota of a host?*
a. The microbiota has a passive relationship with its host
b. Resident microbiota contributes directly to the normal development of the defence systems of the host
c. Resident microbiota is identical for each surface on an individual
d. Resident microbiota makes up around 10% of cells of the human body

2 *In microbial ecology, which of the following terms describes the site where microorganisms grow?*
a. Niche
b. Habitat
c. Ecosystem
d. Community

3 *The mouth can act, on occasions, as a reservoir for which of the following pathogens:*
a. *Helicobacter pylori*
b. *Pseudomonas aeruginosa*
c. Respiratory pathogens
d. All of the above

4 *The human body is estimated to be made up of 10^{14} cells; what proportion are microorganisms?*
a. <0.01%
b. 1%
c. 20%
d. 90%

5 *What is the term used to describe the growth of microorganism on a surface?*
a. Microbial community
b. Biofilm
c. Niche
d. Ecosystem

6 *Dental diseases can be a risk factor for which of the following systemic diseases?*
a. Diabetes
b. Cardiovascular disease
c. Inhalational pneumonia
d. All of the above

7 *What proportion of the oral microbiota can be cultured in the laboratory?*
a. 50-70%
b. 30-50%
c. 1-10%
d. 90-99%

8 *The composition of the human microbiota remains relatively stable over time, unless there is a change in environmental conditions. Which term is used to describe this stability?*
a. Microbial symbiosis
b. Microbial homeostasis
c. Dysbiosis
d. Colonisation resistance

CHAPTER 2

The mouth as a microbial habitat

MOUTH AS A MICROBIAL HABITAT

The properties of the mouth make it ecologically distinct from all other surfaces of the body, and this dictates the types of microbe able to persist. As a consequence, not all of the microorganisms that enter the mouth are able to colonise. Moreover, distinct habitats exist even within the mouth, each of which will support the growth of a characteristic microbiota because of their particular biological features. Habitats that provide obviously different ecological conditions include **mucosal surfaces** (such as the lips, cheek, palate and tongue), **teeth** and any introduced orthodontic or prosthodontic appliance (Table 2.1). The properties of the mouth as a microbial habitat are dynamic and will change over the life of an individual. During the first few months of life, the mouth provides only mucosal surfaces for microbial colonisation. The eruption of teeth provides a unique, hard non-shedding surface which enables much larger masses of microorganisms (dental plaque) to accumulate as biofilms. In addition, gingival crevicular fluid (GCF) is produced that can provide additional nutrients permitting the growth of the fastidious microorganisms found subgingivally. The ecology of the mouth will change over time because of the eruption or extraction of teeth, the insertion of orthodontic bands or dentures and any dental treatment including scaling and restorations. Transient fluctuations in the stability of the oral ecosystem may be induced by the frequency and type of food ingested, variations in saliva flow (e.g., certain medications impair saliva flow) and courses of antibiotic therapy.

Features that help to make the oral cavity distinct from other areas of the body are specialised mucosal surfaces, teeth, saliva and gingival crevicular fluid, while prosthetic devices will also create a novel environment. These will now be considered in more detail.

TABLE 2.1 **Distinct microbial habitats within the mouth**	
Habitat	**Comment**
Lips, cheek, palate	• biomass restricted by desquamation • some surfaces have specialised host cell types
Tongue	• highly papillated surface • acts as a reservoir for obligate anaerobes
Teeth	• non-shedding surface enabling large masses of microbes to accumulate (dental plaque biofilms) • teeth have distinct surfaces for microbial colonisation; each surface (e.g., fissures, smooth surfaces, approximal, gingival crevice) will support a distinct microbiota because of their intrinsic biological properties.

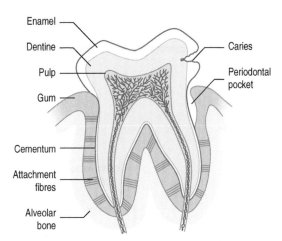

FIGURE 2.1 Tooth structure in health and disease.

MUCOSAL SURFACES

The mouth is similar to other ecosystems in the digestive tract by providing mucosal surfaces for microbial colonisation. The microbial load is relatively low on such surfaces because of the process of desquamation. However, the oral cavity has specialised surfaces which contribute to the diversity of the microbiota at certain sites. The papillary structure of the dorsum of the tongue provides refuge for many microorganisms which would otherwise be removed by mastication and salivary flow. Such sites on the tongue can develop a low redox potential (see later), which encourages the growth of obligately anaerobic bacteria. Indeed, the tongue can act as a reservoir for some of the Gram-negative anaerobes that are implicated in the aetiology of periodontal diseases (Chapter 6) and are responsible for malodour (Chapter 4). The mouth also contains keratinised (as in the palate) as well as non-keratinised stratified squamous epithelium which may influence the intraoral distribution of some microorganisms.

TEETH

The mouth is the only normally accessible site in the body that has hard non-shedding surfaces for microbial colonisation. Teeth do not appear in the mouth until after the first few months of life. The primary dentition is usually complete by the age of 3 years, and at around 6 years of age the permanent teeth begin to erupt; this process is complete by about 12 years of age. Local ecological conditions will vary during these periods of change, which in turn will influence the composition of the resident microbiota at a site.

Teeth (and dentures) allow the accumulation of large masses of microorganisms (predominantly bacteria) and their extracellular products, termed dental plaque. Plaque is an example of a biofilm (see Chapter 5) and, although it is found naturally in health and confers important benefits to the host, it is also associated with disease processes, including dental caries and periodontal disease. In disease, there is a shift in the composition of the plaque microbiota away from species that predominate in health (see Chapter 6).

Each tooth is composed of four tissues: **pulp, dentine, cementum** and **enamel** (Fig. 2.1). The pulp receives nerve signals and blood supplies from the tissues of the jaw via the roots. Thus, the pulp is able to nourish the dentine and to act as a sensory organ by detecting pain. Dentine makes up the bulk of the tooth and functions by supporting the enamel and protecting the pulp. Dentine is composed of bundles of collagen filaments surrounded by mineral crystals. Tubules run throughout the body of the dentine from the pulp to the dentine-enamel and to the dentine-cementum junctions. Enamel is the most highly calcified tissue in the body and is normally the only part of the tooth exposed to the environment. Cementum

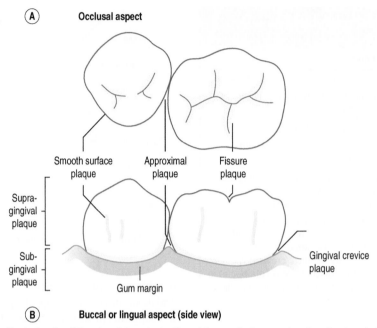

FIGURE 2.2 Diagram illustrating the different surfaces of a tooth and the terminology used to describe dental plaque sampling sites.

is a specialised calcified connective tissue that covers and protects the roots of the tooth. Cementum is important for the anchorage of the tooth; embedded in the cementum are the fibres of the periodontal ligament which anchor each tooth to the periodontal bone of the jaw. With ageing, recession of the gingival tissues can expose cementum to microbial colonisation and increase the risk of root surface caries (see Chapter 6).

The ecological complexity of the mouth is increased further still by the range of habitats found on the tooth. Teeth do not provide a uniform habitat and possess several distinct surfaces (Table 2.1, Fig. 2.2), each of which is optimal for colonisation and growth by different communities of microorganism. This is because of the physical nature of the particular surface and the resulting biological properties of the area. The stagnant areas between adjacent teeth (approximal) and in the gingival crevice afford most protection to colonising microorganisms from adverse conditions in the mouth. Both sites may become anaerobic and, in addition, the gingival crevice region is bathed by the nutritionally rich GCF (see later), particularly during inflammation. Consequently, the approximal region

and the gingival crevice often support a more diverse microbiota. Smooth surfaces are more exposed to the environment and can only be colonised by a limited number of bacterial species adapted to such extreme conditions. Pits and fissures of the biting (occlusal) surfaces of the teeth also offer protection from displacement forces such as saliva flow, and can contain impacted food debris as a source of nutrients. Protected areas on teeth are associated with the largest microbial communities and in general, the most disease.

The relationship between the environment and the microbial community is not unidirectional. Although the properties of the environment dictate which microorganisms can occupy a given site, the metabolism of the microbiota will modify the physical and chemical properties of their surroundings. To exemplify this, early colonisers will consume oxygen and release carbon dioxide and hydrogen to create an environment suitable for obligately anaerobic bacteria. Environmental conditions on the tooth also vary in health and disease (see Fig. 2.1). For example, as caries progresses, the advancing front of the lesion penetrates the dentine. This in turn means that nutritional sources will change and local conditions may become acidic and more anaerobic because of the accumulation of products of bacterial metabolism. Similarly, in disease the gingival crevice develops into a periodontal pocket and the flow of GCF is increased. These new environments will select for the microbiota most adapted to the prevailing conditions. This is a dynamic relationship with each change in the local environment invoking a new response by the resident microorganisms, which may drive a shift in the composition and metabolism of the microbiota.

SALIVA

The mouth is kept moist and lubricated by saliva which flows to form a thin film (approximately 0.1 mm deep) over all the internal surfaces of the oral cavity. Saliva enters the oral cavity via ducts from the major paired parotid, submandibular and sublingual glands as well as from the minor glands of the oral mucosa (labial, lingual, buccal and palatal glands) where it is produced. There are differences in the chemical composition of the secretions from each gland, but the complex mixture is termed 'whole saliva'. Saliva is mainly composed of water (99%) plus proteins (0.3%), inorganic molecules (0.2%), lipids and hormones. The average salivary flow rate is less than 1 mL per minute, but around 1.0 to 1.5 litres are produced daily. Saliva is multifunctional and plays a role in mastication, taste, digestion, swallowing and lubrication, as well as wound healing. Saliva also helps to maintain the integrity of teeth by protecting against demineralisation and promoting remineralisation, clearing food and by buffering potentially damaging acids produced by dental plaque following the metabolism of dietary carbohydrates. Bicarbonate is the major buffering component in saliva, but phosphates, peptides and proteins are also involved. The mean pH of saliva is between 6.75 and 7.25, although the pH and buffering capacity will vary with flow rate. Within the mouth, the flow rate and the concentration of components such as proteins, calcium and phosphate have circadian rhythms, with the slowest flow of saliva occurring during sleep. Thus, it is important to avoid consuming sugary foods or drinks before sleeping because the protective functions of saliva will be lowered at this time.

The major organic constituents of saliva are proteins and glycoproteins, including amylase, proline-rich proteins, statherin, histatins, cystatins, immunoglobulins and mucins. Over 2000 proteins (the salivary **proteome**) have been identified in whole saliva, although the function of many of these is still unknown.

Saliva plays a major role in both promoting colonisation and in removing microorganisms from the mouth. Saliva contains approximately 10^8 viable microorganisms per mL, which are derived from oral surfaces such as dental plaque and the tongue, but these organisms are unable to maintain themselves in saliva by cell division alone because they are lost at an even faster rate by **swallowing**, which is an important host defence mechanism. Paradoxically, saliva also plays an important role in facilitating microbial colonisation and the subsequent growth of microorganisms in the mouth. In these ways, saliva plays a pivotal role in determining which microorganisms form part of the resident oral microbiota, and which are inhibited and removed. Microbial attachment will be described in more detail in Chapters 4 and 5. Proteins and glycoproteins present in saliva can influence the oral microbiota by:

- adsorbing to the tooth surface to form a conditioning film (the acquired pellicle), which protects oral surfaces and provides receptors to which only certain microbes are able to attach (Chapter 5);
- acting as primary sources of nutrients (carbohydrates and proteins) for the resident microbiota;
- aggregating exogenous microorganisms, thereby facilitating their clearance from the mouth by swallowing; and
- inhibiting the growth of some exogenous microorganisms.

A comparison has been made of the proteome of whole saliva and plasma, and approximately 27% of the saliva proteins overlap with the plasma proteome. Perhaps importantly for the future, nearly 40% of plasma proteins that have been proposed as potential biomarkers for systemic diseases, such as cancer, cardiovascular disease and stroke, can be detected in saliva, which opens up the possibility of designing diagnostic kits for use with saliva to detect early signs of disease elsewhere in the body.

Other nitrogenous compounds provided by saliva include urea and numerous amino acids. Oral microorganisms require amino acids for growth, but not all

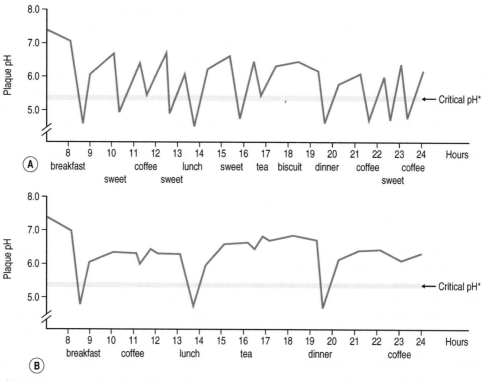

FIGURE 2.3 Schematic representation of the changes in plaque pH in an individual who (A) has frequent intakes of fermentable carbohydrate during the day, or (B) limits their carbohydrate intake to main meals only. *The critical pH is the pH below which demineralisation of enamel is enhanced.

of these are present free in saliva, and are obtained from salivary proteins and peptides by the action of microbial proteases and peptidases. The concentration of free carbohydrates is low in saliva, and most oral bacteria produce glycosidases to degrade the side-chains of host glycoproteins (see Fig. 5.11). The metabolism of amino acids, peptides, proteins and urea can lead to the net production of alkali, which contributes to the rise in pH following acid production after the dietary intake of fermentable carbohydrates (Fig. 2.3).

Antimicrobial factors, including lysozyme, lactoferrin and the sialoperoxidase system, are present in saliva (see later; Table 2.2) and play key roles in controlling bacterial and fungal colonisation of the mouth. Antibodies detected include secretory IgA (sIgA), which is the predominant class of immunoglobulin; IgG and IgM are also present, but in lower concentrations. A range of peptides with antimicrobial activity, including histidine-rich polypeptides (histatins), cystatins and defensins are also present in saliva. A fuller description of these antimicrobial peptides and a discussion of their role in controlling the resident oral microbiota can be found later in this chapter. The properties of saliva are fundamental to the maintenance of a healthy mouth, consequently, it is often referred to as the 'defender of the oral cavity'.

KEY POINTS

Saliva plays a fundamental role in maintaining oral health, being involved in lubrication, food clearance and buffering of microbial acids. It reduces demineralisation and promotes remineralisation of dental tissues. Saliva promotes the attachment and growth of selected microorganisms, as well as delivering components of both the innate and adaptive host response to restrict colonisation by other microbes.

TABLE 2.2 Specific and non-specific host defence factors of the mouth

Defence factor	Main function
Non-specific:	
Saliva flow and gingival crevicular fluid flow	Physical removal of loosely attached microorganisms
Mucin/agglutinins	Aggregation and physical removal of microorganisms
Lysozyme-protease-anion	Cell lysis
Lactoferrin	Iron sequestration
Apo-lactoferrin	Cell killing
Sialoperoxidase system	Hypothiocyanite production (neutral pH) Hypocyanous acid production (low pH)
Histatins	Antifungal with some antibacterial activity
Defensins (α- & β-)	Antimicrobial & immunomodulatory activity
Cystatins, SLPI & TIMP	Cysteine, serine & metalloprotease inhibitors
Chitinase & chromogranin	Antifungal
Cathelicidin	Antimicrobial
Calprotectin	Antimicrobial
Specific:	
Intraepithelial lymphocytes & Langerhans cells	Cellular barrier to penetrating bacteria and/or antigens
sIgA	Prevents microbial adhesion & metabolism
IgG, IgA, IgM	Prevent microbial adhesion; opsonins; complement activators
Complement	Activates neutrophils
Neutrophils/macrophages	Phagocytosis

IgA, Immunoglobulin A; *IgG*, immunoglobulin G; *IgM*, immunoglobulin M; *sIgA*, secretory Immunoglobulin A; *SLPI*, secretory leukocyte protease inhibitor; *TIMP*, tissue inhibitors of metalloproteinases.

GINGIVAL CREVICULAR FLUID (GCF)

Serum components can reach the mouth by the flow of a serum-like fluid through the junctional epithelium of the gingivae (Fig. 2.6). The flow of this GCF is relatively slow at healthy sites, but the rate increases in gingivitis and rises by many fold in advanced periodontal diseases. The GCF flow is part of the inflammatory response to the accumulation of biofilm around the gingival margin. GCF can influence the microbial ecology by:

- removing non-adherent microbial cells;
- introducing components of the host defences, especially antibodies and neutrophils; and
- acting as a novel source of nutrients for the resident microorganisms.

Many bacteria from subgingival plaque are proteolytic and interact synergistically to break down host proteins and glycoproteins to provide peptides, amino acids and carbohydrates for growth. Essential cofactors for growth, including haemin for black-pigmented anaerobes, can also be obtained from the degradation of haeme-containing molecules such as transferrin, haemopexin and haemoglobin.

The increased production of GCF during disease is associated with a rise in the pH of the periodontal pocket from approximately 6.90 in health to between 7.25 and 7.75 during inflammation in gingivitis and periodontal disease. Even such a modest change in pH can alter the competitiveness of individual bacteria, which can affect the proportions of bacteria, especially as the growth of some of the putative periodontal pathogens is favoured by an alkaline environment (Fig. 2.4). In addition, the activity of some proteases associated with the virulence of these opportunistic pathogens is enhanced at alkaline pH (7.5 to 8.0).

GCF contains components of the host defences, which play an important role in regulating the microbiota of the gingival crevice in health and disease. In contrast to saliva, IgG is the predominant immunoglobulin, with IgM and IgA present, as are complement proteins. GCF contains leukocytes, of which 95% are neutrophils, the remainder being lymphocytes and monocytes. A number of antimicrobial peptides and enzymes can be detected in GCF, including collagenases and elastases, which are derived both from phagocytic host cells (such as neutrophils) and subgingival bacteria. These enzymes can degrade host

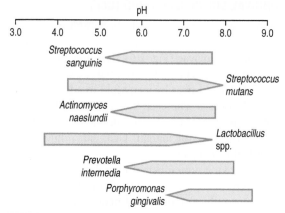

FIGURE 2.4 A diagrammatic representation of the pH range for growth of some oral bacterial species.

tissues and, therefore, contribute to tissue destruction (see Chapter 6). The composition of GCF is under evaluation for potential diagnostic markers of active periodontal breakdown for use in the clinic as chairside kits.

IMPLANTS AND PROSTHETIC DEVICES

As well as the oral tissues of the host, other surfaces that can support colonisation and growth of microorganisms include restorative materials, dental implants and orthodontic and prosthodontic appliances that are placed in the mouth. Such surfaces are rapidly coated with a conditioning film (see Chapter 5) originating from saliva or GCF, and generally it is to this conditioning film that the microorganisms attach. In addition, surface irregularities in the introduced biomaterial can provide sites for entrapment of microorganisms, and often the removal of these microorganisms is difficult because of limited access to the sites by host defence factors. Frequently, infection of oral tissues may follow the microbial colonisation of these biomaterial surfaces particularly if there is suboptimal oral hygiene. In the case of acrylic dentures, microbial colonisation, particularly by the fungus *Candida,* is associated with chronic erythematous candidosis (see Chapter 8). The upper denture fitting surface is generally poorly cleansed by saliva, and *Candida* growing on this surface provide a constant source of potentially infectious agents to the palate.

In recent years, an increasing number of dental implants are being placed in the mouths of patients to replace missing teeth and restore function. Titanium is perhaps the most frequently used biomaterial for implants because on its physical properties and inert nature. A key feature of titanium is the rapid development of titanium oxide on its surface that promotes osseointegration when placed within the bone, and this interaction with bone cells is a favourable process. However, microbial cells can also adhere to titanium and most frequently these are the microorganisms found in subgingival plaque. In healthy sites, bacteria belonging to the genera *Actinomyces, Streptococcus, Neisseria, Prevotella* and *Selenomonas* can be detected. In cases where growth of pathogens is favoured, inflammation of the tissues surrounding the implant may arise leading to periimplantitis (see Chapter 7).

KEY POINTS

The properties of the mouth that make it distinct from other microbial habitats in the body include the presence of teeth, saliva and gingival crevicular fluid (GCF).

Teeth are unique because they are non-shedding surfaces thereby permitting the accumulation of large masses of microorganisms and their products (dental plaque biofilms), especially at stagnant sites that offer protection from oral removal forces. Similarly, a range of biomaterials used to restore the dentition provide novel non-shedding surfaces and environments for significant levels of biofilm to form.

Saliva and GCF provide components of the host defences and are also important sources of nutrients for microorganisms, while saliva also acts as a buffer to maintain a favourable pH for oral health. Saliva also supports the growth of many resident bacteria that have properties that are beneficial to the host.

FACTORS AFFECTING THE GROWTH OF MICROORGANISMS IN THE ORAL CAVITY

Many factors influence the growth of microorganisms, and those of particular relevance to the oral cavity will be considered in the following sections.

TEMPERATURE

The human mouth is kept at a relatively constant temperature (35° to 36°C), which provides stable conditions suitable for the growth of a wide range of microorganisms. Periodontal pockets with active disease (inflammation) have a higher temperature (up to 39°C) compared with healthy sites. Even such relatively small rises in temperature can significantly alter bacterial gene expression and possibly the competitiveness of individual species.

REDOX POTENTIAL/ANAEROBIOSIS

Despite the accessibility of the mouth to air with an oxygen concentration of approximately 20%, the oral microbiota comprises few, if any, truly aerobic (oxygen-requiring) species. The majority of organisms are either facultatively anaerobic (can grow in the presence or absence of oxygen) or obligately anaerobic (require reduced conditions, as oxygen is toxic to these organisms). In addition, there are some capnophilic (CO_2-requiring) and microaerophilic species (requiring low concentrations of oxygen). Anaerobiosis is frequently described in rigid terms, and oral microorganisms are separated into aerobes and anaerobes on their ability to grow in the presence or absence of oxygen. However, a wide spectrum of oxygen tolerance exists among these organisms and sharp distinctions cannot be made between these groups.

Oxygen concentration is the main factor limiting the growth of obligately anaerobic bacteria. Oxygen is the commonest and most readily reduced electron acceptor in the majority of microbial habitats, and its presence results in the oxidation of the environment. Anaerobic species require reduced conditions for their normal metabolism; therefore it is the degree of oxidation-reduction (redox potential; Eh) at a site that governs the survival and relative growth of these organisms. In general, the distribution of anaerobes in the mouth will be related to the redox potential at a particular site, although some survive at overtly aerobic habitats by existing in close partnership with oxygen-consuming species. Obligate anaerobes also possess specific molecular defence mechanisms which enable them to cope with low levels of oxygen; these are described in Chapter 4.

The redox potential falls during plaque development on a clean enamel surface from an initial Eh of over +200 mV (highly oxidised) to −141 mV (highly reduced) after 7 days. The development of plaque in this way is associated with a specific succession of colonising microorganisms (Chapters 4 and 5). Early colonisers will use O_2 and produce CO_2, although later colonisers may produce H_2 and other reducing agents such as sulphur-containing compounds and volatile fermentation products. Thus, as the Eh is gradually lowered, sites become suitable for the survival and growth of a changing pattern of organisms, and particularly obligate anaerobes.

The Eh of the gingival crevice is normally around +70 mV but falls during inflammation associated with gingivitis to around −50 mV, while even lower values will occur in advanced periodontal disease (ca. −300 mV). Gradients of O_2 concentration and Eh will exist in the oral cavity, particularly in thick biofilms, and so dental plaque will be suitable for the growth of bacteria with a range of oxygen tolerances. The metabolism or properties of particular bacteria will be influenced by the Eh of the environment. The activity of intracellular glycolytic enzymes and the pattern of fermentation products of *Streptococcus mutans* varies under strictly anaerobic conditions. During glycolysis, sugars are converted into lactate under aerobic conditions, but formate, acetate and ethanol are generated in anaerobic environments. Therefore the perturbation of the redox potential at a site could have a significant impact on the composition and metabolism of the microbial community. This approach is being pursued as a strategy to control subgingival plaque in periodontal disease, for example, by using redox agents to raise the Eh and make conditions unfavourable for strictly anaerobic bacteria (see Chapter 6).

pH

Many microorganisms require a pH around neutrality for growth and are sensitive to extremes of acidity or alkalinity. The pH of most surfaces in the mouth is regulated by saliva; the mean pH for unstimulated whole saliva is between 6.75 and 7.25, thereby providing an optimal pH for microbial growth.

The mean pH varies at different oral sites in health. The highest pH is found on the palate (mean pH = 7.34 ± 0.38) and the lowest on the buccal mucosa (mean pH = 6.28 ± 0.36). The pH of the palate in patients with dentures tends to be lower than in control subjects, although the palatal pH is even higher in patients with lichen planus than healthy controls.

Shifts in the proportions of bacteria within dental plaque can occur following fluctuations in environmental pH. After sugar consumption, the pH in plaque can fall rapidly to below pH 5.0 by the production of acids (predominantly lactic acid) by bacterial metabolism (see Fig. 2.3); the pH then recovers slowly to resting values. Depending on the frequency of sugar intake, the bacteria in plaque will be exposed to varying challenges of low pH. Many of the predominant plaque bacteria that are associated with healthy sites can tolerate brief conditions of low pH, but are inhibited or killed by more frequent or prolonged exposures to acidic conditions, as occurs in subjects who commonly consume sugar-containing snacks or drinks between meals (see Fig. 2.3). This can result in the selection and enhanced growth of acid-tolerant (aciduric) species, especially mutans streptococci, *Bifidobacterium* and *Lactobacillus* species (see Fig. 2.4). Such bacteria are normally absent or only minor components in dental plaque at healthy sites, and this change in the bacterial composition of plaque predisposes a surface to dental caries. The acid tolerance of these bacteria is achieved by the possession of particular metabolic strategies and the induction of a specific set of stress response proteins (see Chapter 4).

In contrast, the pH of the gingival crevice can become alkaline during the host inflammatory response in periodontal disease, probably as a result of bacterial metabolism, e.g., ammonia production from urea and from the deamination of amino acids. The pH of the healthy gingival crevice is approximately 6.90 and rises to between 7.2 and 7.4 during disease, with a few patients having pockets with an even higher pH. This degree of change can increase the competitiveness of some putative pathogens, for example, by favouring the growth of pathogenic anaerobes such as *P. gingivalis* that have a pH optimum for growth of around 7.5 (see Fig. 2.4).

NUTRIENTS

Populations within a microbial community are dependent solely on the habitat for the nutrients essential for their growth. Therefore, the association of an organism with a particular habitat is direct evidence that all of the necessary growth-requiring nutrients are present. In Chapter 3 it will become apparent that the mouth can support a microbiota of great diversity and richness, and satisfy the requirements of many nutritionally-demanding bacterial populations.

(i) Endogenous nutrients

The persistence and diversity of the resident oral microbiota is caused primarily by the metabolism of the endogenous nutrients provided by the host, rather than by exogenous factors in the diet. The main source of endogenous nutrients is saliva, which contains amino acids, peptides, proteins and glycoproteins (which also act as a source of sugars and amino-sugars), and vitamins. In addition, the gingival crevice is supplied with GCF, which not only delivers components of the host defences, but also provides potentially novel nutrients, such as albumin and other host proteins and glycoproteins, including haeme-containing molecules. This explains the differences in the microbiota of the gingival crevice compared with other oral sites (Chapters 4 and 5).

The importance of endogenous nutrients can be gauged from the persistence of a relatively diverse microbiota in the mouths of humans and animals fed by intubation (stomach tube). The proportions of the *S. mitis*-group of bacteria increase in the saliva of children on a starvation diet before bone marrow transplantation, and in these cases the streptococci satisfy their nutritional and energy requirements primarily from the metabolism of host glycoproteins. In addition, the oral microbiota of animals with dietary habits ranging from insectivores and herbivores to carnivores is broadly similar at the genus level.

Oral microorganisms interact synergistically to break down these endogenous nutrients as few species have the full enzyme complement to independently fully catabolise these structurally complex molecules. Individual organisms possess different but overlapping patterns of enzyme activity (glycosidases, proteases, peptidases, etc.), so that they cooperate and interact with species with complementary degradative activities to achieve complete breakdown of these substrates (Chapter 4).

The oral microbiota may be influenced by changes in hormone levels, for example, during puberty and in pregnancy. The hormones could be used as a novel nutrient source by fastidious bacteria, including some obligately anaerobic species, such as *Prevotella* species. An increase in *Prevotella intermedia* and *Prevotella nigrescens* during pregnancy has been reported in some (but not all) studies, and these changes have been associated with the characteristic gingival inflammation seen during the second trimester (pregnancy gingivitis) (see Chapter 6).

(ii) Exogenous (dietary) nutrients

Superimposed upon these endogenous nutrients is the complex array of foodstuffs ingested periodically in the diet. There was no major difference in the oral microbiota when saliva was compared between healthy subjects on omnivore, ovo-lacto-vegetarian and vegan diets, confirming the importance of endogenous nutrients to the persistence of oral microorganisms, although there were diet-specific biomarkers that could discriminate among the individuals on the basis of their diet.

Fermentable carbohydrates are the only class of compound that markedly influences the ecology of the mouth. These carbohydrates can be broken down to acids, although additionally, sucrose can be converted by bacterial enzymes (glucosyltransferases [GTF], and fructosyltransferases [FTF]) into two main classes of exopolymer (glucans and fructans) which can be used to consolidate attachment or act as extracellular nutrient storage compounds, respectively (Chapter 4).

The frequent consumption of dietary carbohydrates is associated with a shift in the proportions of the microbiota of dental plaque. The levels of acid-tolerating species, especially mutans streptococci and lactobacilli increase, while the growth of acid-sensitive species (e.g., some strains of *Streptococcus sanguinis* and *S. gordonii*) is inhibited. The metabolism of plaque changes so that the predominant fermentation product becomes lactate. Such alterations to the microbiota and its metabolism can predispose a site to dental caries.

Dairy products (milk, cheese) have limited influence on the ecology of the mouth. Milk can modify the structure of the enamel pellicle *in vivo*, producing a distinct globular structure. Cheese has been shown to increase salivary flow rates and to rapidly elevate plaque pH following a sucrose rinse.

Nitrate in green vegetables influences the host environment and microbiota. Nitrate derived from the diet is concentrated by salivary glands so that salivary concentrations are higher than plasma. This nitrate is reduced to nitrite by oral facultatively anaerobic bacteria, which reduces blood pressure and stimulates

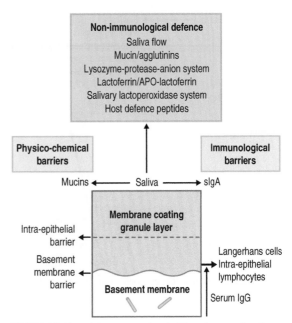

FIGURE 2.5 Host defences associated with oral mucosal surfaces.

mucus production. Nitrite is then acidified in the stomach and converted to nitric oxide, which also has beneficial functions for the host and is also antimicrobial (see Chapter 4).

HOST DEFENCES

The health of the mouth is dependent on the integrity of the mucosa and enamel, which act as physical barriers to prevent penetration by microorganisms or antigens (Fig. 2.5). The host has a number of additional defence mechanisms which play essential roles in maintaining the integrity of these oral surfaces, and these are listed in Table 2.2 and their spheres of influence are indicated diagrammatically in Figs 2.5 and 2.6. These defences are divided into innate (non-specific) and adaptive (specific) immunity. The former do not require prior exposure to an organism or antigen for activity and so provide a continuous, broad spectrum of protection.

(i) Innate immunity

As discussed earlier, the flow of saliva can remove loosely adherent bacteria from oral surface. Desquamation ensures that the microbial load on most

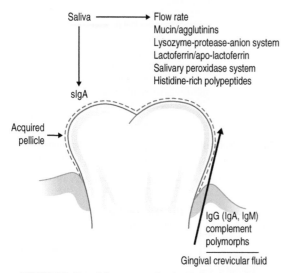

Saliva ──────► Flow rate
            Mucin/agglutinins
            Lysozyme-protease-anion system
            Lactoferrin/apo-lactoferrin
            Salivary peroxidase system
            Histidine-rich polypeptides

sIgA

Acquired ──►
pellicle

IgG (IgA, IgM)
complement
polymorphs

Gingival crevicular fluid

FIGURE 2.6 Host defences associated with the tooth surface.

mucosal surfaces is controlled. The ability of microorganisms to attach firmly to oral surfaces and evade removal from the mouth by swallowing is a fundamental survival strategy. Saliva also contains an array of molecules that can regulate the oral microbiota. **Mucins** are high-molecular-weight glycoproteins containing more than 40% carbohydrate that can agglutinate microorganisms. Their protein backbone has oligosaccharide side chains of different lengths and composition; some of these side chains are branched and sialic acid and fucose are common terminal sugars. Two chemically distinct mucins have been identified in human saliva and are termed mucin glycoproteins 1 and 2 (MG1 and MG2, respectively); MG1 has a molecular weight greater than 103 kDa whereas MG2 is only 130 to 150 kDa. These mucins not only agglutinate oral bacteria, but they can also interact with exogenous pathogens such as *Staphylococcus aureus* and *Pseudomonas aeruginosa*, as well as viruses (e.g. influenza virus), which facilitates their removal by swallowing. Mucin binding to bacteria appears to involve blood group reactive components such as *N*-acetylgalactose and sialic acid. Mucins such as MG2 may interact with other salivary components, including secretory IgA, to enhance their antimicrobial activities. A related molecule (salivary agglutinin; molecular weight 340 kDa) is also highly glycosylated and carries

blood group active antigens, and is similar to another defence glycoprotein present in the lung.

Lysozyme is a 14 kDa basic protein that can aggregate both Gram-positive (including streptococci) and Gram-negative (including periodontal pathogens) bacteria, and can also lyse bacteria by hydrolysing peptidoglycan, the component that confers rigidity to their cell walls. At acidic pH, the lytic action of lysozyme is enhanced by monovalent anions (bicarbonate, fluoride, chloride or thiocyanate) and proteases found in saliva. **Chitinase** has been detected in saliva and may function by attacking yeast cell walls. Iron is essential for microbial growth and the host will avidly sequester this cation using high-affinity, iron-binding proteins such as **lactoferrin** (MW = 75 kDa). Iron-free lactoferrin (**apolactoferrin**) can be bactericidal to a range of bacteria, although direct binding of the protein to the cell surface is necessary. Lactoferrin is a multifunctional protein having bacteriostatic, bactericidal, fungicidal, antiviral and antiinflammatory and immunomodulatory properties.

The salivary peroxidase enzyme system (**sialoperoxidase**) produces hypothiocyanite at neutral pH or hypothiocyanous acid at low pH in the presence of hydrogen peroxide (generated by *Streptococcus sanguinis* and *S. mitis*), and both inhibit glycolysis by plaque bacteria. Myeloperoxidase is found in polymorphonuclear leucocytes (PMNLs), which migrate into the gingival crevice as part of the inflammatory host response to plaque accumulation and may contribute to the total peroxidase activity measured in saliva.

A complex mixture of over 45 **antimicrobial peptides** (also referred to as **host defence peptides** because their effects can also be immunomodulatory) has been identified in saliva and some are also found in GCF. Examples of such antimicrobial peptides include histatins and defensins. Antimicrobial peptides are small, cationic peptides (often <50 amino acids) that can act synergistically with other innate defence molecules to not only inhibit exogenous pathogens, but also to provide a means by which the host can exert some control over the resident oral microbiota. These peptides also bind and neutralise potentially inflammatory molecules found on the surface of microbes (such as lipopolysaccharide [LPS]) and are chemotactic for host defence cells (neutrophils and lymphocytes). In this way antimicrobial peptides can play an important immunomodulatory role.

Histatins are a family of histidine-rich, basic peptides found in human parotid and submandibular/sublingual salivary glands. The major histatins found in saliva are histatins 1, 3 and 5. There are numerous other histatins, the majority of which are degradation fragments of two parent molecules, histatin 1 and histatin 3. Individual histatins may have distinct roles, or may function optimally under specific conditions. Histatins can also inhibit host and bacterial proteases and adhesins, and prevent induction of cytokines by bacterial outer membrane proteins. Overall, these peptides have a broad spectrum of antifungal and antibacterial activity, and have properties that may serve to link the innate and the acquired immune system.

Defensins are a family of antibacterial peptides with a broad spectrum of antibacterial, antifungal and antiviral (including human immunodeficiency virus [HIV]) activity. Some are expressed constitutively (e.g., human β-defensin-1) in salivary glands, whereas others are induced by bacteria and inflammatory mediators. Human β-defensins (HBDs) protect mucosal surfaces, including the gingivae, buccal mucosa and the tongue. HBDs can be associated with mucin, which may protect them from degradation and facilitate their contact with mucin-aggregated bacteria. HBDs have also been detected in saliva, GCF and gingival junctional epithelium, probably because of release from host phagocytic and other defence cells such as neutrophils, macrophages, monocytes and dendritic cells. **Cathelicidin** (LL-37 peptide) is another antimicrobial peptide that is secreted by epithelial cells and is also found in neutrophils. LL-37 can bind inflammatory molecules such as bacterial lipopolysaccharides, and it also acts as a chemoattractant for monocytes, T-cells and neutrophils. This has led to the proposal that LL-37 and other antimicrobial peptides might function as **alarmins**; that is, they activate other components of the innate and adaptive immune response. **Cystatins** are a diverse group of cysteine protease inhibitors; their roles include the control of proteolytic activity, either from the host, such as proteases released during inflammation, or from microorganisms. Other inhibitory proteins include:

- **secretory leucocyte proteinase inhibitor** (SLPI), which inhibits several proteases involved in inflammatory tissue destruction. SLPI also has antimicrobial and antiviral properties;
- **tissue inhibitors of metalloproteinases** (TIMPs);
- **calprotectin** (a calcium- and zinc-binding protein which can inhibit bacterial growth);
- **parotid secretory protein, PSP,** (PSP belongs to a family of oral and airway proteins that are related to Palate, Lung and Nasal epithelial Clone, PLUNC). PSP has multiple functions including the ability to aggregate bacteria and bind LPS; and
- **chromogranin A** (with antifungal properties).

Synthetic analogues of antimicrobial peptides are being investigated in novel strategies to inhibit specific oral microbes, and as immunomodulatory therapeutics.

KEY POINTS

> The mouth has many components of the innate host defences. These include: mucins, agglutinins, lysozyme, lactoferrin, sialoperoxidase, histatins, defensins, cathelicidin and cystatins. These molecules often work together synergistically.

(ii) Adaptive immunity

Components of the specific host defences (intra-epithelial lymphocytes and Langerhans cells, immunoglobulins: IgG and IgA) are found on and within the mucosa (see Fig. 2.5), where they act as barriers to penetrating antigens. The predominant immunoglobulin in the healthy mouth is secretory IgA (sIgA), which is produced by plasma cells in the salivary gland. Secretory IgA is composed of IgA heavy and light chains (300 kDa), secretory component (70 kDa) and the J chain (15 kDa). The J chain connects the two IgA molecules into a dimer, whereas the secretory component stabilises the molecule and reduces its susceptibility to attack by acids or general proteases. Secretory IgA can agglutinate oral bacteria, modulate enzyme activity and inhibit the adherence of bacteria to the buccal epithelium and to enamel. Secretory IgA is only weakly complement-activating and opsonising and is therefore less likely to cause damage to tissues by any indirect effect of an inflammatory response. Other components (IgG, IgM, IgA and complement) can be found in saliva but are almost entirely derived from GCF (Table 2.2) which also contains leukocytes, of which approximately 95% are neutrophils.

Specific antibody production can be stimulated by bacterial antigens associated with plaque at the gingival margin or on the oral mucosa. Salivary antibodies have been detected with activity against a range of oral bacteria, including streptococci, whereas circulating antibodies (particularly IgG) to a variety of oral microbial antigens are present, even in health. In the absence of inflammation, the naturally low levels of complement and neutrophils would reduce antibody-mediated phagocytosis, but antibodies might function by interfering with colonisation or by inhibiting metabolism. Combinations of the adaptive and innate host defence factors can function synergistically. For example, lysozyme and sIgA can react with salivary agglutinins (mucins) and be presented directly to immobilised cells. Other synergistic combinations include mucins or sIgA and salivary peroxidase.

Perhaps surprisingly, despite this rich array of antimicrobial factors, the mouth still supports a diverse microbiota, which confers many beneficial functions to the host.

KEY POINTS

> The mouth has components of the adaptive immune response. The predominant immunoglobulin is secretory IgA in saliva, whereas IgG is present in GCF along with complement and neutrophils.

HOST GENETICS

The oral microbiota can show considerable variation in composition both within and between individuals, which makes it difficult to study the effect of host genetics. The Human Microbiome project resulted in the identification of a 'core microbiome' that is common to all individuals, with the recognition that there can be considerable variation in the other genera present (accessory genome). Certain ethnic groups might harbour distinct microbial signatures. In a study of the microbiota in saliva and dental plaque of people living in the United States, potential pathogens belonging to the genera *Filifactor*, *Staphylococcus*, *Mycoplasma* and *Treponema* were found in higher levels in Chinese and Latin American populations than in other ethnic groups.

Studies of periodontal disease have suggested that gender, host genetics and ethnicity can influence disease susceptibility and possibly also affect the microbiota. The reasons for this are unknown but may reflect some variation in the local immune response. Interestingly, it would seem that the presence of some periodontal pathogens in individuals from different ethnic backgrounds is influenced by the length of time the parents have lived in their new host country, suggesting an important role for environmental factors. For example, in a US study, fewer potential periodontal pathogens were detected in children whose parents had been living in America for longer. Genetic polymorphisms associated with interleukin-1 (IL-1), or other cytokines, can increase the likelihood of detecting certain key periodontal pathogens and predispose individuals to periodontitis.

Young adults from Northwest Africa more commonly harbour *Aggregatibacter* (formerly *Actinobacillus*) *actinomycetemcomitans*, which is implicated in aggressive periodontitis (see Chapter 6). Adolescents who carried the serotype *b* strain had an 18-fold increased risk of developing localised aggressive periodontitis.

The subgingival microbiota of twins has also been compared. The microbiota of twin children living together was more similar than that of unrelated children of the same age. Further analysis showed that the microbiota of identical twins was more similar than that of fraternal twins, again suggesting some genetic influence. No differences in the number of species shared, nor in the composition of the oral microbiota, was found when supragingival and subgingival biofilms from monozygotic and dizygotic adult twin pairs were compared.

HOST LIFESTYLE

The lifestyle of an individual can have a profound impact on their personal oral microbiome. As was mentioned earlier, and which will be discussed in detail in Chapters 4 and 6, a diet that includes the frequent intake of dietary sugars results in the biofilm having regular and prolonged exposures to low pH (see Fig. 2.3). Such conditions select and enrich for bacteria that preferentially grow under acidic conditions, resulting in the biofilm having higher proportions of acid-producing and acid-tolerating species such as mutans streptococci, bifidobacteria and lactobacilli. This also increases the risk for developing dental caries. Smoking is a risk factor for periodontal diseases, and cross-sectional studies of the subgingival microbiota of periodontally-healthy smokers found more obligate anaerobes, more periodontal pathogens (e.g., *Filifactor alocis*, *Dialister* sp., *Fusobacterium nucleatum*, etc.) and fewer beneficial oral bacteria than matched non-smokers. Cessation of smoking can lead to a reduction in the levels or prevalence of these periodontal pathogens. Similarly, smoking also perturbs the subgingival microbiota in patients with implants, leading to a selection of putative periodontal pathogens, thereby increasing the risk of periimplantitis or periimplant mucositis.

CONCLUDING REMARKS

Despite the potential for regular environmental perturbations in some of the host and environmental factors described previously, once established at a site, the oral microbiota remains relatively stable in composition and proportions over time. This stability is termed **microbial homeostasis** and is discussed further in Chapter 5.

KEY POINTS

> The mouth provides conditions able to support the growth of a diverse collection of microorganisms (the oral microbiota), despite the presence of a complex array of components of the innate and adaptive host defences. The resident microbiota is provided with a wide range of endogenous and exogenous nutrients, together with sufficient heterogeneity in pH and redox potential, to accommodate microbes with a variety of requirements. The lifestyle of the individual (e.g., diet, and smoking) can adversely influence the composition of the oral microbiota.

CHAPTER SUMMARY

The mouth is not a uniform habitat for microbial growth and colonisation. A variety of surfaces produce distinct habitats because of their physical nature and biological properties. These include a diversity of mucosal surfaces, teeth and introduced restorative biomaterials. In the case of the latter two surfaces,

substantial biofilm formation (dental plaque) can arise by virtue of them being non-shedding surfaces.

The surfaces of the mouth are lubricated by saliva, whereas the gingival crevice is bathed with GCF. Both fluids will remove weakly attached microorganisms through their flushing action, and they deliver components of the innate and adaptive immune response that help regulate bacterial and fungal colonisation. Saliva and GCF contribute to the acquired pellicle and are also primary sources of nutrients for oral microorganisms. Consortia of different bacterial species with complementary patterns of glycosidase and protease activities are required to break down host glycoproteins. In this manner, saliva and GCF play pivotal roles in the microbial ecology of the mouth. Dietary components have less of an influence on the composition of the microbiota of the mouth, although the frequent intake of fermentable carbohydrates can lead to increases in acidogenic and acid-tolerating (aciduric) organisms that are potentially cariogenic because of the low pH generated from their catabolism, whereas dietary nitrate can be converted to nitrite and acidified nitric oxide, which have important beneficial properties for the host. Other factors that influence the growth of microorganisms in the mouth include the Eh (redox potential) and pH of a site, the integrity of the host defences and the lifestyle of the individual.

There is a dynamic interaction between the oral environment and the composition and metabolism of the resident oral microbiota. Therefore a substantial change in a key environmental parameter that affects microbial growth can disrupt the natural balance of the microbiota and select for organisms that are potentially pathogenic.

FURTHER READING

Baker OJ, Edgerton M, Kramer JM, et al. Saliva-microbe interactions and salivary gland dysfunction. *Adv Dent Res.* 2014;26:7-14.

De Filippis F, Vannini L, La Storia A, et al. The same microbiota and a potentially discriminant metabolome in the saliva of omnivore, ovo-lacto-vegetarian and Vegan individuals. *PLoS ONE.* 2014;9:e112373.

Devine DA, Cosseau C. Antimicrobial host defense peptides in the oral cavity. *Adv Appl Microbiol.* 2008;63:281-322.

Feller L, Altini M, Khammissa RA, et al. Oral mucosal immunity. *Oral Surg Oral Med Oral Pathol Oral Radiol.* 2013;116: 576-583.

Gorr S-U. Antimicrobial peptides in periodontal innate defense. *Front Oral Biol.* 2012;15:84-98.

Kakubovics NS. Saliva as the sole nutritional source in the development of multispecies communities in dental plaque. *Microbiol Spectr*. 2015;3:doi:10.1128/microbiolspec.

Kapil V, Haydar SMA, Pearl V, et al. Physiological role for nitrate-reducing oral bacteria in blood pressure control. *Free RadicBiol Med*. 2013;55:93-100.

Loo JA, Yan W, Ramachandran P, et al. Comparative human salivary and plasma proteomes. *J Dent Res*. 2010;89:1016-1023.

Marsh PD, Do T, Beighton D, et al. Influence of saliva on the oral microbiota. *Periodontol 2000*. 2016;70:80-92.

Mason MR, Nagaraja HN, Joshi V, et al. Deep sequencing identifies ethnicity-specific bacterial signatures in the oral microbiome. *PLoS ONE*. 2013;8:e77287.

Papapostolou A, Kroffke B, Tatakis DN, et al. Contribution of host genotype to the composition of health-associated supragingival and subgingival microbiomes. *J Clin Periodontol*. 2011;38:517-524.

Siqueira WL, Dawes C. The salivary proteome: Challenges and perspectives. *Proteomics Clin Appl*. 2011;5:575-579.

Tsigarida AA, Dabdoud SM, Nagaraja HN, et al. The influence of smoking on the peri-implant microbiome. *J Dent Res*. 2015;94:1202-1217.

van't Hof W, Veerman EC, Nieuw Amerongen AV, et al. Antimicrobial defense systems in saliva. *Monogr Oral Sci*. 2014;24:40-51.

Yoshizawa JM, Schafer CA, Schafer JT, et al. 2. Salivary biomarkers: Towards future clinical and diagnostics utilities. *Clin Microbiol Rev*. 2013;26:781-791.

MULTIPLE CHOICE QUESTIONS

Answers on p. 249

1 *The major buffering system in saliva is made of which of the following?*
- a. Bicarbonate
- b. Phosphates
- c. Peptides
- d. Proteins

2 *Microorganisms are unable to maintain themselves in saliva by cell division alone because of which of the following factors?*
- a. Chewing
- b. Gingival crevicular fluid (GCF) flow
- c. Swallowing
- d. Reduced saliva flow

3 *Which of the following are not innate host defence peptides?*
- a. sIgA
- b. Cystatins
- c. SLPI
- d. TIMP

4 *Which of the following is not part of the adaptive host response in the mouth?*
- a. IgG
- b. IgM
- c. IgA
- d. Lysozyme

5 *Which of the following is not a factor by which saliva influences the microbiota of the mouth?*
- a. Formation of a conditioning film
- b. Providing proteins and glycoproteins for bacterial growth
- c. Providing a neutral pH and acting as a buffer for microbial growth
- d. Delivering neutrophils and complement to kill microorganisms

6 *Which is the class of enzyme responsible for removing carbohydrates from the side chains of salivary mucins?*
- a. Glucosyltransferase
- b. Glycosidase
- c. Fructosyltransferase
- d. Amylase

7 Lactobacillus *species prefer to grow at which pH?*
- a. Neutral pH
- b. Acidic pH
- c. Alkaline pH
- d. All of the above

8 *Which is the predominant immunoglobulin in saliva?*
- a. IgA
- b. Secretory IgA
- c. IgG
- d. IgM

9 *The mouth is freely supplied with air; therefore, which of the following statements is* false?

a. The majority of oral microorganisms are aerobes

b. The majority of oral microorganisms are facultatively anaerobic

c. The oral microbiota includes many obligately anaerobic bacteria

d. The oral microbiota includes bacteria that are capnophilic

10 *Which of the following is the main source of nutrients for the oral microbiota?*

a. Dietary sugars

b. Dietary nitrate

c. Dairy products

d. Salivary glycoproteins

CHAPTER 3

The resident oral microbiota

The resident oral microbiota is diverse and consists of a wide range of viruses, mycoplasmas, bacteria, yeasts and even on occasions, protozoa and *Archaea*. The latter are prokaryotes that are distinct from bacteria and include methanogens. This microbial diversity is a reflection of the numerous and varied habitats present in the mouth that are supplied with a range of endogenous and exogenous nutrients. In addition, in biofilms such as dental plaque, gradients develop in parameters of ecological significance, such as oxygen tension and pH, providing conditions suitable for the growth and survival of microorganisms with a wide spectrum of requirements. Under such conditions, no single bacterial population has a particular advantage and numerous species can coexist. Plaque also functions as a true microbial community, and numerous examples of synergistic metabolic interactions occur. This will enable some fastidious bacteria to survive and grow when part of a consortium under conditions that they would be not be able to tolerate if in pure culture or in a more homogeneous environment. There are over 700 prokaryote species that have been isolated from the human oral cavity; approximately 49% are officially named, 17% unnamed (but cultivable) and 34% are known only as uncultivated phylotypes.

Before the microbial community at individual sites in the mouth can be considered in detail (Chapters 4 and 5), the types and properties of the organisms found commonly in health and disease will be described. Firstly, however, it is beneficial to discuss the principles of microbial classification and identification, and describe briefly some of the methods used. **Classification** is the arrangement of organisms into groups (taxa) on the basis of their similarities and differences. In contrast, **identification** is the process of determining whether a new isolate belongs to a particular taxon. The aim of classification is to define these taxa at the **genus** or **species** level. Traditionally, a hierarchical system is used for the naming of bacteria, so that groups of closely-related organisms form a species, and related species are placed in a genus and so on (Table 3.1). Species are designated by Latin or 'Latinised' binomials (e.g., *Streptococcus mutans*; the genus is *Streptococcus* and the species is *mutans*, Table 3.1). If an isolate does not belong to an existing taxon, then a new species can be proposed. The naming of bacteria to reflect this classification (**nomenclature**) is regulated by international committees. Once an organism has been placed in a species, it may be possible to subtype individual strains; this approach can be valuable in epidemiological studies such as those investigating transmission of organisms between individuals. The interrelationships between these approaches (classification, identification, strain typing) are shown in Fig. 3.1. The process of classification, nomenclature and identification of microorganisms is referred to as **taxonomy**, although, sometimes, the terms classification and taxonomy are used interchangeably.

TABLE 3.1 Hierarchical ranks in microbial classification

Taxonomic rank	Example
Kingdom	*Procaryotae*
Division	*Firmicutes*
Subdivision	low G + C content of DNA
Order	–
Family	*Streptococcaceae*
Genus	*Streptococcus*
Species	*Streptococcus mutans*
Serotype*	*Streptococcus mutans* serotype *c*
Strain*	*Streptococcus mutans* NCTC 10449**

*These ranks are not formally recognised in taxonomy but are of great practical importance.
DNA, Deoxyribonucleic acid; **NCTC*, = National Collection of Type Cultures.

KEY POINTS

The mouth can support the growth of diverse communities of microorganisms.

Over 700 prokaryote species have been isolated from the human mouth. Of these, approximately 49% are officially named, 17% unnamed (but cultivable) and 34% are known only as uncultivated phylotypes. In addition, viruses, mycoplasmas, yeasts, protozoa and *Archaea* are also present.

PRINCIPLES OF MICROBIAL CLASSIFICATION

As stated previously, the purpose of classification schemes is to develop a logical arrangement of organisms based on their similarities and relationships. This requires the determination and comparison of as many characteristics as possible, although in identification schemes, only a few key discriminatory tests may be needed to distinguish between certain organisms. Early classification schemes relied heavily on morphological and simple physiological criteria such as the shape of the cell and the pattern of fermentation of simple sugars (Table 3.2). In effect, these approaches analysed only a fraction of the components encoded by the genetic material of the cell (the **genome**).

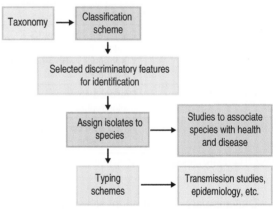

FIGURE 3.1 Diagrammatic representation to distinguish classification, identification and typing of bacterial strains.

Chemotaxonomy, in which there was a broader analysis of more complex components of the cell (for example, the chemical composition of the cell wall or of membrane lipids, whole cell protein profiles, etc.) led to major improvements in classification schemes. The antigenic characteristics of microorganisms can also be compared using immunological techniques (**serology**), in which specific antibodies (polyclonal or monoclonal) are used to detect cell surface antigens.

TABLE 3.2 Some characteristics used in microbial classification and identification schemes

Characteristic	Examples
Cellular morphology	Shape; Gram stain reaction (cell morphology and structure); flagella; spores; size
Colonial appearance	Pigment; haemolysis; shape; size
Carbohydrate fermentation	Acid or gas production
Amino acid hydrolysis	Ammonia production
Pattern of fermentation products	Butyrate; lactate; acetate
Preformed enzymes	Glycosidases (e.g., α-glucosidase)
Antigen	Monoclonal/polyclonal antibodies to cell surface proteins
Lipids	Menaquinones, long-chain fatty acids
DNA	Guanine + Cytosine (G + C) ratio; 16S rRNA gene sequence; whole genome sequence
Enzyme profile	Presence/absence; electrophoretic mobility
Peptidoglycan	Amino acid composition e.g., lysine

DNA, Deoxyribonucleic acid; *RNA,* ribonucleic acid.

Contemporary classification schemes are based more on determining the genetic relatedness among strains, for example, by comparing the sequence of **16S ribosomal ribonucleic acid (RNA) genes** (16S rRNA). Within the rRNA gene of bacteria and fungi, some stretches of deoxyribonucleic acid (DNA) sequence are conserved, whereas other regions are highly variable and reflect evolutionary divergence. Bacterial rRNA genes tend to be around 1500 base pairs long, which is short enough for rapid sequencing using automated DNA sequencing equipment and long enough to provide valuable discriminatory information to demonstrate similarities and differences among strains. The conserved regions can be used as a template for the design of 'universal' polymerase chain reaction (PCR) oligonucleotide primers to amplify the rest of the 16S rRNA gene, which can then be sequenced to identify differences in the variable regions. The sequences can be compared with those from other microorganisms, and those held in nucleotide databases, so that the relationship of an isolate to a known species can be determined and **evolutionary (phylogenetic) trees** can be developed. The technique is relatively rapid and has facilitated the analysis of a far wider range of bacteria than was previously possible. Comparison of 16S rRNA gene sequences has revolutionised the field of microbial taxonomy and has clarified the classification of many previously heterogeneous groups of oral bacteria, such as the streptococci (Table 3.3) and anaerobic Gram-positive rods formerly grouped as *Eubacterium* species (Fig. 3.6). In addition to classifying unknown strains, this approach can also be used to identify isolates and has many advantages over conventional cultural approaches (see later; Fig. 3.2). Likewise, the recent development of next generation bench-top DNA sequencers has enabled research groups to rapidly sequence, at low cost, the entire genome of isolated bacteria (whole genome sequencing [WGS], or next generation sequencing [NGS]). Genome sequences can then be aligned with those of authenticated species in international databases of reference microorganisms. This approach can also be applied to samples taken directly from the environment or from clinical specimens (metagenomics), although the analysis of multiple genomes in a complex sample such as dental plaque does require sophisticated bioinformatic support. Metagenomics is a powerful new approach to determine the composition of microbial communities and is especially advantageous when some of the component species cannot yet be grown in pure culture in the laboratory. Metagenomics is reshaping our understanding of microbial communities and will undoubtedly have a major impact in the future, not only in improving the classification of microorganisms, but also in more accurately analysing clinical samples.

A consequence of classification is the proposal of new species. A species represents a collection of strains

TABLE 3.3 Species of oral streptococci isolated from humans

Group	Species	
mutans-group*	S. mutans	serotypes c, e, f, k
	S. sobrinus	serotype d, g
	S. criceti	serotype a
	S. ratti	serotype b
salivarius-group	S. salivarius	
	S. vestibularis	
anginosus-group	S. constellatus	
	S. intermedius	
	S. anginosus	
mitis-group	S. sanguinis	
	S. gordonii	
	S. parasanguinis	
	S. oralis	
	S. mitis	
	S. cristatus	
	S. oligofermentans	
	S. sinensis	
	S. australis	
	S. peroris	
	S. infantis	
	S. dentisani	
	S. tigurinus	

*mutans streptococci also include S. ferus (isolated from rats), S. macacae and S. downei (serotype h) (isolated from monkeys).

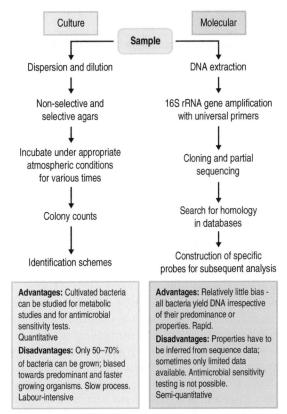

FIGURE 3.2 The main stages in determining the microbial composition of the microbiota of samples from the mouth using either culture or molecular approaches.

that share many features in common, and which differ considerably from other strains. Once a species has been recognised, then a **type strain** is nominated that has properties representative of the species. Type strains are held in national collections, such as the American Type Culture Collection (ATCC), or the National Collection of Type Cultures (NCTC), which is located in the United Kingdom.

A species may be divided into subspecies if minor but consistent phenotypic variations can be recognised. Likewise, groups of strains within a species can sometimes be distinguished by a special characteristic. For example, strains with a special biochemical or physiologic property are termed **biovars** or **biotypes**, whereas strains with a distinctive antigenic composition are described as **serovars** or **serotypes**, and can be recognised using appropriate antibodies. Molecular approaches can also be adapted for subtyping strains within a species. With the exception of direct sequencing, most methods involve PCR amplification and electrophoretic profiling of amplicons or digested fragments of these. In addition, whole genomic DNA can be digested by different restriction enzymes (**endonucleases**), which cut the nucleic acid at specific places. The digests are then electrophoresed in an agarose gel to generate a DNA fingerprint. Different strains will generate different patterns (**restriction fragment length polymorphisms, RFLPs**), although strains that appear to give similar patterns need to be compared after digestion with more than one enzyme. Dedicated fingerprinting computer software is commercially available for analysis of the electrophoretic profiles. For highly complex profiles, restriction fragments may be blotted onto nitrocellulose or nylon membranes and hybridised with a suitably labelled probe to give a simpler profile.

PRINCIPLES OF CONVENTIONAL MICROBIAL IDENTIFICATION

Once organisms have been correctly classified using rigorous techniques, then more simple identification schemes can be devised in which only limited numbers of key discriminatory properties are compared (see Fig. 3.1, Table 3.2). The first stage might involve the reaction of an organism with the Gram stain and the determination of cellular morphology. Bacteria are then described as being, for example, Gram-positive cocci or Gram-negative rods, and so on. Depending on the outcome of that division, simple physiologic tests may be performed, such as the determination of sugar fermentation patterns, the profiles of acidic fermentation products following glucose metabolism or selected enzyme activities. The rapid detection (ca. 4 hours) of constitutively expressed enzymes by concentrated suspensions of bacteria has simplified the identification of some groups of bacteria. Ecologically relevant substrates that detect enzymes such as glycosidases that cleave sugar residues from salivary mucins are now more commonly used to differentiate groups of bacteria that had previously been difficult to separate, for example, oral streptococci. Some of these tests have been incorporated in kits and are available commercially, along with computerised databases, to facilitate identification.

Monoclonal antibodies and nucleic acid (oligonucleotide) probes have been developed for the rapid identification of some species and primarily for those associated with disease. Such antibodies and probes can be labelled with a reporter molecule to enable detection. Examples of these reporters include fluorescent dyes (Fig. 3.3), radiolabels or reporter enzymes such as horseradish peroxidase. These techniques have the advantage that organisms can be detected directly in a clinical sample, such as dental plaque, without the need for lengthy culturing. However, a potential drawback is that these approaches can detect dead as well as viable cells, and they are only applicable for predetermined species for which the reagents are already available.

Conventional microbial identification schemes can only be used when organisms have been isolated and grown in pure culture. Inevitably, the procedure for achieving pure culture (sample dispersion and dilution, growth on selective and non-selective agar plates, incubation conditions, etc.) leads to the introduction of bias towards those microorganisms that grow quickly and easily under laboratory conditions (see Fig. 3.2). Alternative, culture-independent techniques have evolved out of modern molecular approaches, and these are giving a more accurate picture of the diversity (richness) of the microbiota from a wide range of habitats. Many oral bacteria are difficult to grow, and around 30–50% are not currently cultivable in pure culture (these are described as **unculturable** species). Molecular kits are commercially available to identify selected bacteria that are associated with disease, especially for periodontal disease. There is currently a service available from The Forsyth Institute, USA, called HOMINGS (human oral microbe identification using next generation sequencing), which offers species-level identification of around 600 taxa, with a further 100+ genus-level targets, using DNA submitted from oral clinical specimens.

IMPACT OF MOLECULAR MICROBIAL ECOLOGY

As stated previously, the genetic relatedness of microorganisms is now primarily determined by comparisons of **16S ribosomal RNA** (rRNA) **gene** sequences or by **whole genome sequencing** (WGS or NGS). The biggest impact of these approaches has been in the analysis of diverse communities of microorganisms from a number of habitats (**molecular microbial ecology** or **metagenomics**), including the mouth. Comparisons between the number of cells in samples that can be observed by microscopy versus those that can be cultured in the laboratory, even when using the most advanced techniques, have demonstrated that only a proportion of the microbiota at a site can be grown. The culturable fraction can vary from less than 1% of the total cell count in some marine habitats to about 50–70% of the oral microbiota. As mentioned earlier, these bacteria are termed **unculturable** and the

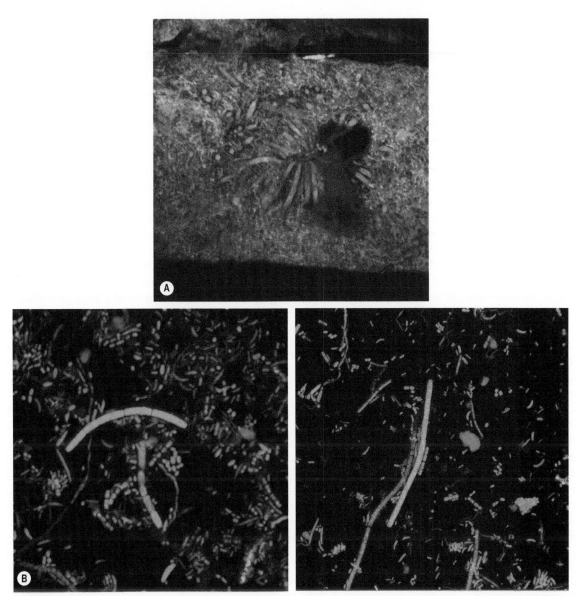

FIGURE 3.3 Examples of currently unculturable bacteria in subgingival plaque visualised using fluorescent in situ hybridisation (FISH) techniques. **(A)** 16S ribosomal ribonucleic acid (rRNA) oligonucleotide probes were used to detect bacteria (green) and *Treponema* species (red). Courtesy of Dr Annette Moter and produced with permission by Springer-Verlag GmbH & Co. (Norris SJ, Paster BJ, Moter A and Gobel UB, The genus *Treponema*, in The Prokaryotes, Third Edition; Berlin: Springer, 2007). **(B)** 16S rRNA oligonucleotide probes were used to detect bacteria (green) and members of the TM7 phylum (blue). Courtesy of Dr Cleber Ouverney and the American Society for Microbiology (see Ouverney et al. *Appl Environ Microbiol* 2003 69:6294–6298).

reasons for this may be ignorance of an essential nutrient or other growth requirement, or because the bacteria have evolved to grow as part of a community of cells, rather than as an isolated pure culture.

Analysis of bacterial 16S rRNA sequences has been crucial in improving bacterial taxonomy. Although such molecular approaches have enabled construction of phylogenetic trees that include currently unculturable organisms, in many cases, a genus and species name still cannot be assigned given the inability to phenotypically characterise the organism. In the case of the oral microbiome, a phylogeny-based database, the Human Oral Microbiome Database (HOMD), was made accessible on the Internet in 2008, and this provides a provisional taxonomic scheme for the unnamed human oral bacteria. Currently, the HOMD indicates that there are 707 bacterial species in the human oral cavity, with 49% of these officially named, 17% unnamed (but can be cultured) and 34% remain unculturable phylotypes. The HOMD groups these 707 species (taxa; species level in this instance) in 16 phyla (the major bacterial taxonomic divisions). Figure 3.4 illustrates the currently accepted predominant genera (and respective phyla) of the oral microbiota based on 16S rRNA gene sequencing. Up to 96% of oral taxa belong to *Firmicutes, Bacteroidetes, Proteobacteria, Actinobacteria, Spirochaetes* and *Fusobacteria*. The remaining 4% of taxa are placed in the phyla *Euryarchaeota, Chlamydiae, Chloroflexi*, SR1, *Synergistetes, Tenericutes, Chlorobi, Gracilibacteria* (GN02), WPS-2 and *Saccharibacteria* (TM7).

Oligonucleotide probes can also be used so that the presence of these organisms can be determined relatively simply in clinical samples using rapid tests, such as PCR or by *in situ* hybridisation, usually with a fluorescent label (FISH, see Fig. 3.3). An important benefit of these PCR-based molecular approaches is their potential to detect organisms that are present in low numbers. Although the properties of these uncultivable organisms cannot be determined using conventional tests (such as sugar fermentation patterns or their antibiotic sensitivity profile), databases of genes exist that can be interrogated to search for homologous sequences with known functions. This can provide insights into potentially important properties of these unculturable organisms, such as their cell wall structure, their virulence attributes, the metabolic

pathways they might use and even their likely resistance to antimicrobial agents.

Two large families of novel bacteria that are unculturable in pure culture have been identified in the mouth (see Fig. 3.3) and are commonly detected in deep periodontal pockets; further details of these will be presented later in this chapter. In addition, some genera contain examples of both culturable and unculturable species. There are around 50 *Treponema* species that, although seen microscopically and detected by molecular approaches, cannot be grown (see Fig. 3.3, A). Similarly, molecular analysis of the microbiota associated with dentoalveolar abscesses and endodontic infections has consistently identified novel groups of bacteria that were not recognised, or were grossly underestimated, in parallel cultural studies (see Fig. 3.2). The existence of unculturable bacteria cannot be ignored because they can form a large proportion of the microbiota and their presence at a site could be clinically significant. It is worth remembering that the aetiological agent of syphilis is the spirochaete, *Treponema pallidum*, which still cannot be grown in the laboratory.

Molecular approaches have also been developed to compare the diversity of oral microbial communities from different sites in health and disease. These approaches originally included microbial community profiling using denaturing gradient gel electrophoresis (DGGE). In this method, total genomic DNA is extracted from clinical samples, amplified by PCR using universal primers for bacterial 16S rRNA genes, and products resolved on polyacrylamide gels in a denaturing gradient. DGGE profiles can be analysed using appropriate software, and novel or discriminatory bands can be excised from the gel, cloned, and sequenced, enabling a presumptive identification to be made. An alternative technique employed checkerboard DNA–DNA hybridisation using labelled whole genomic probes and nylon membranes to simultaneously screen multiple clinical samples for around 40 different preselected microbial species. Subsequently, a DNA-based microarray was developed which could detect 300 of the most prevalent oral bacteria. Termed the Human Oral Microbe Identification Microarray (HOMIM), it was based on 16S rRNA gene sequence hybridisations on a slide and allowed a much wider screen of the microbiota in clinical samples. New

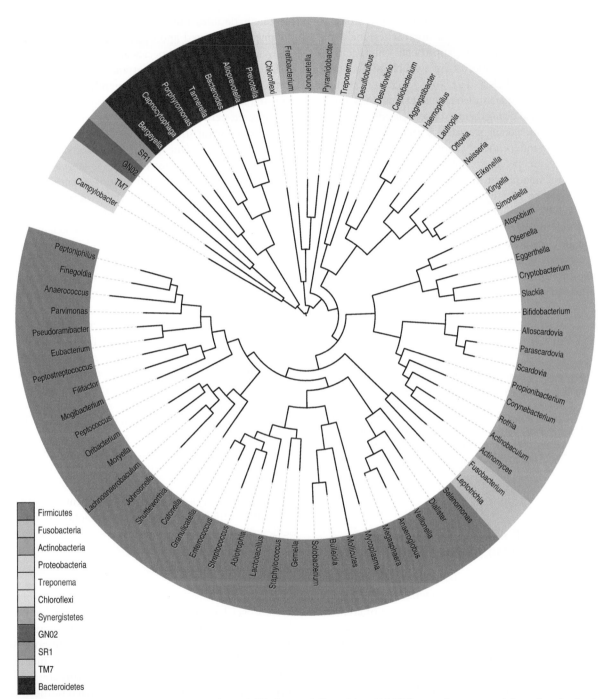

FIGURE 3.4 Phylogenetic tree based on comparison of 16S ribosomal ribonucleic acid (rRNA) genes from representatives of predominant human oral bacterial genera, constructed by maximum likelihood estimation. The authors express their gratitude to Professor William Wade (Queen Mary University of London) for the production of this figure, which was constructed using the Interactive Tree of Life (Letunic and Bork. *Bioinformatics* 2006;23:127-8; Letunic and Bork. *Nucleic Acids Res.* 2011;39:W475-W478).

PCR-based sequencing tools for community profiling, have superseded many of these approaches, including whole genome sequencing approaches (**metagenomics**). A number of platforms are available to undertake metagenomic analysis and key to the success of all these is the ability to compartmentalise individual PCR amplicons, thereby allowing them to be sequenced without the need for prior cloning steps (see Chapter 4).

Culture-independent approaches are radically changing our perception of the diversity of the resident oral microbiota in health and disease. Work is underway to identify the signature DNA sequences of all of the microorganisms in the mouth (culturable and unculturable) and develop kits or services to enable clinicians to rapidly screen for the presence or absence of hundreds of species, thereby leading to the promise of improved diagnostic and treatment opportunities.

KEY POINTS

> Knowledge of the oral microbiota depends on accurate and robust classification systems from which simpler identification schemes can be developed. Both processes have been revolutionised by the advent of molecular approaches, especially those based on 16S rRNA gene and whole genome sequence analysis. Comparisons of data from culture and molecular approaches suggest that around 30–50% of the oral microbiota is currently classed as being 'unculturable'.

DIFFICULTIES ARISING FROM RECENT ADVANCES IN MICROBIAL CLASSIFICATION

Although recent advances have led to improvements in the classification of oral bacteria, they also pose a number of challenges when interpreting or comparing early data when a previous (and sometimes flawed) nomenclature was in use. The classification of many groups of oral bacteria has changed greatly in a relatively short time period, with many new genera and species described. A species highlighted in an early study may have subsequently been reclassified and hence renamed, and so new and old terminologies coexist in the scientific literature. For example, *Streptococcus sanguis* was described in scientific papers for many decades but, as of 1989, its description became more limited and organisms that were previously identified as this species are now known to be sufficiently different as to warrant a distinct species epithet, e.g., *S. gordonii*. Consequently, some strains reported in earlier studies as *S. sanguis* might not have the same properties as strains more recently identified as *S. sanguis sensu stricto*. Furthermore, Latin names originally given to some of the oral streptococci have been shown to be erroneous, and so *S. sanguis* is now termed *S. sanguinis*. For similar reasons, *S. parasanguis*, *S. rattus*, *S. cricetus* and *S. crista* have been renamed as *S. parasanguinis*, *S. ratti*, *S. criceti* and *S. cristatus*, respectively. Thus, great care has to be taken when interpreting older (and indeed not so old) scientific literature.

Microbial taxonomy is a dynamic area with existing species being reclassified because of the application of more stringent tests, together with the recognition of genuinely newly discovered species from sites such as periodontal pockets and infected root canals. The emphasis paid to the classification and identification of the oral microbiota is necessary because without valid subdivision and accurate identification of isolates, the specific association of species with particular diseases (**microbial aetiology**) cannot be determined. Likewise, it has to be accepted that further changes in microbial classification schemes will occur in the future, with new genera and species being identified.

The properties of the main groups of microorganism found in the mouth (the oral microbiota) will now be described.

GRAM-POSITIVE COCCI

STREPTOCOCCUS

Streptococci have been isolated from all sites in the mouth and comprise a large proportion of the resident cultivable oral microbiota. Oral streptococci are generally alpha-haemolytic (partial haemolysis) on blood agar, and early workers called them viridans streptococci. However, haemolysis is not a reliable distinguishing property of these streptococci, and many oral species contain strains showing all 3 types of haemolysis (alpha, beta and gamma). Streptococci can be distinguished from staphylococci and micrococci by lacking the enzyme catalase. Oral streptococci are clustered into four groups (see Table 3.3) and will now be described.

Mutans group (mutans streptococci)

There is great interest in the mutans streptococci because of their potential role in the aetiology of dental caries. *Streptococcus mutans* was originally isolated from carious human teeth by Clarke in 1924 and shortly afterwards, was recovered from a case of infective endocarditis (growth of bacteria on damaged heart valves; Chapter 11). Little attention was paid to this species until the 1960s when it was demonstrated that caries could be experimentally-induced and transmitted in animals artificially infected with strains resembling *S. mutans*. The name of this species derives from the fact that cells can lose their coccal morphology and often appear as short rods or as coccobacilli. Nine serotypes have been recognised (*a–h*, and *k*), based on serological specificity of carbohydrate antigens located in the cell wall, although some serotypes are found only in animals. Subsequent work showed that sufficient differences existed between clusters of these serotypes to warrant subdivision into seven distinct species (Table 3.3); these species are described collectively as **mutans streptococci**. Mutans streptococci are recovered almost exclusively from hard, non-shedding surfaces in the mouth, such as teeth or dentures, and can act as opportunistic pathogens, being isolated from cases of infective endocarditis (Chapter 11). Mutans streptococci are regularly isolated from dental plaque at carious sites, but their prevalence is low on sound enamel.

The specific epithet, *S. mutans*, is now limited to human isolates previously belonging to serotypes *c, e, f* and *k*. This is the most commonly isolated species of mutans streptococci, and epidemiological studies have implicated *S. mutans* as one of the main causative organisms in the aetiology of enamel and root surface caries (see Chapter 6). The next most commonly isolated species of the mutans streptococci group is *S. sobrinus* (previously, *S. mutans* serotypes *d* and *g*) and is also associated with human dental caries. Less is known about the role of *S. sobrinus* in disease because some studies do not attempt to distinguish between these species, and some commonly used selective agar media for the isolation of mutans streptococci contain bacitracin, which can be inhibitory to the growth of both *S. sobrinus* and *S. criceti* (formerly *S. cricetus*, and previously termed *S. mutans* serotype *a*). Some people harbour more than one species of mutans streptococci in their mouth.

The antigenic structure of mutans streptococci has been studied in detail to establish serological typing schemes and for the development of a prospective caries vaccine (see Chapter 6). Mutans streptococci possess cell wall carbohydrate antigens, lipoteichoic acid, lipoproteins and cell wall or cell wall-associated proteins. Antigen I/II (also termed antigen B, SpaP or Pac) has generated considerable interest because it is (a) a major adhesin involved in the initial adherence of *S. mutans* to the tooth surface (see Chapter 5) and (b) a possible component of a subunit caries vaccine (see Chapter 6). Some strains of *S. mutans* carry a collagen-binding gene, and these strains have been isolated from patients with cerebral microbleeds.

Mutans streptococci make extracellular soluble and insoluble polysaccharides (glucan, mutan and fructan) from sucrose that are associated with dental plaque maturation (see Chapters 4 and 5) and cariogenicity (see Chapter 6). The glucans and fructans are produced by glucosyltransferases and fructosyltransferases, respectively. Mutan is a highly insoluble glucan that is only produced by mutans streptococci, whereas the fructan is unusual in having an inulin-like structure. These polymers contribute to the characteristic colonial morphology of mutans streptococci when growing on sucrose-containing agar plates (Fig. 3.5, B). Mutans streptococci can also synthesise intracellular polysaccharides when there is excess sugar, and these can act as carbohydrate reserves and be converted to acid during periods when dietary carbohydrates are in limited supply. Mutans streptococci can scavenge dietary sugars very efficiently and rapidly convert them to acidic fermentation products (mainly lactate). Significantly, mutans streptococci are able to grow and survive under the acidic conditions they generate by the induction of specific molecular stress responses (see Chapter 4 and Fig. 2.4). Mutans streptococci can communicate with other mutans streptococci by the release of diffusible signalling molecules that can induce genetic competence (an ability to take up extracellular DNA) and acid tolerance in neighbouring cells.

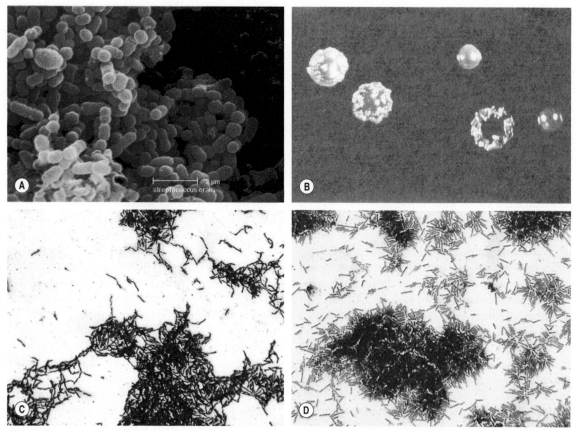

FIGURE 3.5 Examples of Gram-positive bacteria found in the mouth. (**A**) The cell morphology of *Streptococcus oralis* when viewed by scanning electron microscopy (SEM). (**B**) The colony morphology of *Streptococcus mutans* growing on sucrose-containing agar. (**C**) Gram stain of *Actinomyces israelii*. (**D**) Gram stain of *Eubacterium yurii*. Gram-stained images were kindly provided by Owain Dafydd Thomas, Cardiff and Vale UHB. SEM was kindly provided by Wendy Rowe, Cardiff University.

Salivarius group

This group comprises *S. salivarius* and *S. vestibularis*. Strains of *S. salivarius* are commonly isolated from most areas of the mouth, although they preferentially colonise mucosal surfaces, especially the tongue. *Streptococcus salivarius* produces large quantities of an unusual extracellular fructan (polymer of fructose with a levan structure) from sucrose (see Chapter 4), as well as a levanase that can degrade this type of fructan. This levan gives rise to characteristically large mucoid colonies when *S. salivarius* is grown on sucrose-containing agar. *Streptococcus salivarius* also produces extracellular soluble and insoluble glucans from sucrose; some strains have urease activity. *Streptococcus salivarius* is isolated only rarely from diseased sites and is not considered a significant opportunistic pathogen.

Streptococcus vestibularis is isolated mainly from the vestibular mucosa of the human mouth. These bacteria do not produce extracellular polysaccharides from sucrose, but do produce a urease (which can generate ammonia and hence raise the local pH) and hydrogen peroxide (which can contribute to the sialoperoxidase system [see Chapter 2], and inhibit the growth of competing bacteria).

Anginosus group

Representative species of this group, *Streptococcus constellatus* (subspecies *constellatus*, subspecies *viborgensis* and subspecies *pharyngis*), *S. intermedius* and

S. anginosus (subspecies *anginosus* and subspecies *whileyi*), are readily isolated from dental plaque and from mucosal surfaces and are important causes of serious, purulent disease in humans, including maxillofacial infections. Members of the anginosus group are commonly found in abscesses of internal organs, especially of the brain and liver, and have also been recovered from cases of appendicitis, peritonitis, meningitis and endocarditis. *Streptococcus intermedius* is isolated mainly from liver and brain abscesses, whereas *S. anginosus* and *S. constellatus* are derived from purulent infections from a wider range of sites. *Streptococcus intermedius* can produce a cytotoxin, intermedilysin, which may also interfere with neutrophil function and enable the cell to evade the host defences during abscess formation. This group does not make extracellular polysaccharides from sucrose.

Mitis group

The application of molecular phylogenetic techniques (involving the determination of 16S rRNA gene sequences) has resolved many of the previous anomalies in the classification of this group, resulting in the identification of new species.

Streptococcus sanguinis and *S. gordonii* are early colonisers of the tooth surface, and both produce extracellular soluble and insoluble glucans (see Chapter 4) from sucrose that contribute to biofilm formation. Both species can generate ammonia from arginine. *S. sanguinis* produces a protease that can cleave sIgA (IgA protease), whereas *S. gordonii* can bind salivary α-amylase enabling these organisms to break down starch. Amylase-binding may also mask bacterial antigens and allow these bacteria to avoid recognition by the host defences (host mimicry). Both species are composed of several biotypes.

Two of the most common streptococcal species in the mouth are *S. mitis* and *S. oralis*. Strains of *S. oralis* produce neuraminidase (an enzyme that removes sialic acid from oligosaccharide side chains of salivary mucins) and an IgA protease, but cannot bind α-amylase (Fig. 3.5, *A*). *Streptococcus mitis* is subdivided into two biotypes, and these show different distribution patterns in the mouth. Strains of these two species are able to take up extracellular DNA (i.e., they are genetically competent), and this process is facilitated in biofilms like dental plaque where bacteria are in close proximity to one another. Consequently, it is perhaps not surprising that there is considerable genetic and phenotypic heterogeneity when the properties of large numbers of *S. mitis* and *S. oralis* strains are compared. Some, but not all, strains of these two species are able to produce extracellular glucan from sucrose.

Other members of this group include *S. parasanguinis* (formerly *S. parasanguis*) that has been isolated from clinical specimens (throat, blood, urine). Strains can hydrolyse arginine but not urea, and can bind salivary α-amylase, but cannot produce extracellular polysaccharides from sucrose. *Streptococcus cristatus* is characterised by the presence of tufts of fibrils on their cell surface. Newer species have been described including *S. oligofermentans*, *S. sinensis*, *S. australis*, *S. infantis*, *S. peroris*, *S. tigurinus* and *S. dentisani*. The significance of some of these species to the ecology of the mouth has yet to be determined, but species such as *S. tigurinus* and *S. sinensis* can act as opportunistic pathogens, having been isolated from cases of infective endocarditis.

Members of the mitis group are opportunistic pathogens, particularly in infective endocarditis (see Chapter 11). *Streptococcus pneumoniae* can be isolated from the nasopharynx and is a significant opportunistic pathogen, which can acquire and transfer antibiotic resistance genes amongst other members of the mitis group.

OTHER GRAM-POSITIVE COCCI

Strains that were originally described as being nutritionally variant streptococci (NVS) have been isolated from the mouth when appropriate isolation media are used. These have been reclassified as *Granulicatella adiacens* (previously *S. adiacens* and *Abiotrophia adiacens*) and *Abiotrophia defectiva* (previously *S. defectivus*). *Granulicatella adiacens* is common in the mouth and is an early coloniser of the tooth surface, although it is overlooked in most studies because of the need for isolation media to be supplemented with growth factors such as cysteine or pyridoxal. These bacteria often exhibit satellitism, seen as an enhanced growth pattern around colonies of certain other bacteria that produce these cofactors. Other Gram-positive cocci include *Gemella* species (*G. haemolysans* and *G. morbillorum*), although cells sometimes appear Gram-negative on staining.

Anaerobic Gram-positive cocci are commonly recovered from dental biofilms, especially from carious dentine, infected pulp chambers and root canals (see Chapter 6), advanced forms of periodontal disease (see Chapter 6) and from dental abscesses (see Chapter 7). These bacteria are also recovered from deep-seated abscesses elsewhere in the body and are usually isolated in mixed culture (polymicrobial infections). The taxonomy of this group of organisms has been clarified. Originally, strains were placed in the genus, *Peptostreptococcus*, and representative species included *P. micros, P. magnus* and *P. anaerobius*. However, *P. micros* and *P. magnus* have been moved to new genera and are now called *Parvimonas micra* and *Finegoldia magna*, respectively, whereas oral strains of *P. anaerobius* are now designated *Peptostreptococcus stomatis*.

Enterococci have been recovered in low numbers from several oral sites when appropriate selective media have been used; the most frequently isolated species is *Enterococcus faecalis*. Enterococci can be isolated from the mouths of immuno-compromised and medically-compromised patients, and have been isolated from periodontal pockets that fail to respond to therapy and from infected root canals. Lancefield group A streptococci (*S. pyogenes*) are not usually isolated from the mouth of healthy individuals, although they can often be cultured from the saliva of people suffering from streptococcal sore throats and may be associated with a particularly acute form of gingivitis (see Chapter 6).

Staphylococci and micrococci are also not commonly isolated in large numbers from the oral cavity, although the former are found in denture plaque, as well as in immunocompromised patients and individuals suffering from a variety of oral infections (see Chapters 7 and 11). These bacteria are not usually considered to be members of the resident oral microbiota, but they may be present transiently, and they have been isolated from some sites with root surface caries and from some periodontal pockets that fail to respond to conventional therapy. This is in sharp contrast to other surfaces of the human body in close proximity to the mouth, such as the skin surface and the mucous membranes of the nose, where they are among the predominant components of the microbiota. This finding emphasises the major differences that must exist in the ecology of these particular habitats.

Microorganisms from the mucosal surfaces of the skin and nose must be passed consistently into the mouth and yet these organisms are normally unable to colonise or compete against the resident oral microbiota.

GRAM-POSITIVE RODS AND FILAMENTS

ACTINOMYCES

Actinomyces species form a major portion of the microbiota of dental plaque, particularly at approximal sites and the gingival crevice. These bacteria have been associated with root surface caries, and their numbers increase during gingivitis (see Chapter 6). Cells of *Actinomyces* species appear as short rods but are often pleomorphic in shape; some cells show a true branching morphology, whereas those of *A. israelii* can sometimes appear to be filamentous (Fig. 3.5, *C*). Some species (particularly *A. naeslundii*) are heavily fimbriated (cell surface structures involved in attachment), whilst others have relatively smooth surfaces. Some newly described species have been identified in a variety of clinical specimens (*A. radingae, A. neuii, A. johnsonii, A. europaeus, A. graevenitzii, A. funkei, A. dentalis* and *A. turicensis*), including infective endocarditis and abscesses, but the source and habitat of these species is not yet fully understood. *Actinomyces radicidentis* has been isolated from endodontic infections.

The most common Gram-positive bacillus in plaque is *Actinomyces naeslundii*, which was originally subdivided into two genospecies (*A. naeslundii* genospecies 1 and genospecies 2). *Actinomyces naeslundii* genospecies 2 is now classified as *A. oris*. Some strains of *A. naeslundii* produce an extracellular slime and a fructan from sucrose with a levan-like structure as well as enzymes that can hydrolyse fructans. Some strains also produce urease (this enzyme may have a role in modulating pH in plaque) and neuraminidase (can modify receptors in the enamel acquired pellicle). Two types of fimbriae can be found on the surface of cells of *A. naeslundii*. Each type serves a specific function, and are implicated either in cell-to-cell contact (coaggregation) or in cell-to-surface interaction (see Chapter 5). *Actinomyces viscosus* is a closely related species found in animals.

Actinomyces israelii can act as an opportunistic pathogen causing a chronic inflammatory condition called actinomycosis (see Fig. 3.5, *C* and Chapter 7). The disease is usually associated with the orofacial region, but it can disseminate to cause deep-seated infections at other sites in the body such as the abdomen. Strains of *A. israelii* characteristically form granules and these may contribute to the ability of these organisms to disseminate around the body by affording physical protection from the environment, from the host defences and from antibiotic treatment. *Actinomyces israelii* has also been found in cervical smears of women using intrauterine contraceptive devices.

Strains originally classified as *A. israelii* serotype II have now been designated as a separate species, *A. gerencseriae*, which is a common but minor component of the microbiota of the healthy gingival crevice, and it has also been isolated from abscesses. Strains of *A. gerencseriae* can also form protective 'granules' (see previous comments on *A. israelii*). *Actinomyces georgiae* is facultatively anaerobic and is also found occasionally in the healthy gingival crevice. Other species include *A. odontolyticus* and *A. meyeri*; the former has been associated with early caries lesions whereas the latter has been found in low numbers from the gingival crevice in health and disease, and from brain abscesses.

EUBACTERIUM AND RELATED GENERA

Until recently, *Eubacterium* was a poorly defined genus that contained a variety of obligately anaerobic, filamentous bacteria that often appear Gram-variable when stained (Fig. 3.5, *D*). Many strains are asaccharolytic and, therefore, can appear non-reactive in classification schemes and may also be difficult to cultivate. When recovered and identified, these asaccharolytic species can comprise over 50% of the anaerobic microbiota of periodontal pockets and are common in dentoalveolar abscesses. Molecular taxonomic approaches have identified many new bacterial genera (Fig. 3.6), and oral eubacteria are now restricted to *Eubacterium saburreum*, *E. yurii*, *E. infirmum*, *E. sulci*, *E. saphenum*, *E. minutum*, *E. nodatum* and *E. brachy*. New genera include *Mogibacterium* (e.g., *M. timidum*, *M. vescum* and *M. pumilum*), *Pseudoramibacter* (e.g., *P. alactolyticus*) and *Slackia* (e.g., *S. exigua*), all of which have been recovered from infected root canals. Other new genera include *Cryptobacterium* (e.g., *C. curtum*),

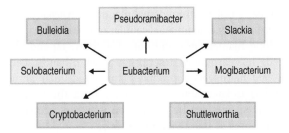

FIGURE 3.6 Recent changes in the nomenclature of bacteria originally grouped together as *Eubacterium* species.

Shuttleworthia (e.g., *S. satelles*), *Solobacterium* (e.g., *S. moorei*) and *Bulleidia* (e.g., *B. extructa*). Many of these bacteria have also been found in periodontal pockets and/or abscesses, but the full clinical significance of these organisms has yet to be determined.

LACTOBACILLUS

Lactobacilli are commonly isolated from the oral cavity, especially from dental plaque and the tongue, although they usually comprise less than 1% of the total cultivable microbiota in the healthy mouth. These bacteria are highly acidogenic and acid tolerant, and their proportions and prevalence increase in advanced enamel and root surface caries lesions. A number of homofermentative and heterofermentative species have been identified, producing either lactate, or lactate and acetate, respectively, from glucose. The most common species are *L. casei*, *L. rhamnosus*, *L. fermentum*, *L. acidophilus*, *L. salivarius*, *L. plantarum*, *L. paracasei*, *L. gasseri* and *L. oris*, but most studies still merely group them as 'lactobacilli' or *Lactobacillus* species. Simple tests with selective media have been designed for estimating the numbers of lactobacilli in patients' saliva to give an indication of the cariogenic potential of a mouth. Some lactobacilli are being considered as possible oral probiotic strains (see Chapter 6).

OTHER GENERA

Propionibacterium species (e.g., *P. acnes*, *P. propionicus*) are obligately anaerobic bacteria that are found in dental plaque. *Propionibacterium propionicus* has been isolated from cases of actinomycosis and lacrimal canaliculitis (infection of the tear duct). *Corynebacterium matruchotii* and *Rothia dentocariosa* are also regularly isolated from dental plaque. *Corynebacterium matruchotii* has an unusual cellular morphology having a long filament growing out of a short, fat rod-like cell, thus earning its description of 'whip-handle' cell. *Rothia mucilaginosa* produces an extracellular slime and is isolated almost exclusively from the tongue. *Rothia* species can be isolated on very rare occasions from cases of infective endocarditis.

Bifidobacteria have undergone several changes in nomenclature; oral bifidobacteria include *Bifidobacterium dentium* and *B. longum*. Two former species of bifidobacteria have been reclassified as *Scardovia inopinata* and *Parascardovia denticolens*, but their role in the mouth has yet to be determined. Other related taxa include *Alloscardovia omnicolens* and *Parascardovia denticolens* (which has been detected in occlusal caries). Many bifidobacteria are acidogenic and acid-tolerating, which supports proposals that they may play a role in dental caries. Non-oral species of bifidobacteria can be found in denture plaque from patients with denture stomatitis, including *B. breve*, but *B. dentium* (although present in dental plaque) could not be isolated from the palate in a healthy edentulous mouth.

Some bacteria previously classified as *Actinomyces* have been placed in the new genera, *Arcanobacterium* (e.g., *A. bernardiae*) and *Actinobaculum*. Bacteria originally described as 'anaerobic lactobacilli' have been placed in new genera such as *Olsenella*, e.g., *Olsenella uli*, which has been isolated from periodontal pockets, and *Atopobium* species (e.g., *Atopobium rimae* and *A. parvulum*).

Filifactor alocis is an asaccharolytic and obligately anaerobic Gram-positive short rod-shaped bacterium that is considered to be a potentially important periodontal pathogen. It has also been found in endodontic infections, periimplantitis and aggressive forms of periodontal disease. As with other putative periodontal pathogens, *F. alocis* is proteolytic and can also utilise arginine, generating ornithine and ammonia (thereby contributing to the rise in pH seen in the inflamed periodontal pocket); other amino acids used include lysine and cysteine. *Filifactor alocis* is also more tolerant of oxidative stress than Gram-negative periodontal pathogens, and it may be able to modulate neutrophil function; both properties would aid its survival in the periodontal environment.

KEY POINTS

Gram-positive bacteria are commonly distributed on most surfaces of the mouth. The predominant genera are *Streptococcus* and *Actinomyces*; representative species are found at healthy sites, although many can also act as opportunistic pathogens. For example, mutans streptococci are implicated in dental caries whereas the anginosus-group and the mitis group of streptococci are recovered commonly from abscesses and infective endocarditis, respectively; *Actinomyces israelii* is implicated in actinomycosis.

GRAM-NEGATIVE COCCI

Neisseria are aerobic or facultatively anaerobic Gram-negative cocci that are isolated in low numbers from most sites in the oral cavity. These bacteria are among the earliest colonisers of teeth and make an important contribution to plaque formation by consuming oxygen and creating conditions that permit obligate anaerobes to grow. Some *Neisseria* species can produce extracellular polysaccharides, and some streptococcal strains can metabolise these polymers, effectively using them as external carbohydrate reserves. The taxonomy of this group remains confused, but common species include *N. subflava*, *N. mucosa*, *N. flavescens* and *N. pharyngis*. *Moraxella catarrhalis* is a commensal of the upper respiratory tract, but it is also a well-established opportunistic pathogen; many strains produce a β-lactamase that can lead to complications during antibiotic treatment.

Veillonella are small, strictly anaerobic Gram-negative cocci (Fig. 3.7, *A*); several species are recognised: *Veillonella parvula*, *V. dispar*, *V. atypica*, *V. denticariosi* (more common in carious dentine), *V. tobetsuensis* (isolated from the tongue) and *V. rogosae* (more common in caries-free individuals). *Veillonella* species have been isolated from most surfaces of the oral cavity although they occur in highest numbers in dental plaque. *Veillonella* species lack glucokinase and fructokinase and are therefore unable to metabolise carbohydrates. Instead, they utilise several intermediary metabolites, in particular lactate, as energy sources and, consequently, play an important role in the ecology of dental plaque and in the aetiology of dental caries. Lactic acid is the strongest acid produced

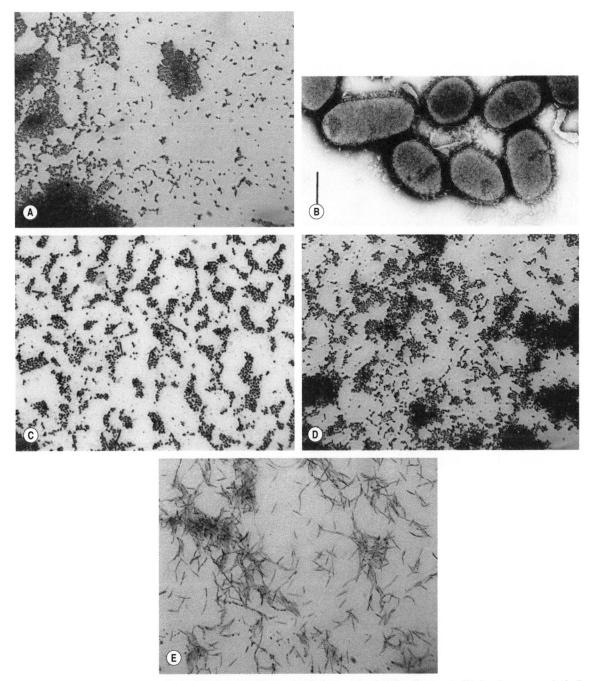

FIGURE 3.7 Examples of Gram-negative bacteria found in the mouth. (**A**) Gram stain of *Veillonella parvula*, (**B**) *Porphyromonas gingivalis*, when viewed by SEM. (**C**) Gram stain of *Porphyromonas gingivalis*. (**D**) Gram stain of *Prevotella nigrescens*. (**E**) Gram stain of *Fusobacterium nucleatum*. Gram-stained images were kindly provided by Owain Dafydd Thomas, Cardiff and Vale UHB. SEM was kindly provided by Barry Dowsett, Porton, and false-colour applied by Wendy Rowe, Cardiff University.

in quantity by oral bacteria and is implicated in the dissolution of enamel (dental caries; Chapter 6). *Veillonella* can convert lactic acid to weaker acids (predominantly propionic acid) and so ameliorate the potential damage of saccharolytic bacteria, such as streptococci. Other Gram-negative cocci include *Anaeroglobus geminatus* and *Megasphaera* species (e.g., *M. micronuciformis*).

GRAM-NEGATIVE RODS

FACULTATIVELY ANAEROBIC AND CAPNOPHILIC GENERA

Haemophili require isolation media that contain the essential growth factors: haemin (X-factor) and/or nicotinamide adenine dinucleotide, NAD (V-factor). The only species of *Haemophilus* found commonly in the mouth is *H. parainfluenzae* (V-factor requiring); *H. parahaemolyticus* is isolated from soft tissue infections of the oral cavity but is probably not a regular member of the oral microbiota.

Organisms previously classified as haemophili have been placed in the genus, *Aggregatibacter*. Examples include *Aggregatibacter aphrophilus*, which can cause brain abscesses and infective endocarditis, *A. segnis,* which is only occasionally isolated from infections, and *A. actinomycetemcomitans* (formerly classified as *Actinobacillus actinomycetemcomitans*), and which is implicated in a particularly aggressive form of periodontal disease in adolescents. Strains are capnophilic, often requiring 5% to 10% CO_2 for growth. Cells have surface layers containing molecules that stimulate bone resorption, as well as serotype-determining polysaccharides. *Aggregatibacter actinomycetemcomitans* produces a range of virulence factors including a powerful leukotoxin, collagenase, immunosuppressive factors and proteases capable of cleaving immunoglobulin G (IgG); in addition, strains can be invasive for epithelial cells. *Aggregatibacter actinomycetemcomitans* is also an opportunistic pathogen, being isolated from cases of endocarditis, brain and subcutaneous abscesses, osteomyelitis and periodontal disease. Recently, a highly virulent clone of *A. actinomycetemcomitans* has been recognised, whose distribution is restricted to certain adolescents with a high risk of aggressive

periodontitis, most of which generally have a North West African origin.

Eikenella corrodens has been isolated from a range of oral infections including endocarditis and abscesses, and has been implicated in periodontal disease. *Capnocytophaga* are CO_2-dependent Gram-negative rods that exhibit a gliding motility. These bacteria are found in subgingival plaque and increase in proportions in gingivitis. A number of species have been recognised including *Capnocytophaga gingivalis*, *C. ochracea*, *C. sputigena*, *C. granulosa*, *C. haemolytica* and *C. leadbetteri*. *Capnocytophaga* are opportunistic pathogens and have been isolated from several infections in immunocompromised patients; some strains produce an IgA1 protease. *Kingella* (e.g., *K. oralis*) is a coccobacillus that has been isolated from several oral sites. The gliding bacterium *Simonsiella* has been isolated from epithelial surfaces of the oral cavity of humans and a variety of animals. These organisms have a unique cellular morphology, being composed of unusually large, multicellular filaments in groups, or multiples of eight cells. There have been reports of *Helicobacter pylori* in dental plaque; this species is microaerophilic and is usually isolated from the stomach where it is associated with gastritis, peptic ulcers and gastric cancer. It may be present in the mouth transiently following reflux from the stomach.

OBLIGATELY ANAEROBIC GENERA

Obligately anaerobic Gram-negative rods comprise a large proportion of the microbiota of dental plaque and the tongue. Many species are difficult to grow or are described as being unculturable; consequently, molecular approaches have been necessary to classify and identify many of these organisms.

Most of the cultivable oral obligate anaerobes belong to the genera *Prevotella* and *Porphyromonas* (Fig. 3.7, *B* and *D*). Some organisms from these genera produce colonies with a characteristic brown or black pigment when grown on blood agar (Fig. 3.8). The pigment acts as a defence mechanism to protect the cells from the toxic effects of oxygen. These organisms are referred to collectively as black-pigmented anaerobes. Haemin is an essential growth factor for these organisms and is obtained in the host from the

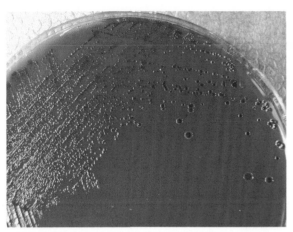

FIGURE 3.8 Colony pigmentation of *Porphyromonas gingivalis* on blood agar. Image was kindly provided by Owain Dafydd Thomas, Cardiff and Vale UHB.

catabolism of haeme-containing molecules such as haemoglobin.

Prevotella species are moderately saccharolytic (i.e., able to ferment carbohydrates); species that produce pigmenting colonies include *P. intermedia*, *P. nigrescens*, *P. melaninogenica*, *P. loescheii*, *P. pallens*, *P. fusca*, *P. scopos* and some strains of *P. denticola*. *Prevotella intermedia* and *P. nigrescens* (see Fig. 3.7, *D*) are difficult to distinguish using simple physiological tests, but importantly *P. intermedia* is associated with periodontal disease whereas *P. nigrescens* is isolated more often, and in higher numbers, from healthy sites. There is a large number of oral non-pigmented species including *P. buccae*, *P. buccalis*, *P. oralis*, *P. oris*, *P. oulora*, *P. veroralis*, *P. dentalis*, *P. enoeca*, *P. bergensis*, *P. multisaccharivorax*, *P. marshii*, *P. baroniae*, *P. shahii*, *P. multiformis*, *P. salivae*, *P. micans*, *P. maculosa*, *P. histicola* and *P. zoogleoformans*. The majority of these species can, on occasions, be isolated from dental plaque, particularly from subgingival sites. Some species are associated with disease and increase in numbers and proportions during periodontal disease and have also been recovered from abscesses (see Chapters 6 and 7). A newly described but related genus is *Alloprevotella*, and examples include *Alloprevotella rava* and *A. tannerae*.

Porphyromonas species are mainly asaccharolytic and use proteins and peptides for growth. *Porphyromonas gingivalis* (see Figs 3.7, *B*, 3.7, *C* and 3.8) is isolated primarily from subgingival sites, especially in advanced periodontal lesions, although it has also been recovered from the tongue and tonsils. Six serotypes are recognised based on capsular polysaccharides (K antigens). *Porphyromonas gingivalis* is highly virulent in experimental infection studies in animals and produces a range of putative virulence factors associated with tissue destruction and subversion of the host defences. These include proteases with specificity for arginine-x bonds and lysine-x bonds (arg-gingipains and lys-gingipains, respectively), that can degrade molecules such as immunoglobulins, complement, and iron- and haeme-sequestering proteins and glycoproteins, as well as host molecules that regulate the host inflammatory response. *Porphyromonas gingivalis* also produces a haemolysin, collagen-degrading enzymes, cytotoxic metabolites and a capsule (see Chapter 6). *Porphyromonas gingivalis* has numerous fimbriae on its cell surface that mediate adherence to oral epithelial cells and to saliva-coated tooth surfaces, and produces large quantities of surface vesicles that can be shed into the environment (see Fig. 3.7, *B*). *Porphyromonas gingivalis* is also linked with systemic diseases including cardiovascular disease (where it has been found in atherosclerotic plaque) and rheumatoid arthritis (it uniquely possesses a peptidylarginine deiminase that can citrullinate host proteins, which can generate autoantibodies) (see Chapter 11). Other species include *Porphyromonas endodontalis*, which has been mainly recovered from infected root canals, and *Porphyromonas catoniae*, which is found mainly at healthy sites or in shallow periodontal pockets.

Another major group of obligately anaerobic Gram-negative bacteria belong to the genus *Fusobacterium*. Cells characteristically form long filaments (5 to 25 μm in length; Fig. 3.7, *E*) or pleomorphic rods, and produce butyric acid as their major end product of metabolism. The most common species is *F. nucleatum*, and several subspecies have been recognised, including subsp. *nucleatum*, subsp. *polymorphum* and subsp. *vincentii*. These subspecies may have different associations with health and disease; *F. nucleatum* subsp.

polymorphum is commonly isolated from the normal gingival crevice whereas subspecies *nucleatum* is recovered mainly from periodontal pockets. Other oral fusobacteria include *F. periodonticum*, which is isolated from sites exhibiting periodontal disease. Fusobacteria are often described as being asaccharolytic, although they can take up carbohydrates for the synthesis of intracellular storage compounds composed of polyglucose. Fusobacteria catabolise amino acids such as aspartate, glutamate, histidine and lysine to provide energy. These amino acids can be obtained from the metabolism of peptides if free amino acids are not available. *Fusobacterium nucleatum* is able to remove sulphur from cysteine and methionine to produce ammonia, butyrate, hydrogen sulphide and methyl mercaptan, and these compounds contribute to the malodour associated with halitosis. Fusobacteria are able to aggregate with most other oral bacteria and consequently, are believed to be important bridging organisms between early and late colonisers during biofilm formation (coadhesion and coaggregation, see Chapter 5). *Fusobacterium nucleatum* is commonly isolated from extraoral infections, which might be related to its ability to adhere to and invade epithelial and endothelial cells mediated by an adhesin, FadA. *Fusobacterium nucleatum* is associated with colorectal cancer; FadA is involved in attachment to gut epithelial cells, enabling it to modulate cell signalling pathways resulting in increased expression of oncogenes (see Chapter 11).

Other oral Gram-negative anaerobic and microaerophilic bacterial genera include *Leptotrichia* (species include *L. buccalis, L. hofstadii, L. shahii* and *L. wadei*), *Wolinella* (e.g., *W. succinogenes*) and *Campylobacter* (cells have a spiral morphology), and species include *Campylobacter concisus, C. gracilis, C. showae, C. sputorum, C. curvus* and *C. rectus* (the latter two species were previously classified as *Wolinella curva* and *W. recta*, respectively). *Campylobacter concisus* is isolated in higher proportions from relatively shallow periodontal pockets and healthy subgingival sites, whereas *C. rectus* is found more commonly at sites with active periodontal disease, especially in immunocompromised patients, and some strains produce a cytotoxin. *Selenomonas sputigena, S. noxia, S. flueggei, S. infelix, S. dianae* and *S. artemidis* have been found in plaque from the human gingival crevice.

Some of the species described previously have flagella and are motile. The *Wolinella* and *Campylobacter* species have a single flagellum, whereas *Selenomonas* species are curved to helical bacilli with a tuft of flagella. Another helical or curved Gram-negative oral anaerobe is *Centipeda periodontii* which has numerous flagella spiralling around the cell. Other genera include *Johnsonii* (*J. ignava*) and *Cantonella* (*C. morbi*), which are associated with gingivitis and periodontitis, respectively; *Dialister* (*D. pneumosintes* and *D. invisus*, which can be found in endodontic infections and periodontitis); *Flavobacterium* and *Tannerella forsythia* (commonly isolated from advanced periodontal disease).

Sulphate-reducing bacteria (e.g., those belonging to genera such as *Desulfobacter, Desulfobulbus, Desulfomicrobium* and *Desulfovibrio*) have been isolated on occasions from dental plaque and from periodontal pockets. They obtain energy by oxidising organic acids or hydrogen, while reducing sulphate to hydrogen sulphide, which can contribute to mouth malodour. These bacteria are extremely difficult to grow in the laboratory because of their sensitivity to even trace amounts of oxygen and their requirement for a very low redox potential for growth.

Spirochaetes are numerous in subgingival plaque and can readily be detected using dark-field or electron microscopy. Several morphological types can be distinguished according to cell size and the arrangement of periplasmic flagella (endoflagella). Some oral spirochaetes adhere to surfaces in a polar orientation, and this type of adhesion results in gross alterations to host cell morphology facilitating penetration into underlying tissues. The numbers of spirochaetes are raised in advanced periodontal diseases and are diagnostic for necrotising ulcerative periodontitis (see Chapter 6). However, whether they cause disease or merely increase following infection is still to be resolved. Oral spirochaetes fall within the genus *Treponema*, and a large number of species have been recognised, including *T. denticola, T. socranskii* (subspecies *socranskii*; subspecies *buccale*; subspecies *paredis*), *T. maltophilum, T. amylovorum, T. parvum, T. pectinovorum, T. putidum, T. lecithinolyticum, T. medium* and *T. vincentii* (see Fig. 3.3, A). These species have been isolated from periodontally-inflamed sites and endodontic infections. Little is known about the physiology of these organisms because of difficulties associated with their laboratory cultivation, and as such they are mainly detected using molecular techniques. However, *T. denticola* has been grown using appropriate methods, and has an arginine-specific ('trypsin-like') protease, and can also degrade collagen and gelatin.

As stated earlier in this chapter, only about 50–70% of the microorganisms that can be visualised in the mouth by microscopy can currently be cultivated. This is not only because of ignorance of the growth requirements of these organisms but also because some bacteria have evolved to grow in partnership (physically and nutritionally) with other microbes. New families of unculturable bacteria are being identified by molecular approaches, for example, *Bacteroidales* and *Lachnospiraceae*, whereas some of the unculturable bacteria show sufficient genetic similarity to known cultivable species that they can be placed within a genus, for example, unculturable spirochaetes to the genus, *Treponema* (see Fig. 3.3, *A*). Others represent novel evolutionary lineages, which are found in a number of habitats, and are designated simply by the phyla in which they are grouped. Most oral examples belong to the TM7 phylum, and can be detected in subgingival plaque by fluorescent *in situ* hybridisation (FISH), which involves combining oligonucleotide probes (coupled to a fluorescent tag) with specialised microscopy techniques (epifluorescence or confocal laser scanning microscopy) (see Fig. 3.3, *B*). Some organisms detected by molecular approaches in

samples from subgingival plaque, periodontal lesions and endodontic infections, belong to a new candidate phylum Synergistetes. Advances are now being made in their classification; examples of these organisms include *Jonquetella anthropic*, *Pyramidobacter piscolens* and *Fretibacterium fastidiosum*. Increasing our understanding of the role of these unculturable bacteria in health and disease is now an important goal for oral microbiologists.

MYCOPLASMA

Bacteria belonging to the genus *Mycoplasma* are primarily characterised by the absence of a cell wall, which makes them appear Gram-negative when stained. Because of their small size (<1 μm; they are the smallest of all free-growing cells), they are difficult to visualise by normal light microscopy.

Analysis of *Mycoplasma* genome sequences (16S rDNA) suggests they are most closely related to *Bacillus–Lactobacillus* and *Streptococcus* subgroups of Gram-positive bacteria. Mycoplasma are notoriously slow growing and require specialised microbiological culture media enriched in proteins and with an elevated carbon dioxide atmosphere for growth. *Mycoplasma* are pleomorphic, and several cell shapes can occur depending on the environment.

Mycoplasmas are most prevalent on mucosal surfaces. Oral carriage rates of between 6% and 32% have been reported in humans with a number of species recovered from saliva (*Mycoplasma salivarium, M. pneumoniae, M. hominis*), the oral mucosa (*M. buccale, M. orale, M. pneumoniae*) and dental plaque (*M. pneumoniae, M. buccale, M. orale*). *Mycoplasma orale* and *M. salivarium* have also been isolated from salivary glands where it has been postulated that they play a role in salivary gland hypofunction.

FUNGI

Fungi generally constitute a relatively small proportion of the oral microbiota. The perfect fungi (fungi that divide by sexual reproduction) are rarely isolated from the oral cavity but are occasionally found infecting patients with advanced acquired immunodeficiency syndrome (AIDS). The main perfect fungi causing oral infection are *Aspergillus, Geotrichum* and

KEY POINTS

Oral Gram-negative bacteria are diverse and include species that are facultatively and obligately anaerobic, as well as species that are microaerophilic and capnophilic. *Veillonella* are anaerobic Gram-negative cocci that play an important role in dental plaque by converting lactate to weaker acids. Most of the anaerobic Gram-negative bacilli are found in dental plaque, have an asaccharolytic metabolism and depend on proteins and glycoproteins for their nutrition; some common genera include *Prevotella* and *Fusobacterium*. The diversity of species increases in periodontal disease, and many of these are unculturable at present. The taxonomy of Gram-negative bacteria has been transformed by molecular techniques such as 16S rRNA gene sequencing.

Mucor species. The perfect yeast species seen in healthy individuals may be transient rather than resident members of the oral microbiota. In contrast, the imperfect yeasts, e.g., *Candida* species (which divide by asexual reproduction), are common in the mouth (see Chapter 8). *Candida albicans* is by far the most prevalent species, but a large number of other yeast species have been isolated, including *C. glabrata, C. tropicalis, C. krusei, C. parapsilosis,* and *C. guilliermondii,* as well as species of *Rhodotorula* and *Saccharomyces.* Estimations of carriage rates of *Candida* in the mouth vary markedly because of the different isolation techniques used and the population groups investigated (see Chapter 8). Carriage rates range from 2% to 71% in asymptomatic adults, but this increases, and approaches 100%, in medically-compromised patients or those on broad spectrum antibacterial agents.

Candida are distributed evenly throughout the mouth, but the most common site of isolation is the dorsum of the tongue. The isolation of *Candida* increases with the presence of intra-oral devices such as dentures or orthodontic appliances, particularly in the upper jaw on the fitting surface; *Candida* species can attach tenaciously to acrylic.

ARCHAEA

Archaea have characteristics that make them distinct from either *Bacteria* or *Eukarya* and constitute a distinct branch of the phylogenetic tree of life. *Archaea* are found in complex microbial communities in the gut and mouth, and *Methanobrevibacter oralis* is the main species in the oral cavity, detected in subgingival dental plaque and infected root canals. These organisms obtain energy by the reduction of CO_2 to methane, and associations between methanogens and sulphate-reducing bacteria with *Synergistes* and other putative periodontal pathogens have been reported, suggesting that these bacteria may function as terminal degraders during the catabolism of complex host molecules (see Chapter 5). Other Archaea isolated from the mouth include *Methanobacterium* and *Methanosarcina.*

VIRUSES

A number of viruses can be detected in the mouth using molecular techniques (see Chapter 9). It is now no longer necessary to use time-consuming and often unreliable methods of detection of viruses, such as tissue culture or electron microscopy. Indeed, some viruses have only been detected by the use of molecular approaches and have never been cultured in the laboratory (e.g., hepatitis C virus and hepatitis G virus).

The virus most frequently encountered in saliva and the orofacial area is Herpes simplex type 1 (HSV-1). The vast majority (80% to 90%) of adults in the western world have suffered from primary infection with HSV-1, which when reactivated from its latent form causes secondary infection lesions known as cold sores on the orofacial tissues. Molecular techniques have revealed that HSV-1 is persistent within the oral tissues and can also be detected occasionally by culture in saliva in the absence of any clinical signs or symptoms, which indicates periodic shedding. The virus also remains latent in neural tissue, in particular the trigeminal nerve, where it may be reactivated by a number of factors including UV light or stress. Once reactivated, the genome passes through the peripheral nerves to cause the characteristic blisters on the skin or within the mouth, which rupture to release further virus particles.

Cytomegalovirus is present in most individuals. These viruses have been detected in the saliva of symptomless adults, but their portal of entry into the oral cavity is not clear. Coxsackie virus A2, 4, 5, 6, 8, 9, 10 and 16 have all been detected in saliva and in the oral epithelium. The detection of these viruses has usually been associated with hand, foot and mouth disease or herpangina.

There are more than 100 types of human papilloma virus (HPV), of which types 2 and 4 have been frequently encountered within localised hyperplastic wart-like epithelial lesions of the lips and mouth (verruca vulgaris, condylomata acuminata). HPV types 2, 4, 6, 11 and 16 have also been detected relatively frequently in the oral tissues of HIV–positive patients. Recent studies have explored the possible role of HPV in mouth cancer, and it is now established that types 16 and 18 are the cause of some cases of oropharyngeal carcinoma.

Bacteriophages (viruses for which bacteria are the natural hosts) have been observed in samples of saliva and dental plaque, but few have been isolated. Bacteriophages specific for *S. mutans, Lactobacillus, Actinomyces, Veillonella* and *Aggregatibacter* species have been described. The role of bacteriophage in the microbial ecology of the mouth is not fully understood. Some bacteriophage with activity against non-oral bacteria (e.g., *Proteus mirabilis*) have been detected, and this might contribute to the ability of the resident oral microbiota to exclude exogenous species (colonisation resistance; see Chapter 4). Bacteriophage may also drive molecular diversity in oral biofilms by delivering new gene function in response to antimicrobial therapy or other environmental perturbations.

On rare occasions, potentially pathogenic viruses can be found in the oral cavity, especially in saliva, where their presence may pose a significant cross-infection threat. Although some patients may have obvious disease, many can be asymptomatic. Hepatitis B virus is a specific example of a pathogenic virus that can spread from the saliva of an apparently healthy patient (see Chapter 12). Other viruses that have been detected in saliva include a number of respiratory viruses, human immunodeficiency virus (HIV), measles virus and mumps virus.

PROTOZOA

Protozoa are defined as unicellular eukaryotic microorganisms that lack a cell wall. Two protozoan species frequently recovered from the mouth are *Trichomonas tenax* and *Entamoeba gingivalis*. Their oral prevalence is variable, but estimates report carriage rates of between 4% and 52% in the healthy population. Molecular techniques can be used to detect these organisms and PCR has detected *T. tenax* in 2% of healthy oral cavities, increasing to 21% in patients with periodontal disease.

Both of the above oral protozoan species are motile, and in the case of *T. tenax*, its characteristic tumbling motility is mediated through the presence of four anterior flagella and a fifth recurrent flagellum, attached to an undulating membrane along the length of the cell. *Trichomonas tenax* and *E. gingivalis* are heterotrophic, acquiring their carbon requirements through ingestion of other microorganisms, host leukocytes and dead organic matter within the mouth and, in this sense, they are truly parasitic. Both species are strictly anaerobic and although generally considered to be harmless commensals, there are reports associating their presence with periodontal disease. *Trichomonas tenax* produces cysteine proteinases and metalloproteinases, which could damage host connective tissues. However, whether or not these organisms play an active role in periodontal disease still remains unclear, although it is apparent that their incidence does increase in individuals with poor oral hygiene.

CHAPTER SUMMARY

The healthy mouth supports the growth of a wide range of microorganisms including bacteria, yeasts, mycoplasmas, *Archaea*, viruses and even protozoa. Bacteria are the predominant components of the resident oral microbiota, and a list of the major genera is given in Table 3.4. Many of these bacteria are fastidious in their nutritional requirements, although others are obligate anaerobic and highly sensitive to oxygen, and some have evolved to grow in mixed culture. At present, only about 70% of the organisms in plaque can be isolated in pure culture in the laboratory. Molecular approaches, based on comparisons of 16S rRNA gene sequences and whole genome sequencing, have revolutionised our understanding of the complexity of the resident oral microbiota and resolved many long-standing problems with the classification of several groups of oral bacteria (for an example, see Fig. 3.6). These approaches have identified many new genera and species, including phyla such as TM7 that are unculturable when growth is attempted in pure culture (see Fig. 3.3, *B*). Molecular approaches offer the potential for rapid (and relatively simple) techniques to detect, visualise and identify even the most fastidious of oral microbe in clinical samples. The resultant benefits in classification and detection will increase the likelihood of finding closer associations between particular species or taxa with sites in health and disease.

The high diversity of the oral microbiota reflects the wide range of nutrients available endogenously in the mouth, the varied types of habitat for colonisation, and the opportunity provided by biofilms such as plaque for survival on surfaces. Despite this diversity, many microorganisms commonly isolated from neighbouring ecosystems, such as the skin and the gut, are not found in the mouth, emphasising the unique and selective properties of the mouth for microbial colonisation.

TABLE 3.4 The principal bacterial genera found in the oral cavity

GRAM-POSITIVE		GRAM-NEGATIVE	
Cocci	**Rods**	**Cocci**	**Rods**
Abiotrophia	Actinobaculum	Anaeroglobus	Aggregatibacter
Enterococcus	Actinomyces	Megasphaera	Campylobacter
Finegoldia	Alloscardovia	Moraxella	Cantonella
Gemella	Arcanobacterium	Neisseria	Capnocytophaga
Granulicatella	Atopobium	Veillonella	Centipeda
Peptostreptococcus	Bifidobacterium		Desulfomicrobium
Streptococcus	Corynebacterium		Desulfovibrio
	Cryptobacterium		Dialister
	Eubacterium		Eikenella
	Filifactor		Flavobacterium
	Lactobacillus		Fusobacterium
	Mogibacterium		Haemophilus
	Olsenella		Johnsonii
	Parascardovia		Kingella
	Propionibacterium		Leptotrichia
	Pseudoramibacter		Methanobrevibacter
	Rothia		Porphyromonas
	Scardovia		Prevotella
	Shuttleworthia		Selenomonas
	Slackia		Simonsiella
	Solobacterium		Tannerella
			Treponema
			Wolinella

Not all bacterial genera have been listed. Mycoplasma is also isolated from the mouth.
There are also unculturable bacteria that have yet to be placed in a genus; some belong to the phylum TM7.

FURTHER READING

Aas JA, Paster BJ, Stokes LN, et al. Defining the normal bacterial flora of the oral cavity. *J Clin Microbiol*. 2005;43:5721-5732.

Asam D, Spellerberg B. Molecular pathogenicity of *Streptococcus anginosus*. *Mol Oral Microbiol*. 2014;29:145-155.

Aruni W, Chioma O, Fletcher HM. *Filifactor alocis*: the newly discovered kid on the block with special talents. *J Dent Res*. 2014;93:725-732.

Chen T, Yu WH, Izard J, et al. The Human Oral Microbiome Database: a web accessible resource for investigating oral microbe taxonomic and genomic information. *Database*. 2010;doi:10.1093/database/baq013; Article ID baq013.

Dewhirst FE, Chen T, Izard J, et al. The Human Oral Microbiome. *J Bacteriol*. 2010;192:5002-5017.

Edlund A, Santiago-Rodriguez TM, Boehm TK, et al. Bacteriophage and their potential roles in the human oral cavity. *J Oral Microbiol*. 2015;7:27423.

Han YW. *Fusobacterium nucleatum*: a commensal-turned pathogen. *Curr Opin Microbiol*. 2015;23:141-147.

Henderson B, Ward JM, Ready D. *Aggregatibacter (Actinobacillus) actinomycetemcomitans*: a triple A* periodontopathogen? *Periodontol 2000*. 2010;54:78-105.

Ghannoum MA, Jurevic RJ, Mukherjee PK, et al. Characterization of the oral fungal microbiome (mycobiome) in healthy individuals. *PLoS Pathog*. 2010;8(6):e1000713.

Human Microbiome Project Consortium. Structure, function and diversity of the healthy human microbiome. *Nature*. 2012;486(7402):207-214.

Könönen E, Wade WG. *Actinomyces* and related organisms in human infections. *Clin Microbiol Revs*. 2015;28:419-442.

Li L, Redding S, Dongari-Bagtzoglou A. *Candida glabrata:* an emerging oral opportunistic pathogen. *J Dent Res*. 2007;86:204-215.

Matarazzo F, Ribeiro AC, Faveri M, et al. The domain *Archaea* in human mucosal surfaces. *Clin Microbiol Infect*. 2012;18:834-840.

Murphy EC, Frick I-M. Gram-positive anaerobic cocci – commensals and opportunistic pathogens. *FEMS Microbiol Rev*. 2013;37: 520-553.

Nair RG, Salajegheh A, Itthagarun A, et al. Orofacial viral infections – an update for clinicians. *Dent Update*. 2014;41:518-520, 522-524.

Nakayama K. *Porphyromonas gingivalis* and related bacteria: from colonial pigmentation to the type IX secretion system and gliding motility. *J Periodontal Res*. 2015;50:1-8.

Nguyen-Hieu T, Khelaifia S, Aboudharam G, et al. Methanogenic archaea in subgingival sites: a review. *APMIS*. 2013;121:467-477.

Sharma A. Virulence mechanisms of *Tannerella forsythia. Periodontol 2000*. 2010;54:106-116.

Visser MB, Ellen RP. New insights into the emerging role of oral spirochaetes in periodontal disease. *Clin Microbiol Infect*. 2011;17: 502-512.

Wade WG. The oral microbiome in health and disease. *Pharmacol Res*. 2013;69:137-143.

Whitmore SE, Lamont RJ. The pathogenic persona of community-associated oral streptococci. *Mol Microbiol*. 2011;81:305-314.

The Human Oral Microbiome Database (HOMD) provides comprehensive information on the microorganisms found in the human oral cavity. This is an ongoing project and the database will be continuously updated. The database can be accessed at: <www.homd.org>

MULTIPLE CHOICE QUESTIONS

Answers on p. 249

1 *Classification of microorganisms is the process of which of the following?*
a. Grouping microorganisms logically based on their similarities and differences
b. Giving microorganisms a name
c. Developing an identification scheme
d. Describing the colonial appearance of a bacterial strain

2 *Bacteria that are dependent for their growth on carbon dioxide are referred to as what?*
a. Obligately anaerobic
b. Facultatively anaerobic
c. Aerobic
d. Capnophilic

3 *Strains of* Streptococcus salivarius *produce large quantities of what type of exopolymer from sucrose?*
a. Heteropolysaccharide
b. Fructan (inulin-structure)
c. Fructan (levan structure)
d. Glycogen

4 *Which of the following is a bacterium that is capnophilic?*
a. *Capnocytophaga gingivalis*
b. *Porphyromonas gingivalis*
c. *Fusobacterium nucleatum*
d. *Veillonella atypica*

5 *Which of the following species produce colonies with a brown or black pigment on blood agar?*
a. *Aggregatibacterium actinomycetemcomitans*
b. *Porphyromonas gingivalis*
c. *Prevotella oralis*
d. *Eikenella corrodens*

6 *Oral spirochaetes fall within which genus?*
a. *Bacteroides*
b. *Centipeda*
c. *Treponema*
d. *Selenomonas*

7 *Which of the following protozoa are found in the mouth?*
a. Paramecium
b. *Trichomonas tenax*
c. *Entamoeba histolytica*
d. *Giardia lamblia*

8 *Initial tests on colonies that are alpha-haemolytic on blood agar provide the following results: Gram-positive cocci in chains; negative catalase reaction; produce ammonia from arginine; bind alpha-amylase; produce glucan from sucrose. What is the most likely identification of these bacteria?*
a. *Streptococcus mutans*
b. *Streptococcus vestibularis*
c. *Streptococcus gordonii*
d. *Streptococcus intermedius*

9 Which of the following species is the most commonly isolated Gram-positive facultatively anaerobic bacillus isolated from dental biofilms?

a. *Actinomyces naeslundii*

b. *Actinomyces israelii*

c. *Lactobacillus casei*

d. *Bifidobacterium dentium*

10 Which of the following is the Gram-negative anaerobic coccus that is found most commonly in high numbers in the mouth?

a. *Neisseria subflava*

b. *Veillonella parvula*

c. *Eikennela corrodens*

d. *Megasphaera micronuciformis*

CHAPTER 4

Distribution, development and benefits of the oral microbiota

The foetus in the womb is normally sterile, but from birth the baby is exposed to, and colonised by, a wide variety of microorganisms. These are derived predominantly from the mother, but only a small proportion are able to establish in the infant mouth. The biological and physical properties of each habitat determine which organisms will attach and grow, and dictate which will be major or minor components of the human microbiota at each site. This results in different surfaces having distinct and characteristic microbiotas.

ACQUISITION OF THE RESIDENT ORAL MICROBIOTA

Microbial acquisition depends on the transmission of microorganisms to the site of potential colonisation. Initially, in the mouth, this is by passive inoculation mainly from the mother, but also from other individuals in close proximity to the baby and from ingested milk and water. The mode of delivery of the baby influences the microbiota of the newborn. Conventionally delivered babies harbour bacterial communities that are similar to the vaginal microbial community of the mother. These include representatives of genera such as *Lactobacillus*, *Prevotella* and *Atopobium*. In contrast, babies delivered by Caesarean section have bacterial communities that resemble the skin microbiota, and include many *Staphylococcus* species. The oral microbiota of breastfed babies differs from that of formula-fed infants during the first months of life. Lactobacilli (especially *L. plantarum*) are more common in breastfed infants, and this may influence the subsequent development of the infant oral microbiota, as these organisms have been shown to inhibit the growth of mutans streptococci and *Candida albicans*.

Over time, further episodes of transmission occur, especially via saliva, but the properties of each site exert selective pressures, and the microbiota becomes more differentiated and characteristic of each surface. The ability to type (fingerprint) strains (see Chapter 3, Fig. 3.1) has enabled confirmation of the transfer of *Streptococcus salivarius*, mutans streptococci and some other oral bacterial species from mother to child via saliva (**vertical transmission**). There is little evidence of father-infant (or father-mother) transmission of mutans streptococci, although **horizontal transmission** between spouses, and vertical transmission within family units, can occur with some periodontal pathogens, such as *Porphyromonas gingivalis* and *Aggregatibacter actinomycetemcomitans*. Oral bacteria have been shown to be transferred through repeated intimate kissing between partners, although this does not necessarily lead to colonisation.

PIONEER COMMUNITY AND MICROBIAL SUCCESSION

The mouth is highly selective for microbial colonisation. Very few of the species common to the oral cavity of adults, and even fewer of the large number of bacteria found in the environment, are able to become established in the mouth of the newborn. The first microorganisms to colonise are termed **pioneer species**, and collectively they make up the **pioneer microbial community**. These pioneer species continue to grow and colonise until environmental resistance (physical and chemical) is encountered. In the mouth, physical factors that promote removal include the shedding of epithelial cells (desquamation), and the shear forces from chewing and saliva flow, whereas nutrient availability and unfavourable conditions of redox potential (Eh; see Chapter 2) or pH, and the antibacterial properties of saliva, are chemical barriers that can limit growth.

One genus or species is usually predominant during the development of the pioneer community. In the mouth of babies, the predominant cultivable organisms are streptococci, and in particular *S. salivarius, S. mitis* and *S. oralis*. Many of the pioneer species possess immunoglobulin A1 (IgA$_1$) protease activity, which may enable producer organisms to evade the effects of this important mucosal defence factor. Over time, the metabolic activity of the pioneer community modifies the environment providing conditions suitable for colonisation by a succession of other populations. This may be by:

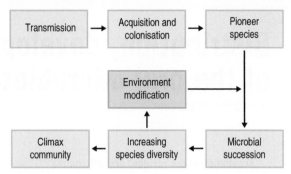

FIGURE 4.1 Ecological stages in the establishment of a microbial community. As microbial diversity increases, the metabolism of the pioneer species modifies the local environment making conditions suitable for secondary colonisers.

- modifying or exposing new receptors for attachment (cryptitopes, see Chapter 5),
- changing the local pH, or by reducing oxygen levels and lowering the redox potential, Eh, or
- generating additional nutrients, for example, as end products of metabolism (lactate, succinate) or breakdown products (peptides, haemin) that can be used by other organisms as part of a food chain.

As outlined previously, the pioneer community influences the pattern of **microbial succession**. This involves the progressive development of the pioneer community (containing few species) through several stages in which the number of microbial groups increases, until equilibrium is reached; this is termed the **climax community** and generally has a high species diversity (Fig. 4.1). Succession is associated with a change from a site possessing few niches (roles; see Chapter 1) to one with a multitude of potential niches. A climax community reflects a highly dynamic situation between the host, the environment and the microbiota, and must not be regarded as a static state.

The oral cavity of babies contains only mucosal surfaces for colonisation. The pioneer populations consist mainly of aerobic and facultatively anaerobic bacterial species; streptococci are commonly isolated after the first few days, and *S. oralis, S. mitis* biovar 1 and *S. salivarius* are numerically dominant (Table 4.1). The diversity of the streptococcal microbiota increases with time; after one month, all babies are colonised by at least two species of *Streptococcus*, with *S. salivarius* and *S. mitis* biovar 1 being most common

TABLE 4.1 **Streptococcal species cultured from the mucosal surfaces of babies**

Streptococcus	PERCENTAGE VIABLE COUNT		
	AGE		
	1–3 days	2 weeks	1 month
S. oralis	41	24	20
S. mitis biovar 1	30	28	30
S. mitis biovar 2	4	1	1
S. salivarius	10	30	28
S. sanguinis	4	3	2
S. anginosus	3	5	5
S. gordonii	1	2	4

TABLE 4.2 **The effect of tooth eruption on the composition of the cultivatable Gram-negative oral microbiota in young children**

Bacterium	PERCENTAGE ISOLATION FREQUENCY	
	MEAN AGE	
	3 months	32 months
Prevotella melaninogenica	76	100
non-pigmented Prevotella	62	100
Prevotella loescheii	14	90
Prevotella intermedia	10	67
Prevotella denticola	ND	71
Fusobacterium nucleatum	67	100
Fusobacterium spp.	ND	71
Selenomonas spp.	ND	43
Capnocytophaga spp.	19	100
Leptotrichia spp.	24	71
Campylobacter spp.	5	43
Eikenella corrodens	5	57
Veillonella spp.	63	63

21 children were sampled, both when they were edentulous (mean age = 3 months) and dentate (mean age: 32 months).
ND, Not detected.

(Table 4.1). *Actinomyces odontolyticus* can be isolated from oral mucosal surfaces in infants as young as two months. In contrast, the prevalence of *S. sanguinis*, mutans streptococci and *A. naeslundii* increase once teeth have erupted.

The diversity of the pioneer oral community continues to increase during the first few months of life, and Gram-negative obligately anaerobic bacteria begin to colonise. In culture-based studies, *Prevotella melaninogenica* was the most frequently isolated obligate anaerobe, being recovered from 76% of edentulous infants (mean age: 3 months; range: 1 to 7 months) (Table 4.2). Other commonly isolated bacteria were *Fusobacterium nucleatum* (present in 67% of infants), *Veillonella* spp. (63%) and non-pigmented *Prevotella* spp. (62%) (Table 4.2); the number of culturable anaerobes in a single mouth varied from 0 to 7 species.

In a longitudinal study of the development of the microbiota during the eruption of the primary dentition, Gram-negative obligately anaerobic bacteria were isolated more commonly, and a greater diversity of species were recovered from around the gingival margin of newly erupted teeth (mean age of the infants: 32 months) (Table 4.2). These findings confirm that the eruption of teeth has a significant ecological impact on the oral environment and its resident microbiota.

During the first year of life, members of the genera *Neisseria*, *Veillonella*, *Actinomyces*, *Streptococcus*, *Lactobacillus* and *Rothia* are commonly isolated, particularly after tooth eruption. Culture-independent (molecular) methods have detected, on occasions, some of the obligately anaerobic species implicated in periodontal diseases from tooth and tongue samples from young children (aged 18 to 36 months). *Porphyromonas gingivalis*, *Tannerella forsythia* and *A. actinomycetemcomitans* were detected in the mouths of approximately 10% to 30% of 18-month-old infants. The proportions of putative periodontal pathogens, such as *P. gingivalis*, *T. forsythia* and *Treponema denticola*, in biofilms from mucosal surfaces (especially the tongue and teeth) were found to increase over time in children aged 3 to 12 years. When present, these bacteria are usually at very low levels and, therefore, are not of any clinical relevance. However, these bacteria can be carried and could at some point exploit either a change in local environmental conditions or a suppression of the host defences, to outcompete species associated with oral health, thereby predisposing such sites to disease. An appreciation of this dynamic relationship between the host and the oral microbiota is central to understanding the aetiology of most dental diseases.

KEY POINTS

> The mother is the main source of the oral microbiota of the newborn infant.
>
> The biological properties of the mouth dictate which microorganisms are able to colonise successfully and which will be predominant.
>
> Each oral surface will support a distinct but characteristic microbiota. There is a dynamic relationship between the host environment and the composition and activity of the oral microbiota.

ALLOGENIC AND AUTOGENIC MICROBIAL SUCCESSION

The establishment of a climax community at any oral site involves a series of phases of development during which the complexity of the microbiota increases (**microbial succession**; see Fig. 4.1). Two distinct types of succession have been identified (Fig. 4.2). In **allogenic succession**, factors of non-microbial origin are responsible for an altered pattern of community development. For example, the frequency of detection of mutans streptococci and *S. sanguinis* increases markedly once hard, non-shedding surfaces appear in the mouth. Such a situation would arise following tooth eruption, or after the insertion of dentures or removable orthodontic appliances, or acrylic obturators in children with cleft palate.

The increase in number and diversity of obligate anaerobes once teeth are present is an example of **autogenic succession** in which community development is influenced by microbial factors (see Fig. 4.2). The metabolism of the aerobic and facultatively anaerobic pioneer species lowers the redox potential in plaque and creates conditions suitable for colonisation by strict anaerobes (see Chapter 5). Other examples of autogenic succession are the development of food chains and food webs, whereby the metabolic end product of one organism becomes a primary nutrient for another:

$$\text{complex substrate} \xrightarrow{\substack{\text{primary} \\ \text{feeder}}} \text{product} \xrightarrow{\substack{\text{secondary} \\ \text{feeder}}} \text{simpler product}$$

A further example of autogenic succession is the exposure of new receptors for bacterial adhesion (cryptitopes; see Chapter 5) following microbial modification of host macromolecules.

The gross composition of the oral microbiota can remain relatively stable over time at individual sites (microbial homeostasis), especially when analysed at the genus or species level. Species that comprise the resident human microbiota often display large numbers of clones, and these can vary over time. Clones of some species appear to persist for long periods at a site, whereas others appear to be transient, and undergo replacement by fresh clones. This may be a strategy to help such species evade the host defences.

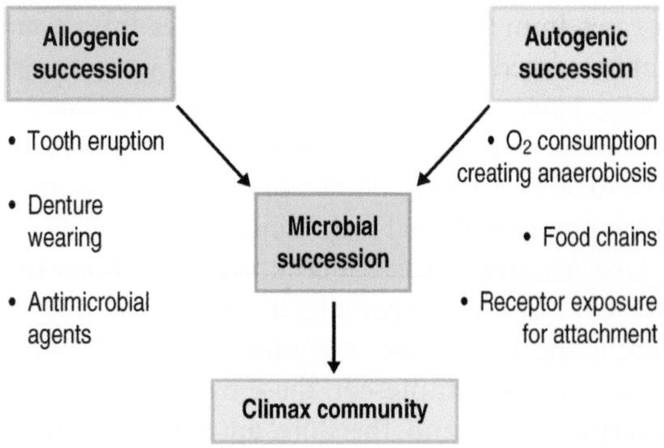

FIGURE 4.2 Role of autogenic and allogenic succession in the development of oral microbial communities.

KEY POINTS

> The mouth is usually sterile at birth. The acquisition of the normal oral microbiota starts at birth and follows a specific ecological progression from a small number of pioneer species, especially *S. salivarius, S. mitis* and *S. oralis*, to a diverse climax community containing many obligately anaerobic and nutritionally fastidious bacteria. This development involves both allogenic and autogenic succession; in allogenic succession, community development is influenced by non-microbial factors whereas microbial factors are responsible for autogenic succession. Once established, the microbiota remains relatively stable over time (microbial homeostasis), unless there is a significant change in the local environment.

AGEING AND THE ORAL MICROBIOTA

The development of the oral microbiota continues with age. Following tooth eruption, the isolation frequency of spirochaetes and black-pigmented anaerobes increases. In one culture-based study, black-pigmented anaerobes were recovered from 18% to 40% of children aged 5 years and were subsequently found in over 90% of teenagers aged 13 to 16 years. The increased prevalence of spirochaetes and black-pigmented anaerobes during puberty might be because of hormones entering the gingival crevice and acting as a novel nutrient source for these bacteria. The rise in *Prevotella intermedia* in plaque during the second trimester of pregnancy has also been ascribed to the elevated serum levels of oestradiol and progesterone which can satisfy the naphthoquinone requirement for growth of this organism. Increases in the numbers of black-pigmented anaerobes have also been observed in women taking oral contraceptives. However, other studies failed to show similar associations between black-pigmented anaerobes and pregnancy. Interestingly, the recent application of more sensitive molecular techniques has detected these organisms in prepubertal children, implying that hormonal changes cannot be the only factor affecting the prevalence of these fastidious bacteria.

In adults, the composition and proportions of the resident oral microbiota remain reasonably stable over time, and this microbiota coexists in relative harmony with the host. This stability (termed **microbial homeostasis**; Chapter 5, see Fig. 5.18) is not a passive response to the environment, but is because of a dynamic balance being achieved from numerous inter-bacterial and host-bacterial interactions. The diversity of the oral microbiota in a healthy individual is typically in the order of several hundred species.

Some variations in the oral microbiota have been discerned in later life and can be attributed to both direct and indirect effects of ageing (Fig. 4.3). In the case of the latter, variations can occur if the habitat or environment is severely perturbed. For example, the risk of cancer rises with age, and cytotoxic therapy or myelosuppression combined with the disease itself is associated with the increased carriage of *Candida albicans* and non-oral opportunistic pathogens such as

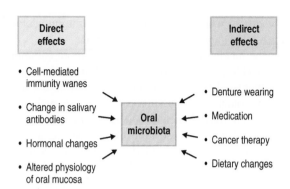

FIGURE 4.3 Direct and indirect effects of ageing on the oral microbiota.

enterobacteria (e.g., *Klebsiella* spp., *Escherichia coli*, *Pseudomonas aeruginosa*) and *Staphylococcus aureus*. The wearing of dentures also increases with age and this also promotes colonisation by *C. albicans*. In edentulous older subjects who wear dentures, the dorsum of the tongue harbours the most diverse microbiota, with many Gram-negative anaerobic bacteria being present (e.g., *Veillonella*, *Fusobacterium*, *Prevotella* species and spirochaetes). Periodontal pathogens such as *Tannerella forsythia*, *Porphyromonas gingivalis* and *Treponema denticola* can also be detected. Many elderly subjects take a variety of medications, the side effects of which can reduce the flow of saliva and thereby perturb the normal balance of the resident oral microbiota.

Direct age-related changes to the oral microbiota have been detected, including significantly higher proportions and isolation frequencies of lactobacilli and staphylococci (mainly *S. aureus*) in the saliva of healthy subjects aged 70 years and the increased isolation of yeasts in those aged 80 years or more. Cell-mediated immunity declines with age, but the precise effect of old age on the innate and adaptive host defences of the mouth has yet to be established definitively. Serum IgM antibody titres to selected oral and gut commensal bacteria are lower in older subjects. These antibodies represent the initial response by the host to infection, and such a decrease in titre may be one explanation for the increased susceptibility to disease seen in the elderly. Age-related changes in salivary antibodies have also been reported. In general, activities of specific salivary IgG and IgM antibodies decreased in the elderly, whereas specific secretory Immunoglobulin A (sIgA) antibodies increase with age.

The incidence of oral candidosis is more common in the elderly, and this has been attributed not only to the increased likelihood of denture wearing, but also to physiological changes in the oral mucosa, malnutrition and to trace element deficiencies. There have been reports of increased isolation of enterobacteria from the oropharynx of the elderly, but this seems to be related in many cases to the health of the individual rather than to their age per se, with the highest incidences being in the most debilitated individuals. One of the fundamental problems in determining whether or not the oral microbiota changes in old age is that the chronologic age of a person does not always equate to their physiological age!

Social habits change with age and can perturb the balance of the oral microbiota. The regular intake of dietary carbohydrates or acidic drinks can lead to the enrichment of aciduric (acid-tolerating) and cariogenic species such as mutans streptococci and lactobacilli. Furthermore, mutans streptococci and *S. sanguinis* are not generally detected in the mouths of individuals who have full dentures when these surfaces are not worn, although both groups of bacteria can reappear when these 'hard surfaces' are inserted again. Smoking has been shown to affect the composition of the microbiota and is a significant risk factor for periodontal diseases. Smoking is associated with the increased prevalence of members of the genera: *Parvimonas*, *Fusobacterium*, *Porphyromonas*, *Treponema* and *Campylobacter* and a reduction in *Veillonella*, *Neisseria* and *Streptococcus* species. However, a combination of non-surgical treatment and smoking cessation counselling resulted in a reversal of some of these trends, with lower levels of some periodontally-associated pathogens, including *Filifactor alocis*, *Dialister pneumosintes*, *Parvimonas micra* and *T. denticola*, and an increase in some beneficial bacteria.

KEY POINTS

> The composition of the oral microbiota changes during the life of an individual. These changes correlate with significant alterations to the biology of the mouth, such as eruption (or loss) of teeth, denture wearing, changes in immune status and lifestyle (diet, smoking, etc.).

METHODS OF DETERMINING THE COMPOSITION OF THE RESIDENT ORAL MICROBIOTA

There are a number of challenges when attempting to determine the composition of the oral microbiota. These range from the basic problem of removing the majority of the microorganisms from their habitat (many of which, are by necessity, bound tenaciously as biofilms to a surface or to each other, and the site may be difficult to access) to their eventual identification (Table 4.3; see Chapter 3). The main approaches to determining the microbial composition of the oral microbiota are illustrated in Figure 4.4, while the main differences between culture-dependent and culture-independent approaches have previously been highlighted in Figure 3.2 (see Chapter 3). Some of the issues are discussed in more detail in the following sections.

SAMPLE ACQUISITION

The quality of the original sample is fundamental to the outcome of the subsequent determination of the composition of the oral microbiota irrespective of whether culture-dependent or culture-independent (molecular-based) methods are used. The microbiota can vary in composition over relatively small distances and so large plaque samples or a number of pooled samples from different sites can be of little value because important site-specific differences will be obscured. Consequently, small samples from discrete sites are preferable, but the method of sampling will depend on the anatomy and properties of the site to be studied.

The oral mucosa can be sampled by swabbing, direct impression techniques or by removing epithelial cells by scraping or scrubbing with a blunt instrument into a container. Microbial counts can then be related to a fixed area or to an individual epithelial cell. Saliva can be collected by expectoration into a sterile container; the saliva flow can be at a normal resting rate (unstimulated) or it can be stimulated by chemical means or by chewing. Although a greater volume is collected by stimulation, such samples will also contain many more organisms that have been dislodged from oral surfaces; microbial counts are expressed as colony forming units (CFUs) per millilitre of saliva.

There is no universally accepted way of sampling dental plaque. The accessible smooth surfaces of enamel

TABLE 4.3 **Some properties of the oral microbiota that contribute to the difficulty in determining its composition**	
Property	**Comment**
High species diversity	The oral microbiota, and especially dental plaque, consists of a diverse number of microbial species, some of which are present only in low numbers.
Surface attachment/ coaggregation (coadhesion)	Oral microorganisms attach firmly to surfaces and to each other and, therefore, are difficult to remove and have to be dispersed efficiently without loss of viability.
Obligate anaerobes	Many oral bacteria die if exposed to air for prolonged periods, and special precautions are needed to preserve their viability.
Fastidious nutrition/ unculturable	Some bacteria are difficult to grow in pure culture and may require specific cofactors etc. for growth. Some groups (e.g., certain spirochaetes; TM7 group) cannot as yet be cultured in the laboratory. Some bacteria have evolved to grow in coculture with other species.
Slow growth	The slow growth of some organisms makes enumeration time consuming (e.g., they may require14–21 days incubation).
Identification	The classification of many oral microorganisms still remains unresolved or confused; simple criteria for identification are not always available (particularly for some obligate anaerobes). Molecular methods are being used more commonly to identify oral microorganisms.

pose few problems and a range of dental instruments have been used. Dental probes, scalers, dental floss and abrasive strips have been used to remove biofilm from approximal surfaces between teeth. Fine probes, pieces of wire, blunt hypodermic needles and toothpicks have been used to sample plaque from fissures, although the amount of biofilm removed can depend on the anatomy of the site. Subgingival plaque is difficult to sample because of the inaccessibility and anaerobic nature of the site. High numbers of obligately anaerobic bacteria are found in the gingival crevice and periodontal pocket, most of which will lose their viability if exposed to air (atmospheric oxygen). In disease, the anatomy of the site means that those organisms at the base of the pocket, near the advancing front of the lesion, are likely to be of most relevance (see Chapter 6). Again, it is important to avoid removing plaque from other areas within the pocket so as not to obscure significant relationships between particular bacteria and disease. A common approach is to insert paper points into pockets, but these will not remove all of the firmly adherent organisms from the root of the tooth. Samples have also been taken by irrigation of the site and retrieval of the material through syringe needles; however, this method will inevitably remove plaque from the whole depth of the pocket. A particularly sophisticated method employed a broach kept withdrawn in a cannula that was flushed constantly with oxygen-free nitrogen. The broach was used to sample plaque only when the cannula was in position near the base of the pocket. After sampling, the broach was retracted into the cannula and withdrawn. Another approach has been to use a curette or scaler after the supragingival area has been cleared. The scaler tips can be detached and placed immediately in gas-flushed tubes containing anaerobic transport fluid for delivery to the laboratory. Alternatively, when periodontal surgery is needed, plaque has been removed from extracted teeth or from surfaces exposed when gingival flaps are reflected. The samples can be used either for culture-based studies or nucleic acid can be extracted for molecular analyses.

KEY POINTS

A variety of methods can be used to take samples from oral surfaces. The choice will reflect the anatomy of the site. Small samples from discrete sites are preferable. It is important to appreciate, particularly when comparing studies in which different sampling procedures have been used, that the results will, to a certain extent, reflect the method adopted.

TRANSPORT AND DISPERSION OF SAMPLES

Samples should be transported to the laboratory for processing as quickly as possible for culture-based

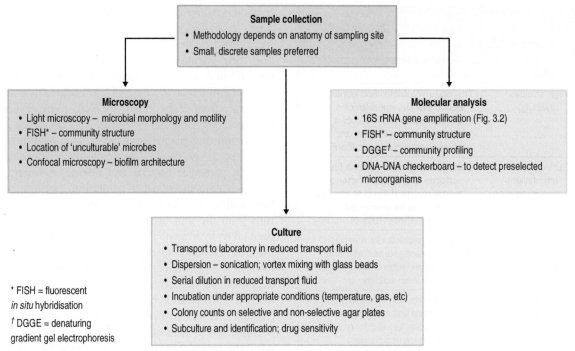

FIGURE 4.4 Stages in the microbiological analysis of the oral microbiota. Culture, microscopy and molecular approaches can be used to characterise the oral microbiota.

studies. Specially designed transport fluids containing reducing agents to maintain a low redox potential will reduce the loss of viability of anaerobic organisms during delivery to the laboratory.

Clumps and aggregates of bacteria must be dispersed efficiently (ideally to single cells) before dilution and plating of the specimen. Plaque poses a particular problem in this respect because, by definition, it is a biofilm containing a diverse range of microorganisms bound tenaciously to one another. One of the most efficient methods, particularly for subgingival plaque, is to vortex samples with small, sterile glass beads, ideally in a tube filled with inert gas. Mild sonication produces the maximum number of particles from a specimen, but it exerts a selective effect by specifically damaging spirochaetes and some other Gram-negative bacteria, particularly *Fusobacterium* species.

CULTIVATION

For decades, culture-based methods were the only approaches available to determine which microorganisms were present. Such methods are labour intensive

and relatively expensive. Following dispersal, samples are serially diluted in a suitable fluid (usually a transport fluid designed to preserve the viability of obligately anaerobic bacteria) and aliquots are spread on to a number of freshly prepared, pre-reduced (i.e., already anaerobic) agar plates and incubated to allow cells to form microbial colonies. These media are designed to grow either (a) the maximum number of bacteria (e.g., blood agar) or (b) only a limited number of species (**selective media**) to recover minor components of the microbiota. For example, the addition of vancomycin to blood agar plates will inhibit most Gram-positive bacteria, whereas a high sucrose concentration encourages the growth of oral streptococci, and plates with a low pH favour lactobacilli. It should be emphasised that these media are selective and not specific for any type of microbe. The identity of the colonies on these plates must be confirmed; colonial appearance or mere growth on a particular medium is not diagnostic. Media need to be incubated for different times and under different atmospheric conditions depending on the bacteria being cultivated. For example, 7 to 14 days incubation at 37°C in an anaerobic jar or anaerobic cabinet filled with a gas mix containing $CO_2/H_2/N_2$ will be needed to grow some obligate anaerobes. In contrast, *Neisseria* require only 2 days incubation in air, whereas other organisms are capnophilic (CO_2-loving) and grow optimally in 10% CO_2 in air. Some laboratory media are supplemented with growth factors to enable certain fastidious organisms to grow (Chapter 3). At present, only about 50–70% of the resident oral microbiota can be cultured in the laboratory.

ENUMERATION AND IDENTIFICATION

After appropriate incubation, bacteria form visible colonies that can be counted, and their concentration in the original sample is determined by mathematically compensating for the dilution steps; data are typically expressed as CFUs. Representative colonies are subcultured to check for purity and for subsequent identification; isolates can also be tested for antimicrobial susceptibility. Colony counting assumes that:

(a) cells of the same microorganism produce colonies with an identical morphology;

(b) cells of different species produce distinct morphologies; and

(c) one colony arises from a single cell.

Generally, these assumptions hold true except for (c), as colonies may arise from small aggregates of cells; this emphasises the need for efficient dispersion of samples. It is also advisable to take several examples of a particular colony type to ensure that some species are not overlooked because of their appearance being similar to a numerically dominant organism. One stratagem to determine the predominant microbiota involves identifying 30 to 50 random colonies, irrespective of their morphology, rather than selecting only those colony types that appear different.

The first level of discrimination involves the Gram staining of subcultured colonies; bacteria are then grouped according to whether their cells are Gram-positive or Gram-negative, and are rod- or coccal-shaped. This dictates which tests will be necessary to achieve speciation. Some bacteria can be identified using simple criteria, for example, sugar fermentation tests or the detection of preformed enzymes using commercial kits. Other bacteria require a more sophisticated approach and, more commonly now, molecular

tests (e.g., polymerase chain reaction [PCR] or whole genome sequencing) are used to identify these challenging species (see later section).

MICROSCOPY

Dark-field illumination or phase contrast techniques have been used to quantify the numbers of motile bacteria (including spirochaetes) directly in dental plaque (particularly from subgingival sites). Such organisms are related to the severity of some periodontal diseases, and this approach has been used in the clinic to monitor sites undergoing treatment. However, most of the putative pathogens cannot be recognised by morphology alone. To overcome this problem, cells can be identified by reaction with antisera (monoclonal or specific polyclonal), oligonucleotide probes or tagged with a fluorescent label (see Figs 3.3 and 4.4).

Scanning and transmission electron microscopy have proved useful in studying plaque formation and have also been used to show that bacteria invade gingival tissues in aggressive forms of periodontal disease. Electron microscopy requires samples to be processed before viewing, and this can distort the structure of plaque. Non-invasive techniques such as confocal laser scanning microscopy are now widely used, with and without the use of specific probes (antibody or oligonucleotide), to determine the true architecture of plaque and the location of selected bacteria within the biofilm (see Fig. 3.3 and Chapter 5). Confocal microscopy involves the generation of numerous focused images throughout the depth of an untreated specimen (optical sections); image analysis software is then used to combine these sections and reconstruct the three-dimensional structure of the original specimen (for an example, see Fig. 4.7). Confocal microscopy has shown that plaque has a more open architecture than previously indicated by electron microscopy.

IN SITU MODELS

As a result of some of the methodological problems outlined previously, various devices have been developed that can be worn in the mouth by volunteers, containing model surfaces for microbial colonisation, and which can be removed from the mouth for sampling. The microbiology of fissure plaque has been studied using artificial or natural fissures mounted in a crown or in an occlusal filling. Removable pieces of enamel or denture acrylic have been placed on natural teeth or dentures in a desired position and have been used for studies of the structural development of dental plaque. Removable appliances have the additional advantages that experiments can be performed on the surfaces when out of the mouth that would not be permitted on natural teeth, such as the effect of regular sugar applications, or the evaluation of novel antimicrobial agents.

MOLECULAR APPROACHES

The limitations and bias of culture approaches can be avoided by applying molecular analyses for microbial detection and identification, and these are being increasingly applied to determining the composition of the oral microbiota (see Fig. 4.4). Most commonly, 16S ribosomal ribonucleic acid (rRNA) gene sequences are amplified by PCR using universal bacterial oligonucleotide primers. The 16S rRNA gene represents a suitable target for identification of bacteria as the sequences of certain regions tend to be highly conserved for a given species, and identification can be achieved using suitably designed oligonucleotide primers that are specific to conserved sites, yet flank sequences that differ between bacterial species. Originally, the approach would have involved first separating the PCR amplicons by cloning before sequencing individual clones and then making comparison to existing sequences in international databases. Other methods include the extraction of nucleic acid from clinical samples followed by hybridisation with probes for approximately 40 predetermined species on a membrane, in a deoxyribonucleic acid (DNA)-DNA checkerboard approach. Species diversity can be compared by running gradient gels in which the mixture of DNA is separated by size, and diversity is gauged by the number of bands observed.

In recent years, a more powerful metagenomic methodology has emerged that circumvents the requirement for laborious cloning steps. High-throughput sequencing is now the preferred metagenomic approach for analysing microbial communities, and currently there are several different methods that may be used. Essentially, all high-throughput sequencing approaches involve initial DNA extraction from the microbial community. This extracted DNA is fragmented and short adaptor sequences are ligated on

either end of the fragments. The DNA is then denatured into single-stranded DNA and captured through use of immobilised primers specific for one of the adapter sequences. There are different platforms now available to sequence the DNA. The most common are the Roche 454, which uses a pyrosequencing chemistry, and Illumina (e.g., MiSeq and HiSeq), which is based on a reversible dye terminator chemistry. The 454 platform provides longer read lengths of the DNA but is being superseded by the Illumina platform; the read length is not quite so long, but the Illumina platform provides greater output and currently at lower costs. The technology in this area is changing and evolving rapidly and has revolutionised our ability to determine what is present in a clinical sample. However, the sequencing is still only as good as the quality of the sample that is taken, and these approaches still have some limitations and biases, for example, the primers do not work equally well for all species, and it is more difficult to lyse certain organisms. Dedicated software packages can be used to correctly assemble the sequence reads and then compare them with those held in databases such as the Human Oral Microbiome Database (HOMD) (Chapter 3). In this manner, not only can the composition of entire microbial communities be ascertained, but also the detection of species currently classed as being unculturable. Metatranscriptomics is being developed to analyse the messenger RNA (mRNA) synthesised by microbial communities so as to determine the gene expression profile of these consortia. This approach is not concerned with which organisms are present, but is focused on what they are doing (i.e., their function) at the time of sampling. Other approaches are being applied to determine the function and activity of the microbiota, and these include metaproteomics (total community proteins that are expressed) and metabolomics (metabolic products that are produced by a microbial community). The way that different molecular approaches can be used in a complementary manner to determine the microbial composition and metabolic activity of a microbial community is shown in Figure 4.5. Molecular analyses also facilitate detection and location of microorganisms by combining fluorescent *in situ* hybridisation (FISH) and confocal laser scanning microscopy (CLSM) (see Fig. 3.3 and Fig. 4.7).

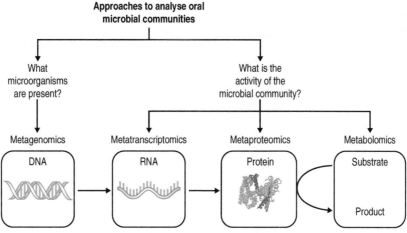

FIGURE 4.5 Complementary molecular approaches to determine the composition and metabolic activity of oral microbial communities.

There is now a service that is provided by The Forsyth Dental Institute, Boston, USA, that enables nearly 600 oral bacterial species to be identified and to get identification to the genus level for the remaining 129 taxa. The Human Oral Microbe Identification using Next Generation Sequencing (HOMINGS) research tool is based on 16S rDNA analysis of clinical samples using Illumina high throughput sequencing.

KEY POINTS

> There are two main approaches to determine the composition of the oral microbiota:
> - Culture methods: these require the growth of microorganisms on non-selective and selective agar plates under appropriate conditions. Only 50–70% of the oral microbiota can be cultured.
> - Molecular (culture-independent) methods: metagenomic approaches enable the detection of both culturable and non-culturable microorganisms.
>
> The function and activity of the oral microbiota can be determined by metatranscriptomics (RNA profile), metaproteomics (protein profile) and metabolomics (metabolic products produced).

DISTRIBUTION OF THE RESIDENT ORAL MICROBIOTA

The populations making up the resident microbiota of the oral cavity are not found with equal frequency throughout the mouth. Biofilm composition varies on distinct surfaces because of differences in the biological and physical properties of each site. In the following sections the predominant microbiota from several characteristic sites in the oral cavity will be compared (Fig. 4.6, Table 4.5). Details of the main microorganisms are presented in Chapter 3.

LIPS AND PALATE

The lips form the border between the skin microbiota (which consists predominantly of staphylococci, micrococci and Gram-positive rods such as *Corynebacterium* and *Propionibacterium* spp.) and that of the mouth (which contains many Gram-negative species and few of the organisms commonly found on the skin surface). Facultatively anaerobic streptococci comprise a large part of the microbiota on the lips. *Veillonella* and *Neisseria* have also been found, but only in very low numbers (<1% of the total cultivable microbiota). *Streptococcus vestibularis* is recovered most commonly from the 'gutter' between the lower lip and the gums, and occasionally black-pigmented anaerobes and fusobacteria have been detected; culture-based studies detect only between 3 and 9 species from this region. *Candida albicans* can colonise damaged lip mucosal surfaces in the corners of the mouth, potentially causing angular cheilitis (see Chapter 8). Molecular techniques have confirmed the presence of a range of streptococci on the lips, especially *S. mitis, S.*

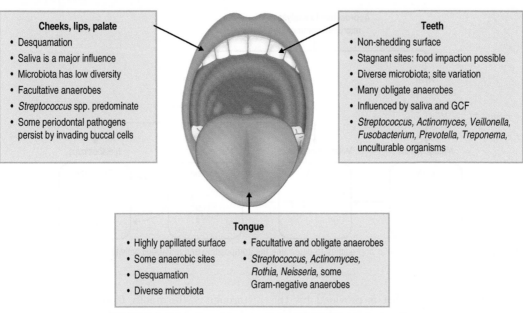

FIGURE 4.6 Distribution of the microbiota at distinct sites in the mouth.

oralis and *S. constellatus*; some obligate anaerobes are also detected occasionally, including *P. melaninogenica*.

The microbiota of the healthy palate can show large variations between subjects, not only in the total colony-forming units recovered (which may reflect differences in the area sampled or the success in removing organisms), but also in the proportions of the individual species. The majority of the culturable bacteria are streptococci and actinomyces; veillonellae, haemophili and Gram-negative anaerobes are also regularly recovered, but at lower levels (Table 4.4). *Candida* are not regularly isolated from the healthy palate except when dentures are worn; in this situation, the mucosa of the palate can become infected with *C. albicans* (denture stomatitis; see Chapter 8).

Culture-independent molecular approaches have indicated a more diverse microbiota in samples from the palate from healthy adults, including a range of streptococci (*S. mitis, S. oralis* and *S. infantis*), as well as *Gemella* spp., *Neisseria* spp., *Veillonella* spp., *Capnocytophaga gingivalis* and *Prevotella melaninogenica* (and other *Prevotella* spp.). The number of species typically ranged from 4 to 21 per person in a survey of 5 people.

TABLE 4.4   Predominant cultivable microbiota of the healthy human palatal mucosa

Microorganism	Percentage of the total cultivable microbiota (%)	Percentage isolation frequency (%)
Streptococcus	52	100
Actinomyces	15	100
Lactobacillus	1	87
Neisseria	2	93
Veillonella	1	100
Prevotella	4	100
Candida	+*	7

*Present, but in numbers too low to count.

CHEEK

Streptococci are the predominant bacteria cultured from the cheek (buccal mucosa), especially members of the mitis group, and *H. parainfluenzae* is also commonly isolated (Table 4.5). *Simonsiella* spp. are

TABLE 4.5 Proportions of some cultivable bacterial populations at different sites in the normal oral cavity				
Bacterium	**Buccal mucosa**	**Tongue dorsum**	**Supragingival plaque**	**Subgingival plaque**
Streptococcus sanguinis	–	–	●●●	–
S. salivarius	●●	●●●	●	–
S. oralis / S. mitis	●●	●●	●●●●	●●
mutans streptococci	–	–	●	–
Actinomyces naeslundii	●	●●	●●●	●●
Neisseria species	●	●	●	–
Veillonella species	●	●●	●●●	●●
Prevotella species	–	●	●●	●●●
Fusobacterium species	–	●	●●	●●●
Porphyromonas species	–	–	●	●●
Treponema species	–	–	–	●●

– Not normally present at this site
● detected occasionally, but usually in low numbers
●● detected commonly, in moderate numbers
●●● detected frequently, and in substantial numbers
●●●● always detected, and in high numbers

isolated primarily from the cheek cells of humans and animals. Obligate anaerobes are not present in high numbers, although spirochaetes and other motile organisms have been observed by microscopy to be attached to the buccal mucosa. Molecular techniques have confirmed the presence of a range of streptococcal species on buccal cells, as well as *Granulicatella* and *Gemella* spp.; obligate anaerobes are less commonly detected, although *Veillonella* and *Prevotella* spp. can be present. Between 4 and 20 species can be detected in a sample from the buccal mucosa.

Recent studies, in which FISH was combined with confocal microscopy, have shown that some of the species implicated in periodontal disease (*A. actinomycetemcomitans, P. gingivalis, F. nucleatum, P. intermedia, T. forsythia*) can gain refuge within buccal epithelial cells in healthy people, where they persist as intracellular polymicrobial communities (see Fig. 4.7). Furthermore, *F. nucleatum* can transport non-invasive species, such as *S. cristatus*, into human oral epithelial cells via inter-bacterial coaggregation (see Chapter 5). Streptococci were the most common organisms found

intracellularly in about 30% of buccal epithelial cells, followed by *Granulicatella adiacens* and *Gemella haemolysans*. These studies imply that oral mucosal cells could serve as a reservoir for potential periodontal pathogens.

TONGUE

The dorsum of the tongue has a highly papillated surface which provides a large surface area and supports a higher bacterial density and a more diverse microbiota than other oral mucosal surfaces (Table 4.5). Streptococci are the most numerous group of bacteria (approximately 40% of the total cultivable microbiota) with salivarius- and mitis-group organisms predominating. Anaerobic streptococci have also been isolated while *Rothia mucilaginosa* is found almost exclusively on the tongue. Other major groups of bacteria (and their proportions) include *Veillonella* spp. (16%), Gram-positive rods (16%) of which *Actinomyces naeslundii* and *A. odontolyticus* are common and haemophili (15%). Both pigmenting (*Prevotella intermedia, P. melaninogenica*) and non-pigmenting obligate anaerobes can be recovered

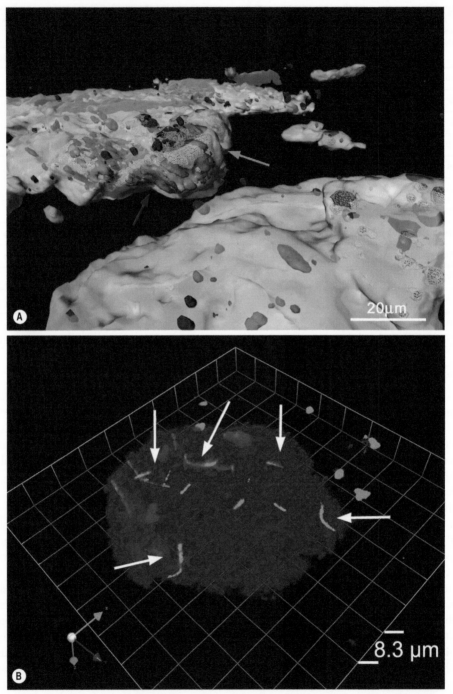

FIGURE 4.7 Intracellular colonisation of buccal epithelial cells. (**A**) Three-dimensional reconstruction of a buccal epithelial cell (BEC). Bacteria recognised only by a universal bacterial probe are shown in solid red, while colocalisation of the *Aggregatibacter actinomycetemcomitans* and universal probes is depicted by a green wireframe over a red interior. Reconstructed BEC surfaces are presented in blue. The red and green colours are muted when bacterial masses are intracellular, and brighter when bacteria appear to project out of the surface. The large mass indicated by red and green arrows is a cohesive unit containing *A. actinomycetemcomitans* in direct proximity to other species. Published with permission: Rudney et al, *J Dent Res* 2005 84:59–63. (**B**) Buccal cell dominated by presumed streptococci that were labelled by a universal bacterial probe (red). The sample also was treated with a *Fusobacterium nucleatum*-specific probe, and the buccal cell shown contained several yellow *F. nucleatum* cells (*arrows*) in close association with cocci. Published with permission: Rudney et al, *J Dent Res* 2005 84:1165–1171.

TABLE 4.6 The predominant cultivable microbiota of the tongue of preschool children		
Bacterium	**Mean proportion (%)**	**Isolation frequency (%)**
Streptococcus anginosus	4.7	42
Streptococcus oralis	3.8	30
Streptococcus mitis	11.8	75
Streptococcus mutans	1.0	8
Streptococcus sobrinus	0.5	2
Streptococcus salivarius	22.3	94
Streptococcus sanguinis	7.6	58
Total streptococci	**51.7**	
Actinomyces naeslundii	4.2	46
Actinomyces odontolyticus	1.1	17
Rothia dentocariosa	0.9	21
Rothia mucilaginosa	5.5	46
Corynebacterium matruchotii	0.1	4
Lactobacillus spp.	0.3	6
Total Gram-positive rods	**12.1**	
Neisseria spp.	20.2	>90
Veillonella spp.	6.3	73
Total Gram-negative cocci	**26.5**	
Prevotella spp.	0.4	15
Fusobacterium spp.	0.6	25
Leptotrichia spp.	0.2	13
Haemophilus spp.	0.6	19
Aggregatibacter spp.	0.1	4
Capnocytophaga spp.	0.1	6
Aerobic Gram-negative rods	2.3	40
Anaerobic Gram-negative rods	1.8	40
Yeasts	1.0	4

Data are from 9 children, aged 8 to 13 months.

from the tongue, and this site is regarded as a potential reservoir (along with the tonsils) for some of the organisms implicated in periodontal diseases. Organisms including lactobacilli, yeasts, fusobacteria, spirochaetes and other motile bacteria have been found in low numbers (<1% of the total microbiota) on the tongue.

Similar findings have been obtained from a comprehensive study of the anterior dorsal surface of the tongue in infants (aged 8 to 13 months). Streptococci accounted for about 50% of the microbiota, and *S. salivarius* and *S. mitis* were the predominant species (Table 4.6). *Rothia mucilaginosa* was recovered from almost half of the samples. High proportions of *Neisseria* (20%) were also found, together with *Actinomyces* (5%) and occasional Gram-negative species including haemophili, fusobacteria, *Prevotella*, *Capnocytophaga* and *Aggregatibacter*.

Molecular studies have demonstrated an even more diverse microbiota from samples from the dorsum of the tongue. DNA–DNA checkerboard techniques found a number of Gram-negative bacteria on the tongue, including *P. melaninogenica, V. parvula* and *C. gingivalis*, whereas other studies commonly detected *Granulicatella* and *Gemella* species. Studies of 16S rRNA gene sequences (see Chapter 3) showed that about 30% of the bacterial populations detected were unique to the tongue, suggesting that the properties of this habitat were distinct from those of other oral surfaces. The most common isolates were *Rothia mucilaginosa, S. salivarius* and a *Eubacterium* spp.; about 16 to 22 species were detected in each tongue sample.

Oral malodour is associated with the microbiota of the tongue (see later). A higher bacterial load, especially of Gram-negative anaerobes (including *Porphyromonas, Prevotella* and *Fusobacterium* spp.), was isolated from the tongue of subjects with high odour. An even more diverse microbiota was found when culture independent molecular methods were applied; species associated with halitosis included *Atopobium parvulum, Dialister* spp., *Eubacterium sulci, Solobacterium moorei*, an uncharacterised *Streptococcus* and members of the uncultivable group, TM7 (see Fig. 3.3, B). Oral malodour involves the production of volatile sulphur compounds by the resident microbiota (see later in this chapter).

TEETH AND DENTURES

The microbial community associated with teeth and dentures is referred to as dental plaque and denture plaque, respectively. Biofilm composition varies on distinct tooth surfaces (such as smooth surface, approximal, fissure or gingival crevice) because of differences in local environmental conditions (see Chapter 2). The terms supragingival and subgingival plaque describe samples taken above and below the gum margin, respectively (see Fig. 2.2). The detailed composition of dental plaque from these sites and dentures is given in Chapter 5. As teeth and dentures are non-shedding surfaces, the highest numbers of microorganisms are found at stagnant sites which afford protection from removal forces.

Gram-positive rods and filaments (mainly *Actinomyces* species) are among the major groups of bacteria cultured from plaque (Table 4.5). Mutans streptococci and members of the mitis and anginosus groups of streptococci are found in highest numbers on teeth, whereas, in contrast to mucosal surfaces, *S. salivarius* is only a minor component of dental plaque. Obligate anaerobes are found in high numbers particularly in the gingival crevice, and oral spirochaetes are almost uniquely associated with this region. Obligate anaerobes are also commonly isolated from dentures. In plaque, there are high proportions of bacteria belonging to groups that cannot, as yet, be cultured in the laboratory.

SALIVA

Although a millilitre of saliva contains up to 10^8 microorganisms, it is not considered to have its own resident microbiota. The normal rate of swallowing ensures that bacteria cannot be maintained in the mouth by multiplication in saliva. The organisms found are derived from other surfaces, especially the tongue (Table 4.5), from which they are displaced by oral removal forces such as saliva and gingival crevicular fluid flow, chewing and oral hygiene procedures. The microbial profile of saliva (in particular, the level of mutans streptococci and/or lactobacilli) has been used as an indicator of the caries susceptibility of an individual, and commercially-available kits for their culture are a convenient means of detecting them. People with high counts of these potentially cariogenic bacteria are considered to be 'at-risk' and can be targeted for intense oral hygiene, antimicrobial therapy and dietary counselling (see Chapter 6).

KEY POINTS

Oral microbial populations are not distributed evenly in the mouth. Large differences occur in the prevalence of individual species at particular oral sites (Table 4.5; Fig. 4.6), resulting in each habitat having a characteristic microbiota. Desquamation ensures that the microbial load on most mucosal surfaces is low, although the papillated surfaces of the tongue promote the accumulation of complex microbial communities, including obligate anaerobes. Dental plaque, especially at stagnant sites on teeth, harbours the most diverse microbiota.

Key factors influencing the distribution of the oral microbiota include pH, nutrient availability, redox potential, and receptors for attachment (see Chapter 2).

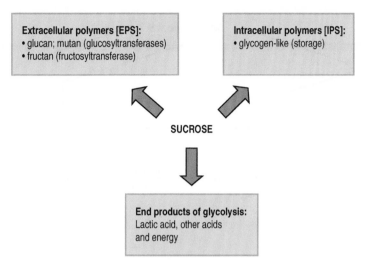

FIGURE 4.8 The metabolism of sucrose by oral bacteria.

METABOLISM OF ORAL BACTERIA

The persistence of the resident oral microbiota is dependent on the ability of microbes to attach to oral surfaces, obtain nutrients and multiply. Nutrients are derived mainly from the metabolism of endogenous substrates present in saliva and gingival crevicular fluid (GCF), and these often require the concerted action of consortia of microorganisms (see Chapter 5; see Figs 5.11 and 5.14). Superimposed on these components are the exogenous nutrients that are supplied intermittently via the diet; the most significant of these for the oral microbiota are fermentable dietary carbohydrates and nitrate. Microbial gene expression will respond to changes in environmental conditions; bacteria are able to sense their environment via membrane-bound two component signal transduction pathways consisting of a sensor histidine kinase and a response regulator. These systems enable bacteria to detect signals and respond to environment changes by specific gene activation or repression. The fluctuating conditions of nutrient supply (feast and famine) and environmental change require the oral microbiota to possess biochemical flexibility. The pattern of metabolism is closely related to whether the resident microbiota displays a pathogenic or commensal relationship with the host.

CARBOHYDRATE METABOLISM

Most attention has been paid to the metabolism of carbohydrates because of the relationship between dietary sugars, acid production and dental caries (Chapters 2 and 6). The metabolic fate of dietary carbohydrates is illustrated in simplified form in Figure 4.8.

Sucrose (a disaccharide of glucose and fructose) is the most widely used dietary sweetening agent, and can be:

- broken down by extracellular bacterial invertases (α-glucosidases) and the resultant glucose and fructose molecules taken up directly by bacteria;
- transported intact as the disaccharide or disaccharide phosphate, and cleaved inside the cell by an intracellular invertase or a sucrose phosphate hydrolase;
- used extracellularly by glycosyltransferases. Glucosyltransferases (GTF) produce both soluble and insoluble glucans (with a release of fructose), which are important in biofilm maturation (see Chapter 5) and in the consolidation of bacterial attachment to teeth. Fructosyltransferases (FTF) produce fructans (and liberate glucose), which can be metabolised by other microorganisms (Fig. 4.9).

Starches, which contain mixtures of amylose and amylopectin, can be broken into their constituent

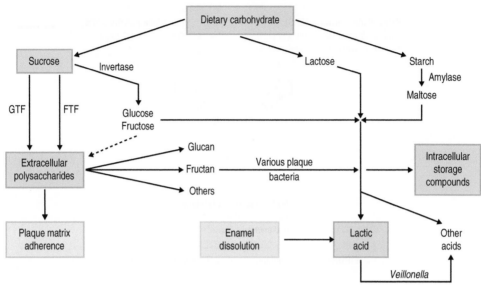

FIGURE 4.9 Simplified diagram to show the metabolic fate of dietary carbohydrates. *GTF*, Glucosyltransferase; *FTF*, fructosyltransferase.

sugars by amylases of salivary and bacterial origin. Some streptococci (*S. gordonii, S. mitis*) are able to bind amylase, which provides them with an additional metabolic capability. *Streptococcus mutans* possesses a spectrum of enzymes with the potential to catabolise dietary starches, including an extracellular pullulanase, which degrades pullulan and debranches amylopectin, as well as an amylase; there is also an extracellular endodextranase and an intracellular exodextranase. Aspects of the metabolism of carbohydrates will be considered in more detail in the following sections.

Sugar transport and acid production

All substrates have to be transported across the cytoplasmic membrane and into the bacterial cell if they are to be used for biomass production or as an energy source. Oral bacteria can transport carbohydrates by:

- the phosphoenolpyruvate phosphotransferase (PEP-PTS) transport system;
- the multiple sugar metabolism (Msm) system; and
- a glucose permease.

The PEP-PTS is a high-affinity sugar transport system for mono- and disaccharides in saccharolytic oral bacteria (*Streptococcus, Actinomyces, Lactobacillus*).

The PEP-PTS is a carrier-mediated, group translocation system involving phosphoryl-transfer from PEP via two non-sugar-specific, general cytoplasmic proteins, histidine protein (HPr) and enzyme I (E1), to a sugar-specific, membrane-bound enzyme II complex (EII), that catalyses the transport and phosphorylation of the incoming sugar. The phosphate group of E1~P, generated from PEP, is transferred to HPr, forming HPr~P, and then to the EII complex.

The PEP-PTS is constitutive for some sugars, such as glucose, mannose and sucrose, but must be induced for the transport of lactose and sugar alcohols such as mannitol and sorbitol. The activity of the PEP-PTS in oral streptococci is modulated by environmental conditions. It is optimal under conditions of carbohydrate-limitation, neutral pH and slow rates of bacterial growth. In contrast, it is repressed under conditions of excess sugar, low pH and high growth rates. This is significant because oral streptococci in dental plaque are continually exposed to transitory conditions of low pH and high sugar concentration.

Many strains of *S. mutans* possess a second system to transport sugars into the cell (the Msm transport system). The Msm system is capable of transporting various common sugars including sucrose, as well as melibiose, raffinose and maltose (a derivative of starch). The exact role of this system in plaque ecology is unknown, but it might be involved in transporting the breakdown products of extracellular polysaccharide degradation during periods between meals when the supply of the more refined dietary monosaccharides and disaccharides is negligible.

At high sugar concentrations, PEP-PTS activity is repressed and sugar transport is augmented by an ATP-dependent glucose permease; this system also functions at high growth rates and at low pH. The sugar is transported into the cell where it is phosphorylated on the inner surface of the membrane. Some bacteria can form glycogen under conditions of carbohydrate-excess to reduce the toxic intracellular levels of glycolytic intermediates. Organisms with this ability, therefore, are able to cope better than most other oral bacteria with the fluctuating feast-and-famine conditions in the mouth in terms of capturing dietary sugars.

The resident oral microbiota can also obtain carbohydrates for biomass and energy from the catabolism of host glycoproteins present in saliva (such as mucins) and in GCF (e.g., transferrin). Bacteria produce a range of glycosidases that can remove sugars sequentially from the oligosaccharide side chains of these glycoproteins, and these can be transported by systems such as the PEP-PTS. Generally, bacteria interact synergistically to fully degrade these molecules (see Chapter 5), as no single organism can optimally produce all the enzymes required. Acid production from these glycoproteins is slow compared with that from exogenous sugars and, consequently, would not cause significant enamel demineralisation.

Streptococcus oralis is highly prevalent, being found on most oral surfaces; it can also act as an opportunistic pathogen and is commonly isolated from cases of infective endocarditis. Sialidase (neuraminidase) and N-acetylglucosaminidase activities are induced when *S. oralis* grows in the presence of glycoproteins, and these enzymes cleave sialic acid and N-acetylglucosamine, respectively, from the oligosaccharide side chains. These sugars are then transported inside the cell, and key intracellular enzymes associated with the catabolism of N-acetyl sugars are also induced. These include N-acetylneuraminate pyruvate lyase, N-acetylglucosamine-6-phosphate deacetylase and glucosamine-6-phosphate deaminase. Only low concentrations of lactate are produced from sialic acid metabolism; the main fermentation products are formate and ethanol.

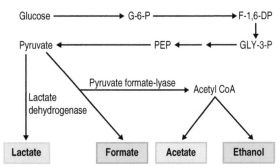

FIGURE 4.10 Formation of end products of sugar metabolism by mutans streptococci. *G-6-P*, Glucose-6-phosphate; *F-1,6-DP*, fructose-1,6-diphosphate; *GLY-3-P*, glyceraldehyde-3-phosphate; *PEP*, phosphoenolpyruvate.

Once sugars have been transported into the bacterial cell, they can be used either in anabolic pathways to generate biomass, or they can be broken down to organic acids (which are subsequently excreted) to generate energy. Acid production has been studied intensively because of its role in the demineralisation of enamel. Bacteria catabolise sugars by glycolysis to pyruvate; the fate of pyruvate will depend on the particular organism and the availability of oxygen. Most oral bacteria metabolise pyruvate anaerobically to organic acids. Oral streptococci convert pyruvate to lactate by lactate dehydrogenase when sugars are in excess, whereas formate, acetate and ethanol are the products of metabolism by mutans streptococci and *S. sanguinis* (but not *S. salivarius*) under carbohydrate limitation (Fig. 4.10). Other bacterial genera produce acetate, butyrate, propionate, and formate as primary products of metabolism.

The mechanism of excretion of lactic acid in *S. mutans* involves translocation of lactate and protons across the cell membrane as lactic acid in a carrier-mediated, electroneutral process. After the addition of a fermentable substrate to cells, lactate begins to accumulate, and protons are pumped out of the cell by an ATP synthase (an F_1F_0-ATPase). This generates a transmembrane pH gradient, which then acts as the driving force to transport lactate as lactic acid out of the cell. Once this process is energised, the ATP synthase is only needed to maintain the pH gradient if protons enter the cell by leakage or in symport with substrates such as amino acids. Thus, once the process is initiated no metabolic energy is needed for lactate efflux, thereby maximising the energy (ATP) return from carbohydrate catabolism.

Different species (and even strains within a species) produce acid at different rates, and vary in the terminal pH reached, and in their ability to survive under such conditions. Generally, mutans streptococci produce acid at the fastest rates whereas lactobacilli generate the lowest environmental pH; both groups are also aciduric and can tolerate conditions of acidity that most other oral bacteria would find inhibitory or even lethal; the biochemical mechanisms behind this tolerance are described later.

Variations are found in the profiles of acids found in plaque at different times of the day. Acetic, succinic, propionic, valeric, caproic and butyric acids are found in human plaque sampled after overnight fasting. These profiles reflect hetero-fermentation and amino acid catabolism. Following exposure to sucrose, the concentration of volatile acids falls whereas lactic acid becomes the predominant fermentation product. Such a switch in metabolism will encourage demineralisation.

Acid tolerance and adaptation to low pH

Although many of the saccharolytic bacteria found in dental plaque can generate a low terminal pH from sugar metabolism, few species can survive such conditions for prolonged periods. One of the prime distinguishing features of cariogenic bacteria such as mutans streptococci and lactobacilli is their ability to tolerate a low pH stress. For example, cells of *S. mutans* were unaffected by exposure for one hour at pH 4.0, whereas less than 0.01% of cells of some streptococcal species survived this treatment.

Microbial survival in acidic environments depends on the ability of a cell to maintain intracellular pH homeostasis. The mechanisms by which *S. mutans* achieves this include:

- proton extrusion via membrane-associated, proton-translocating ATP synthase (H$^+$/ATPase), and
- acid end-product efflux (see previous section).

These mechanisms ensure that the intracellular pH remains higher (i.e., more alkaline) than that of the external environment during acid production. Acid tolerant organisms such as mutans streptococci and lactobacilli have higher levels of ATP synthase activity, and the pH optimum for their activity is lower than for less tolerant species such as *S. sanguinis* or *A. naeslundii*.

TABLE 4.7 **Metabolic strategies adopted by *Streptococcus mutans* to cope with low pH stress**
Metabolic Strategy
• increase in glycolytic activity
• shift to lower pH optimum for glucose transport, glycolysis and proton impermeability
• decrease in activity of specific components of the PEP-PTS sugar transport system
• increased activity of the H$^+$/ATP synthase
• increased capacity to maintain transmembrane pH gradients at lower pH values
• shift to homofermentative metabolism
• synthesis of stress response proteins

Streptococcus mutans undergoes a specific alteration in its physiology to survive an acidic environment (Table 4.7), providing cells with a competitive advantage at low pH over organisms that are associated with enamel health and which lack this response, such as *S. sanguinis*. Other species cope with the stress of a low environmental pH by upregulating genes involved in base production. For example, urease (urea is converted to two molecules of ammonia) expression by *S. salivarius* is enhanced significantly at low pH, whereas the arginine deiminase system (which degrades arginine to ornithine, CO_2 and ammonia) of *S. sanguinis* is active at lower pH values (pH 4.0) than it can grow (pH 5.2) or carry out glycolysis. A number of stress proteins are also upregulated when streptococci are exposed to low pH.

Repeated exposure of oral bacteria to periods of low pH enables some cells to adapt biochemically to acidic conditions and become more acid tolerant. Some non-mutans streptococci survived better and made more acid when grown at an intermediate pH (around pH 5.5) for up to 90 mins and then exposed to low pH (pH 4.0 for one hour).

Polysaccharide production

Oral bacteria are subjected to continual cycles of feast and famine with respect to dietary carbohydrates. As a consequence, the resident microbiota has developed strategies to store these carbohydrates during their brief exposure to these energy sources. These strategies help to avoid the lethal effects of the build-up of intracellular glycolytic intermediates and provide a source of carbon and energy for the subsequent periods of famine. The most common strategy is to store these carbohydrates as intracellular polysaccharides (IPS) (see Figs 4.8 and 4.9), and many species of oral streptococci can synthesise polymers that resemble glycogen ($1,4$-α-glucan), although other polymers might also be formed. IPS metabolism to acid is a virulence factor for *S. mutans*, and mutants defective in this property cause less caries in animal models.

Many species of oral bacteria are also able to synthesise extracellular polysaccharides (EPS) from carbohydrates, especially from sucrose (Table 4.8; see Figs 4.8, 4.9 and Fig. 4.11). The polysaccharides can be soluble or insoluble; the former are more labile and can be metabolised by other bacteria, whereas the latter make a major contribution to the structural integrity of dental plaque (plaque matrix; see Chapter 5) and can consolidate the attachment of bacteria in plaque. Sucrose has a unique property as a substrate in that the bond between the glucose and fructose moieties has sufficient energy on cleavage to support the synthesis of polysaccharide. The polysaccharides formed are either glucans or fructans, and are synthesised by GTFs and FTFs, respectively:

$$n-\text{sucrose} \xrightarrow{\text{glucosyltransferase}} (\text{glucan})_n + n\text{-fructose}$$

$$n-\text{sucrose} \xrightarrow{\text{fructosyltransferase}} (\text{fructan})_n + n\text{-glucose}$$

GTFs are divided into four groups depending on whether they produce a soluble dextran (GTF-S enzymes synthesise predominantly α, 1-6 linked glucan) or an insoluble glucan (GTF-I enzymes synthesise predominantly α, 1-3 polymers), and whether or not they require a dextran primer for activity. *Streptococcus mutans* possesses three GTFs (encoded for by genes: *gtfB*, *gtfC* and *gtfD*) which synthesise α, 1-3- and α, 1-6-linked glucan polymers (Table 4.8). In *S. mutans*, the *gtfB* and *gtfC* genes encode enzymes that produce water-insoluble glucans, consisting primarily of α, 1-3 linkages. These gene products contribute to cell adhesion, plaque formation and structure, and are also essential for the initiation of caries on smooth surfaces of teeth in animal models. In contrast, the *gtfD* gene encodes a primer-dependent enzyme responsible for the formation of glucan, predominantly with α, 1-6 linked

glucose units, that is much more water soluble. The basic structure of some glucans is shown in Figure 4.11.

Streptococcus mutans has a single FTF (produced by the *ftf* gene), which catalyses the incorporation of the fructose component of the sucrose molecule into

Bacterium	Carbohydrate substrate	Type of polymer (with predominant linkages*)
Streptococcus mutans	Sucrose	Water-insoluble and soluble glucans α, 1–3-; α, 1–3- + 1–6-; α, 1–6-.
	Sucrose	Fructan 2, 1–β-
Streptococcus sanguinis[‡]	Sucrose	Water-insoluble glucan α, 1–3- + α, 1–6
	Sucrose	Water-soluble glucan (dextran) α, 1–6-
Streptococcus salivarius[§]	Sucrose	Fructan (levan) β, 2–6-
Actinomyces naeslundii	Sucrose	Fructan (levan) β, 2–6-
	[†]	Heteropolysaccharide (60% N-acetyl glucosamine)
Lactobacillus sp.	[†]	Glucan Heteropolysaccharide
Eubacterium spp.	[†]	Heteropolysaccharide (predominantly acetate) Homopolysaccharide (D-glycero-D-galacto-heptose)
Rothia dentocariosa	Glucose Sucrose	Heteropolysaccharide Levan
Rothia mucilaginosa	[†]	Heteropolysaccharide (hexoses, hexosamines, amino acids)
Neisseria spp.	Sucrose	Glycogen-like

TABLE 4.8 Extracellular polysaccharide-producing bacteria found in the mouth

*Where known.
[†]No specific substrate required.
[‡]Some strains produce a fructan.
[§]Some strains produce a glucan.

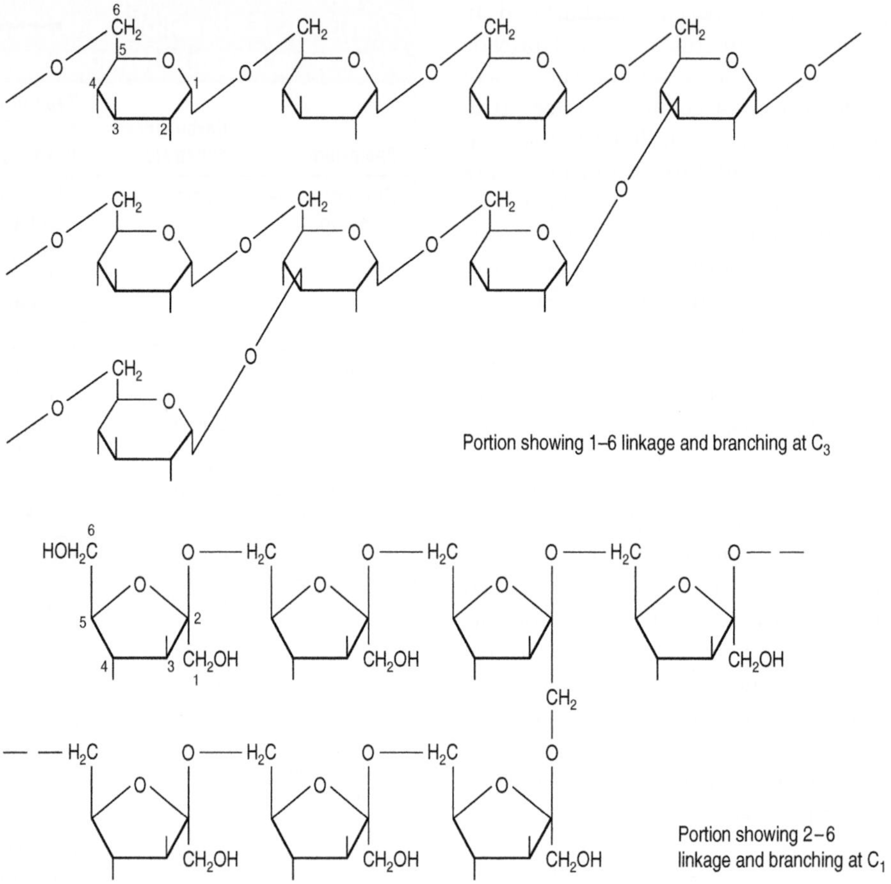

FIGURE 4.11 Structure of part of a glucan chain, showing α, 1-6,- and α, 1-3,- linkages (top), and a fructan, showing an α, 2-6,- linkage (bottom).

a fructan polymer with an inulin-type structure, composed mainly of β,2-1 linked fructose units. Fructans are not involved in adhesion and act more as extracellular carbohydrate storage compounds in plaque biofilms, being broken down to fructose (which can be transported by the PEP-PTS for glycolysis) by fructan hydrolases produced by a range of oral bacteria.

Other streptococci possess different numbers of GTF genes. Four GTF activities have been detected in *S. sobrinus*, including a primer-dependent GTF-I, which synthesises a glucan with predominantly α, 1-3 linked glucose residues. There are two gene products which produce polymers with mixed α, 1-3 and α, 1-6 linked glucose molecules, and a primer-independent GTF-S

producing a linear glucan composed predominantly of α, 1-6 residues. *Streptococcus salivarius* also produces four GTFs, although their properties differ from those described for *S. sobrinus*. In contrast, *S. gordonii* possesses only a single GTF, although this can form both soluble and insoluble glucan depending on the prevailing environmental conditions. *Streptococcus salivarius* also produces a fructan, but in contrast to that of *S. mutans*, it is a levan with a characteristic β,2-6 linkage (Table 4.8). The FTF of *S. salivarius* is cell associated, whereas those of most other organisms are secreted.

Other species that produce extracellular polysaccharides are listed in Table 4.8. The heteropolysaccharides are generally complex in composition; for example, the polymer produced by a strain of *Actinomyces naeslundii* contains N-acetyl glucosamine (62%), galactose (7%), glucose (4%), uronic acids (3%), and small amounts of glycerol, rhamnose, arabinose, and xylose. *Actinomyces naeslundii* also has FTF activity, and synthesises a fructan with a levan-type structure containing mainly β,2-6 linkages. Some of the homopolysaccharides and heteropolysaccharides can be metabolised by other oral bacteria; this aspect will be discussed in Chapter 5.

NITROGEN METABOLISM

Casein can be incorporated into dental plaque and degraded. *Streptococcus sanguinis* has been shown to have both endopeptidase and exopeptidase (amino-terminal and carboxy-terminal) activity that can cleave proteins such as casein into a range of peptide fragments. Exopeptidase activity is mainly cell-associated and upregulated at high pH, whereas endopeptidase activity is extracellular and optimal at neutral pH. *Streptococcus sanguinis* can rapidly release arginine from C-terminal peptides, converting the released arginine to energy (and carbamyl phosphate) via the arginine deiminase pathway. Urea is present in relatively high concentrations (200 mg/L) in saliva, and some oral species (e.g., *A. naeslundii* and *S. salivarius*) possess urease activity, which can convert the urea to carbon dioxide and ammonia. At acidic pH, decarboxylation of amino acids yields carbon dioxide and amines, whereas at high pH, deamination produces ammonia and keto acids, which can be converted to acetic, propionic, and possibly isobutyric and *n*-butyric acids. For example, some periodontal pathogens can convert histidine, glutamine or arginine to acetate and butyrate. In this way, amino acid metabolism might be an important mechanism by which oral microorganisms counter the extremes of pH caused by the catabolism of carbohydrates and urea.

Essential amino acids can be obtained from the environment or synthesised by the cell. Ammonia can be converted into a number of amino acids, for example:

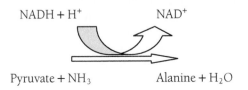

$$NADH + H^+ \qquad\qquad NAD^+$$

$$Pyruvate + NH_3 \qquad Alanine + H_2O$$

Further transamination reactions can provide other essential amino acids. The transport of amino acids such as glutamate and aspartate in *S. mutans* is by a primary transport system driven by ATP hydrolysis, whereas branched-chain amino acids (such as leucine) are taken up by an energised membrane- (proton motive force) driven carrier system. Essential amino acids can also be derived from the metabolism of peptides either inside or outside of the cell. This process is energetically favourable for cells because all of the amino acids present in the peptide are obtained for the same energy cost as the transport of a single amino acid.

Many of the microorganisms from the periodontal pocket are asaccharolytic (i.e., do not gain energy from the conversion of sugars to acidic fermentation products) and proteolytic, and their growth depends on their ability to use the nutrients provided locally by the host. During inflammation, the flow of GCF (see Chapter 2) is increased in response to an increase in biofilm accumulation. GCF delivers several components of the host defences to combat the biofilm, but several of the proteins can also act as potential novel nutrients for these proteolytic bacteria. For example, haemoglobin, transferrin, haemopexin and haptoglobin are present in GCF, and these can provide essential growth factors such as haeme, which select for highly proteolytic periodontal pathogens such as *P. gingivalis*. *Porphyromonas gingivalis* can directly transport and utilise some amino acids; this species prefers to take up short peptides for bioenergetic reasons; such peptides are then broken down within the cell by intracellular peptidases. The main proteases produced by *P. gingivalis* belong to the cysteine proteinase family, with specificity for arginine and lysine residues, and are termed Arg-gingipain (RgpA and RgpB) and Lys-gingipain (Kgp), respectively. RgpA and Kgp have C-terminal adhesin domains, and these can bind to host molecules. For example, *P. gingivalis* preferentially utilises haemoglobin-derived haeme, and this is acquired through the ability of the RgpA-Kgp proteinase-adhesin extracellular complexes to bind and hydrolyse haemoglobin, releasing haeme at the cell surface. Indeed, Kgp has been shown to be essential for the formation of the black pigment associated with *P. gingivalis* colonies on blood agar (see Fig. 3.8); the pigmentation is because of the deposition of haeme, as a μ-oxo dimer on the cell surface, which provides protection from the lethal effects of oxygen (see later this chapter).

In addition to obtaining essential nutrients from GCF, many subgingival organisms are also able to degrade structural proteins and glycoproteins associated with the periodontal pocket epithelium. The production of enzymes such as chondroitin sulphatase, hyaluronidase and collagenase contributes to tissue damage and periodontal pocket formation. Arg-gingipain is also important in virulence and can deregulate and subvert the host inflammatory response by degrading host protease inhibitors designed to control inflammation, and this leads to by-stander damage to the periodontal tissues (see Chapter 6). Gingipains degrade cytokines, components of the complement system and receptors on macrophages and T-cells, thereby perturbing the host defences; they also degrade host receptors, thereby increasing vascular permeability and increasing the influx of neutrophils. The pH optimum of some of these enzymes is at neutral or slightly alkaline pH, which corresponds to that of the inflamed periodontal pocket.

Synergistic interactions occur in the breakdown of host molecules, and mutually beneficial associations occur between organisms with complementary patterns of enzyme activity (see Chapter 5). The endopeptidase activity of *P. gingivalis* can provide appropriate peptides from the catabolism of host molecules for the growth of *F. nucleatum*. Similarly, *F. nucleatum* can support the growth of *P. gingivalis* in oxygenated environments. This might explain why these two species are frequently found together in periodontal pockets. The concept of plaque behaving as a microbial community in terms of the breakdown of complex host molecules and environment modification is developed further in Chapter 5.

Collectively, these findings emphasise the significance of nitrogen metabolism in oral microbial ecology. Host and bacterial proteases are associated directly and indirectly with tissue destruction in periodontal disease, whereas some have argued that caries results not so much from an over-production of acid, but more from a deficiency in base production by plaque bacteria.

OXYGEN METABOLISM

The mouth is an overtly aerobic environment and yet the majority of bacteria are either facultatively anaerobic or obligately anaerobic, especially in dental plaque. Early colonisers tend to be more tolerant of the toxic effects of oxygen metabolism, especially with respect to hydrogen peroxide and hypothiocyanite, than later colonisers, which may depend on interspecies metabolic interactions within the biofilm to cope with oxygen and toxic radicals.

All plaque bacteria, including obligate anaerobes, are able to metabolise oxygen, albeit at different rates. Aerobic bacteria (such as *Neisseria* spp.) may use cytochrome-containing electron transport chains for oxygen reduction and coupled ATP synthesis. In contrast, facultatively anaerobic, lactic acid-producing species have a flavin-containing nicotinamide adenine dinucleotide (NADH) oxidase and NADH peroxidase; similarly, even *T. denticola* (which is highly anaerobic), possesses NADH oxidases and NADH peroxidases, enabling it to scavenge low levels of oxygen in the subgingival environment. Some of these reactions are illustrated below:

$$O^-_2 + O^-_2 + 2H^+ \xrightarrow{\text{superoxide dismutase}} H_2O_2 + O_2$$

$$2H_2O_2 \xrightarrow{\text{catalase}} 2H_2O + O_2$$

$$NADH + H^+ + H_2O_2 \xrightarrow{\text{NADH peroxidase}} NAD^+ + 2H_2O$$

$$2NADH + 2H^+ + 2O_2 \xrightarrow{\text{NADH oxidase}} 2NAD^+ + 2H_2O$$

Although oxygen itself is not toxic, the production of oxygen metabolites can be, and so oral bacteria possess molecular defence mechanisms to prevent or reduce oxidative damage. These mechanisms involve the production of catalase, peroxidases and superoxide dismutase. Thus, oral organisms as metabolically diverse as mutans streptococci and *P. gingivalis* produce protective enzymes; mutans streptococci produce superoxide dismutase, NADH peroxidase and glutathione reductase, whereas *P. gingivalis* has a superoxide dismutase, NADH oxidase and NADH peroxidase. The activities of these enzymes increase when cells of *P. gingivalis* are exposed to oxygen. The characteristic black pigmentation of colonies of *P. gingivalis* growing on blood agar can also provide protection against oxidative damage. When haeme is released from haemoglobin it can react with oxygen to form dimers that accumulate on the cell surface of *P. gingivalis*. These aggregated dimers can provide antioxidant protection, serving as a physical barrier to environmental oxygen, as well as acting as a buffer system to hydrogen peroxide, because of a catalase-like activity inherent to the layer.

Some obligate anaerobes form close physical associations with oxygen-consuming species (e.g., *Neisseria* spp.) to be able to grow in biofilms and survive in the mouth.

ORAL MALODOUR (HALITOSIS)

Oral malodour is a relatively common condition in the adult population and is associated with the metabolism of bacteria located on the tongue. High odour subjects generally have a higher total bacterial load on the tongue and higher numbers of Gram-negative anaerobes, including *Leptotrichia*, *Porphyromonas*, *Prevotella*, *Fusobacterium* and *Treponema* species.

Malodour production is strongly associated with high proteolytic activity and the production of volatile sulphur compounds. The predominant sulphur compounds are hydrogen sulphide [H_2S] and methyl mercaptan [CH_3SH], with lower concentrations of dimethyl sulphide [$(CH_3)_2S$] and dimethyl disulphide [$(CH_3S)_2$]. Hydrogen sulphide is generated principally by the action of L-cysteine dehydro-sulphatase on L-cysteine, whereas methyl mercaptan (methanethiol) is produced by the oxidation of L-methionine. *Fusobacterium* spp. and *Parvimonas micra* produce high concentrations of hydrogen sulphide from glutathione (a tripeptide: L-δ-glutamyl-L-cysteinylglycine), which is present in most

tissue cells and would be available in the periodontal pocket. Tongue scraping to reduce the microbial load at this site can be effective in treating halitosis.

BENEFITS OF THE ORAL MICROBIOTA

It has been emphasised that the presence of a diverse microbiota in the mouth is natural. Humans have coevolved with these resident microbes, and it is clear that this is a genuinely mutualistic relationship. The host provides a warm and nutritious environment for microbial growth, whereas evidence has emerged to show that the natural microbial residents are essential for the normal development of the physiology, nutrition and defences of the host (Fig. 4.12).

COLONISATION RESISTANCE

One of the main beneficial functions of the oral microbiota is its ability to prevent colonisation by exogenous (and often pathogenic) microorganisms (Table 4.9). This property, termed 'colonisation resistance', is because of resident microorganisms being more effective at:

- attachment to host receptors;
- competition for endogenous nutrients;
- creating unfavourable conditions to discourage attachment and retard multiplication of invading organisms; and
- producing antagonistic substances (hydrogen peroxide, bacteriocins, etc.), which are inhibitory to exogenous microbes.

KEY POINTS

The oral microbiota exhibits considerable biochemical flexibility to cope with the oscillating feast-famine conditions in the mouth.

Dietary sugars are rapidly transported into cells (e.g., via the PEP-PTS) by cariogenic bacteria and converted to acidic fermentation products or to extracellular and intracellular polysaccharides. Mutans streptococci have specific strategies to cope with the resultant acid stress conditions.

Subgingival bacteria rely on metabolising proteins and glycoproteins supplied by GCF, often generating base, and raising the local pH to alkaline levels. Many of these proteolytic bacteria are obligately anaerobic, and they have specific mechanisms to cope with oxidative stress.

TABLE 4.9 **Functions of the resident oral microbiota that contribute to colonisation resistance**

Function
Competition for receptors for adhesion
Competition for essential endogenous nutrients and cofactors
Creation of microenvironments that discourage the growth of exogenous species
Production of inhibitory substances (bacteriocins, H_2O_2, bacteriophage, etc.)

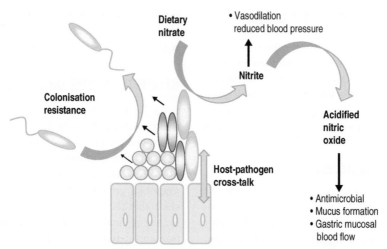

FIGURE 4.12 Benefits associated with the resident oral microbiota. The resident oral microbiota can (a) exclude exogenous microorganisms (colonisation resistance); (b) be involved in cross-talk with the host, and downregulate potential pro-inflammatory activity towards commensal organisms, and (c) reduce dietary nitrate to nitrite, which can be further converted to acidified nitric oxide, and which deliver multiple physiologic benefits to the host.

Colonisation resistance can be impaired by factors that compromise the integrity of the host defences or perturb the stability of the resident microbiota, such as the side effects of cytotoxic therapy or the long-term use of broad-spectrum antibiotics. For example, the latter can suppress the resident bacterial oral microbiota, permitting overgrowth by previously minor populations of microbes such as oral yeasts.

Ways to boost colonisation resistance are being explored by using prebiotics and probiotics. **Prebiotics** are molecules that stimulate the growth and/or activity of those members of the resident microbiota that contribute to the well-being of their host. Prebiotics such as non-digestible fibre compounds (e.g., inulin, oligofructose) have been delivered to the gastrointestinal tract to stabilise the composition and boost the metabolism of the gut microbiota, especially that of beneficial bifidobacteria and lactobacilli. Attempts are now being made to use prebiotics to boost the growth of selected resident oral bacteria. Probiotics are live microorganisms, typically bifidobacteria and lactobacilli, that are claimed to provide health benefits when consumed. They can be consumed in dairy products such as yoghurts, and most applications are again targeted at the gut microbiota. Commonly claimed benefits of probiotics include the decrease of potentially pathogenic gastrointestinal

microorganisms, the reduction of gastrointestinal discomfort, the strengthening of the immune system and the recovery of the intestinal microbiota in subjects who have received antibiotic treatment or who have suffered a gastric illness. Now, probiotic milk, cheese, yoghurts and so on are being developed to provide similar benefits for oral health. There is little evidence that these probiotic microbes are able to colonise the mouth, and unequivocal proof that they deliver benefit is still being actively sought.

Another approach to increase the colonisation resistance of the oral microbiota is by replacement therapy. Examples include the deliberate reimplantation of beneficial resident organisms into the subgingival environment, for example, after periodontal therapy, or by the preemptive colonisation of teeth with either low virulence mutants of *S. mutans* or with harmless plaque organisms that are more competitive than wild-type *S. mutans* strains.

HOST-MICROBE CROSS-TALK

The host is not indifferent to the presence of the diverse microbial communities that reside on its surfaces, many of which produce proinflammatory molecules. The host is able to detect microorganisms, and has evolved systems to tolerate beneficial resident microorganisms without initiating a damaging inflammatory response, while also being able to mount an efficient defence against pathogens. The attachment of bacteria to specific receptors on host cells can trigger substantial changes in gene expression in both the prokaryotic and eukaryotic cells.

Host cell-pattern recognition receptors (e.g., Toll-like receptors) can recognise microbe-associated molecular patterns (e.g., lipopolysaccharide, lipoteichoic acid) and activate multiple signalling pathways, many of which converge on nuclear factor kappa-light-chain-enhancer of activated B cells (NFκB). The host has developed strategies to distinguish between commensal and pathogenic bacteria. Certain oral streptococci have been shown to suppress epithelial cell inflammatory responses by functional modulation of immunity via Toll-like receptor expression and signalling, and also by suppressing inflammatory responses by inhibiting activation of NFκB or by increasing the secretion of antiinflammatory cytokines, such as interleukin-10 (IL-10). Beneficial oral streptococci may also actively stimulate beneficial pathways in epithelial cells, including type I and II interferon responses, promote wound healing, enhance mucin production, and induce positive effects on the cytoskeleton.

NITRATE METABOLISM

The resident oral bacteria play an important role in general health by maintaining key aspects of the gastrointestinal and cardiovascular systems, via the metabolism of dietary nitrate. Nitrate is present in many leafy green vegetables and beets and is absorbed into the bloodstream during digestion. Circulating nitrate is concentrated by the salivary glands, and approximately 25% of dietary nitrate reappears in saliva where it is reduced to nitrite by the oral microbiota. The host is unable to perform this biochemical reduction step and is entirely dependent on the metabolic capability of resident oral bacteria. The bacteria with the greatest nitrate reductase activity are found on the dorsum of the tongue and belong to the genera *Neisseria*, *Veillonella*, *Actinomyces* and *Rothia*. Nitrite affects a number of key physiological processes including the regulation of blood flow, blood pressure, gastric integrity and tissue protection against ischemic injury. Nitrite can be further converted to nitric oxide

in the acidified stomach, and this has antimicrobial properties and contributes to defence against enteropathogens and in the regulation of gastric mucosal blood flow and mucus formation. The deliberate suppression of the oral microbiota using either an antimicrobial mouthwash or a broad-spectrum antibiotic was shown to reduce the microbial conversion of nitrate to nitrite with a loss of the biological benefits of nitrite (including reduced gastric mucus thickness), while blood pressure rose slightly. These observations emphasise the need to preserve a resident oral microbiota with a normal composition and activity to maintain health (see Fig. 4.12).

KEY POINTS

> The natural, resident oral microbiota provides essential benefits to the host, including:
> - colonisation resistance;
> - cross-talk with the host (modulates immune responses, upregulates beneficial host pathways, enhances mucin production); and
> - nitrate reduction to nitrite and nitric oxide.

CHAPTER SUMMARY

The acquisition of the resident oral microbiota begins during delivery of the baby and continues throughout life. The biological properties of the mouth make it highly selective in terms of the types of microorganisms able to colonise. Few of the species found in the mouths of adults and even fewer of the organisms of the general environment are able to establish successfully in infants. Acquisition of the resident microbiota follows a pattern of ecological succession: relatively few organisms (pioneer species) are able to colonise, but their presence enables other species to become established; this process eventually leads to a climax community with a high species diversity. Many species are acquired from the mother by transmission via saliva. The development of a climax community in the mouth can involve both allogenic (non-microbial influenced) and autogenic (microbial influenced) succession.

The composition of the resident microbiota varies at different sites around the mouth, with each site having a relatively characteristic microbial community. Mutans streptococci and *S. sanguinis* have preferences for hard surfaces for colonisation, whereas species such as *S. salivarius* are recovered predominantly from the oral mucosa. The tongue has the highest number of microorganisms per unit area of oral mucosal surface and can act as a reservoir for some Gram-negative anaerobes that are implicated in periodontal diseases and halitosis.

The distribution of microorganisms is related to their ability to adhere at a site, to have their nutritional and environmental requirements (pH and redox potential) satisfied and to grow to form biofilms. To cope with the fluctuating nutritional conditions in the mouth, the resident oral microbiota is biochemically flexible. The primary source of nutrients is the endogenous supply of host proteins and glycoproteins from saliva and GCF. Superimposed on these are carbohydrates (and some proteins) provided by the diet. Carbohydrates can be transported into the bacterial cell by, for example, a high affinity PEP-PTS system, and either converted to organic acids or used to synthesise intracellular storage polysaccharides. Potentially cariogenic bacteria deploy specific molecular strategies that enable them to tolerate the low pH conditions generated following sugar catabolism, and which would be inhibitory to other species. Some disaccharides can be metabolised extracellularly into constituent sugars (for transport) or into extracellular polysaccharides; these polysaccharides can function to consolidate attachment, form a biofilm matrix (see Chapter 5) or used as extracellular storage compounds. The extracellular glucans and fructans are synthesised by glucosyltransferases and fructosyltransferases, respectively.

The metabolism of nitrogen compounds involves a wide range of exopeptidases and endopeptidases; nitrogen metabolism can lead to base production which helps to regulate environmental pH. The catabolism of complex host molecules requires bacteria with complementary patterns of enzyme activity to interact to ensure their complete breakdown. Obligate anaerobes are found commonly at many sites in the mouth. These bacteria survive oxygen exposure by interacting with oxygen-consuming species and by the possession of a number of specific enzyme systems to scavenge oxygen and toxic radicals.

Halitosis occurs through the production of increased levels of malodorous compounds (such as hydrogen sulphide and methyl mercaptan) by proteolytic anaerobic bacteria, many of which are located on the tongue.

The resident oral microbiota is natural and provides several critically important benefits to the host. These include colonisation resistance, modulation of the host response (to reduce inflammation), promotion of wound healing, the reduction of nitrate to nitrite (which regulates blood pressure and other host functions) and nitric oxide (an important antimicrobial agent), induction of host defence peptides and enhancement of mucin production.

FURTHER READING

Aas JA, Paster BJ, Stokes LN, et al. Defining the normal bacterial flora of the oral cavity. *J Clin Microbiol.* 2005;43:5721-5732.

Carlsson J. Growth and nutrition as ecological factors. In: Kuramitsu HK, Ellen RP, eds. *Oral bacterial ecology. The molecular basis.* Wymondham: Horizon Scientific Press; 2000:67-130.

Chen H, Jiang W. Application of high-throughput sequencing in understanding human oral microbiome related with health and disease. *Front Microbiol.* 2014;5:508.

Delima SL, McBride RK, Preshaw PM, et al. Response of subgingival bacteria to smoking cessation. *J Clin Microbiol.* 2010;48:2344-2349.

Devine DA, Marsh PD, Meade J. Modulation of host responses by oral commensal bacteria. *J Oral Microbiol.* 2015;7:26941.

Dominguez-Bello MG, Costello EK, Contreras M, et al. Delivery mode shapes the acquisition and structure of the initial microbiota across multiple body habitats in newborns. *PNAS.* 2010;107:11971-11975.

Douglas CWI, Naylor K, Phansopa C, et al. Physiological adaptations of key oral bacteria. *Adv Microb Physiol.* 2014;65:257-335.

Kapil V, Haydar SM, Pearl V, et al. Physiological role for nitrate-reducing oral bacteria in blood pressure control. *Free Radic Biol Med.* 2013;55:93-100.

Kumar PS. Sex and the subgingival microbiome: Do female sex steroids affect periodontal bacteria? *Periodontol 2000.* 2013;61:103-124.

Kumar PS, Mason MR. Mouthguards: does the indigenous microbiome play a role in maintaining oral health? *Front Cell Infect Microbiol.* 2015;5:article 35. doi:10.3389/fcimb.2015.00035.

Mark Welch JL, Utter DR, Rossetti BJ, et al. Dynamics of tongue microbial communities with single-nucleotide resolution using oligotyping. *Front Microbiol.* 2014;5:article 568. doi:10.3389/fmicrb.2014.00568.

Papaioannou W, Gizani S, Haffajee AD, et al. The microbiota on different oral surfaces in healthy children. *Oral Microbiol Immunol.* 2009;24:183-189.

Paster BJ, Dewhirst FE. Molecular microbial diagnosis. *Periodontol 2000.* 2009;51:38-44.

Percival RS. Changes in oral microflora and host defences with advanced age. In: Percival S, Hart A, eds. *Microbiology and aging: clinical manifestations.* New York: Springer; 2009:131-152.

Pozhitkov AE, Beikler T, Flemmig T, et al. High-throughput methods for analysis of the human oral microbiome. *Periodontol 2000*. 2009;55:70-86.

Quivey RG, Kuhnert WL, Hahn K. Adaptation of oral streptococci to low pH. *Adv Microb Physiol*. 2000;42:239-274.

Sachdeo A, Haffajee AD, Socransky SS. Biofilms in the edentulous oral cavity. *J Prosthodont*. 2008;17:348-356.

Scully C, Greenman J. Halitology (breath odour: aetiopathogenesis and management). *Oral Dis*. 2012;18:333-345.

Takahashi N. Oral microbiome metabolism: From "Who are they?" to "What are they doing?". *J Dent Res*. 2015;94:1628-1637.

Wade WG. The oral microbiome in health and disease. *Pharmacol Res*. 2013;69:137-143.

Yang F, Huang S, He T, et al. Microbial basis of oral malodour development in humans. *J Dent Res*. 2013;92:1106-1112.

MULTIPLE CHOICE QUESTIONS

Answers on p. 249

1 *Who or what is the major source of microorganisms in the newborn?*
   a. The environment of the delivery room (home or hospital)
   b. Midwife, or person delivering the baby
   c. Mother
   d. Both parents

2 *Which of the following are pioneer species that colonise the mouth of the newborn?*
   a. *Streptococcus mutans*
   b. *Streptococcus mitis*
   c. *Actinomyces naeslundii*
   d. *Prevotella denticola*

3 *Pioneer bacterial colonising species can modify the local environment to provide conditions suitable for the growth of later colonisers. Which of the following is not a mechanism that facilitates bacterial succession to increase the diversity of the biofilm?*
   a. Modifying or exposing new receptors for attachment
   b. Consuming oxygen, and lowering the redox potential
   c. Generating potential nutrients, either as end-products of breakdown products metabolism
   d. Lowering the pH by glycolysis

4 *Which of the following anaerobic bacteria is most commonly isolated from young edentulous infants?*
   a. *Prevotella melaninogenica*
   b. *Porphyromonas gingivalis*
   c. *Prevotella denticola*
   d. *Prevotella loescheii*

5 *Which of the following is not a recognised method for sampling plaque biofilms?*
   a. Paper points
   b. Direct impression
   c. Toothpick
   d. Abrasive strip

6 *Which is a suitable genetic target for identification of oral bacteria?*
   a. 18S ribosomal ribonucleic acid (rRNA) gene
   b. Plasmid deoxyribonucleic acid (DNA)
   c. Messenger ribonucleic acid (mRNA)
   d. 16S rRNA gene

7 *Which of the following groups of bacteria that can be cultured from the tongue are present in the highest numbers?*
   a. *Actinomyces*
   b. *Streptococcus*
   c. *Prevotella*
   d. *Fusobacterium*

8 *Which of the following is not a molecular technique for detecting bacteria?*
   a. FISH
   b. PCR
   c. 454 pyrosequencing
   d. TM7

9 *Sucrose can be metabolised in several ways. Which of the following is not a product of sucrose catabolism?*
a. Glucan
b. Lactate
c. Ammonia
d. Intracellular polysaccharide

10 *What are the main proteases of* Porphyromonas gingivalis *termed?*
a. Interpains
b. Gingipains
c. Urease
d. Superoxide dismutase

11 *Urea can be converted to which of the following?*
a. Lactate
b. Acetate, formate and ethanol
c. ammonia and carbon dioxide
d. Hydrogen sulfide

12 *Oral malodour is associated with high proteolytic activity; which of the following molecules is not associated with halitosis?*
a. Hydrogen sulfide
b. Methyl mercaptan
c. Phosphoenolpyruvate
d. Dimethyl sulfide

13 *Which of the following is not an enzyme involved in the scavenging of oxygen or other reactive oxygen species by anaerobic bacteria?*
a. Enolase
b. Catalase
c. Superoxide dismutase
d. Nicotinamide adenine dinucleotide phosphate-oxidase (NADH)

14 *Many of the anaerobic bacteria isolated from the periodontal pocket have which of the following type of metabolism?*
a. Saccharolytic.
b. Asaccharolytic and proteolytic
c. Capnophilic
d. Fermentative

15 *Bacteria such as* Streptococcus mutans *survive in a low pH environment in biofilms by which of the following strategies?*
a. Increase in the activity of their H^+/ATPase enzyme
b. Shift to a heterofermentative metabolism
c. Metabolism of arginine to ammonia
d. Raising the pH optima of glycolytic enzymes

Dental plaque

Dental plaque is the microbial community that develops as a **biofilm** on the tooth surface, embedded in a matrix of polymers of bacterial and salivary origin. Plaque that becomes calcified is referred to as calculus or tartar. The presence of plaque in the mouth can readily be demonstrated by rinsing with a disclosing solution such as erythrosin (Fig. 5.1). The majority of plaque is found associated with the protected and stagnant regions of the tooth surface such as fissures, approximal regions between teeth and the gingival crevice (see Figs 2.2 and 5.1). Plaque is found naturally on the tooth surface and forms part of the host defences by excluding exogenous (and often pathogenic) species (**colonisation resistance**) (see Table 4.9). On occasions, however, plaque can accumulate beyond levels compatible with oral health, and this can lead to shifts in the composition of the microbiota and predispose sites to disease (see Chapter 6). Dental plaque is an example of both a biofilm and a microbial community, and the significance of this will be explained in the following sections.

MICROBIAL BIOFILMS

The vast majority of microorganisms from a range of ecosystems grow on a surface as a **biofilm**. Biofilms are spatially and functionally organised and are enclosed in a matrix of extracellular polymers. If biofilm microbes were simply planktonic (liquid-phase) cells that had adhered to a surface, and the properties of microbial communities were merely the sum of the constitutive populations, then scientific interest in such issues would be limited. However, research has revealed that cells growing as biofilms have unique properties, some of which are of clinical significance (Table 5.1); for example, biofilms are manyfold more tolerant of antimicrobial agents than the same cells growing in liquid culture, making them more difficult to treat, while communities of interacting species can be more pathogenic than pure cultures of the constituent microorganisms.

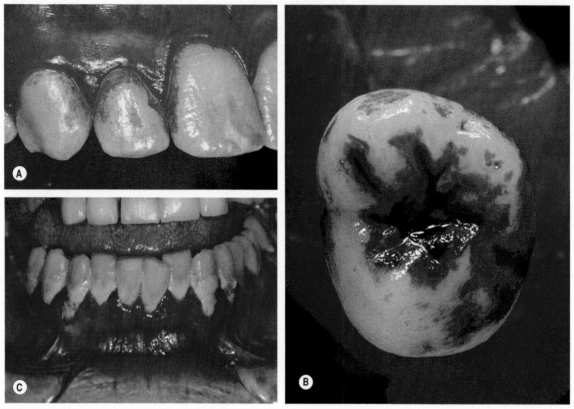

FIGURE 5.1 Dental plaque on human teeth. (**A**) Visualisation of dental plaque after staining with a disclosing solution. Biofilm typically forms at retention and stagnation areas along the gingival margin and between teeth (approximal areas). (**B**) Heavy accumulation of biofilm on the occlusal surface of an erupting third molar; plaque is preferentially located in the fissures. (Taken from Marsh PD, Takahashi N & Nyvad B, Biofilms in caries development, in Dental Caries. The disease and its clinical management, 3rd ed, Fejerskov O, Nyvad B and Kidd EAM, Blackwell, Oxford, 2015; pp. 107-131, published with permission.) (**C**) Unstained plaque on teeth in the mouth.

Originally, biofilms were considered to be dense, compressed accumulations of cells, and this compacted structure was believed to be responsible for many of their novel features. Advances in microscopy have enabled biofilms to be viewed in their natural (hydrated) state *in situ* without any processing of samples (e.g., chemical fixation or embedding techniques) that could distort their structure. Confocal laser scanning microscopy (CLSM) enables optical thin sections to be generated throughout the depth of the biofilm, and these can be combined using imaging software to generate three-dimensional images. The location of specific organisms can be visualised with immunological or oligonucleotide probes by fluorescent *in situ* hybridisation (FISH), while other molecular probes can indicate the viability and metabolic activity of cells. These techniques have shown that biofilms that develop in low-nutrient environments, especially those from aquatic habitats, have a more open structure than predicted from earlier studies using electron microscopy. Channels have been observed in biofilms of environmental bacteria, enabling potentially growth-limiting factors such as nutrients and oxygen to penetrate more extensively than previously thought. The use of microelectrodes and chemical probes have shown that gradients in critical factors (pH, oxygen, etc.) that affect microbial growth can occur over relatively short distances (a few microns, i.e., a few cell diameters) within biofilms. This produces spatial and temporal heterogeneity within the biofilm, enabling

TABLE 5.1 General properties of biofilms and microbial communities

General property	Dental plaque example
Open architecture	Presence of channels and voids
Protection from host defences, desiccation, etc.	Production of extracellular polymers to form a functional matrix; physical protection from phagocytosis
Enhanced tolerance to antimicrobials*	Reduced sensitivity to chlorhexidine and antibiotics; gene transfer of resistance genes
Neutralisation of inhibitors	β-Lactamase production by neighbouring cells to protect sensitive organisms
Novel gene expression*	Synthesis of novel proteins on attachment; upregulation of glucosyltransferases in mature biofilms
Coordinated gene responses	Production of cell-cell signalling molecules (e.g., CSP, AI-2)
Spatial and environmental heterogeneity	pH and O_2 gradients; coadhesion
Broader habitat range	Obligate anaerobes in an overtly aerobic environment
More efficient metabolism	Complete catabolism of complex host macromolecules (e.g., mucins) by microbial consortia
Enhanced virulence	Pathogenic synergism in abscesses and periodontal diseases

*One consequence of altered gene expression can also be an increased tolerance of antimicrobial agents.
CSP, Competence-stimulating peptide. AI-2 (Autoinducer-2).

fastidious bacteria to survive in apparently hostile or incompatible environments (see Table 5.1).

A biofilm lifestyle may affect the properties of an organism in more than one way. Firstly, the attachment of cells to a surface may exert a **direct effect** by inducing expression of a subset of genes. Bacteria are able to sense their environment via membrane-bound two component signal transduction pathways consisting of a sensor histidine kinase and a response regulator. *Pseudomonas aeruginosa* is an environmental bacterium that can also act as an opportunistic pathogen, for example, in cystic fibrosis, and can colonise dental unit water lines. Attachment leads to the upregulation of genes involved in exopolysaccharide (alginate) synthesis within a few minutes of the initial contact of a cell with a surface. Secondly, the growth environment within the biofilm may differ significantly in respect of key factors (pH, oxygen and nutrient concentration) compared with the surrounding (planktonic) environment. Again, this may result in altered gene expression, and hence an altered phenotype, but as an **indirect effect** of growing in a biofilm. Likewise, organisms in a biofilm will be growing more slowly, because of a particular nutrient limitation or an unfavourable pH, and this will also affect the properties of a cell. Biofilm bacteria are phenotypically distinct from their planktonic equivalents, and one particularly important aspect of this is an increased tolerance of biofilm cells to antimicrobial agents. Conventionally, the sensitivity of bacteria to antimicrobial agents is determined on cells grown in liquid culture by the measurement of the minimum inhibitory concentration (MIC) or minimum bactericidal concentration (MBC) against relevant antimicrobial agents. An extreme example was the finding that *P. aeruginosa* growing on urinary catheter material had an MIC that was between 500 to 1000 times greater to the antibiotic, tobramycin, compared with the same cells in liquid (planktonic) culture. Given the decreased sensitivity of an organism on a surface to antimicrobial agents, it has been argued that it would be more appropriate to determine the biofilm-inhibitory concentration (BIC) and biofilm-killing concentration (BKC) or biofilm-eradicating concentration (BEC). As yet, these proposals have not been widely accepted, and there are no generally agreed methods by which these concentrations could be determined.

Microorganisms in biofilms are described as being tolerant to antimicrobial agents. This is because the cells return to being susceptible when the biofilm is dispersed, indicating that the tolerance is phenotypic rather than genotypic. However, microorganisms within a biofilm can become genotypically resistant to antibiotics as biofilms provide ideal conditions for the transfer of resistance genes, e.g., via plasmids, among neighbouring cells in close proximity to one another (horizontal gene transfer).

The mechanisms behind this increased tolerance include the limited penetration of an antimicrobial agent into the depths of the biofilm; for example, positively-charged antibiotics such as aminoglycosides will bind to negatively-charged polymers that are components of the extracellular matrix (diffusion-reaction theory). Agents may also bind to and inhibit the organisms at the surface of the biofilm, leaving cells in the depths of the biofilm relatively unaffected, that is, the agent is exhausted or quenched at the surface (see later, Fig. 5.15). The drug target may be modified or not expressed during growth on a surface, or the organism may use alternative biochemical strategies thereby diminishing the potential impact of the active agent. Cells also grow much slower in a mature biofilm and, as a consequence, are much less susceptible to antimicrobials than faster growing cells. The environment in the depths of a biofilm may also be unfavourable for the optimal action of some antimicrobial agents. In multi-species biofilms, a microorganism can be protected if neighbouring cells produce a neutralising or drug-degrading enzyme.

KEY POINTS

- Most microorganisms grow as a biofilm on a surface.
- A biofilm describes microorganisms attached to a surface, often as part of a multi-species community, embedded in a polymeric matrix.
- The phenotype of microorganisms in a biofilm is different from when they grow in liquid culture.
- Microorganisms in biofilms are more tolerant of antimicrobial agents, environmental stresses and the host defences.

BIOFILMS IN THE MOUTH

Dental plaque was probably the first biofilm to have been studied in terms of either its microbial composition or its sensitivity to antimicrobial agents. In the seventeenth century, Antonie van Leeuwenhoek pioneered the approach of studying biofilms by direct microscopic observation when he reported on the diversity and high numbers of animalcules present in scrapings taken from around human teeth. He also conducted early studies on the novel properties of surface-grown cells when he failed to kill plaque bacteria on his teeth by prolonged rinsing with wine-vinegar,

although the organisms were killed if they were first removed from his molars and mixed with vinegar *in vitro*.

Dental plaque displays all of the characteristic features of a typical biofilm (see Table 5.1). Compared with other habitats, dental plaque is relatively accessible for sampling and can even be grown on relevant removable surfaces for subsequent investigation and experimentation in the laboratory (in situ models; see Chapter 4). A large proportion of the microorganisms in dental plaque can be identified, while the phenotype of such microbes (adhesins, metabolic potential, cell–cell interactions) is well-characterised. Extensive biofilms also develop on dentures and the tongue. On other mucosal surfaces, bacteria attach to epithelial cells and may develop a surface-associated phenotype, but desquamation ensures that extensive biofilms cannot develop. Another dentally relevant biofilm develops on the tubing used in dental unit water supply systems (DUWS); this will be discussed in Chapter 12 (see Fig. 12.5), but the principles governing the formation and properties of these biofilms will be similar to those described next for dental plaque.

MECHANISMS OF DENTAL PLAQUE FORMATION

The development of a biofilm such as dental plaque can be subdivided arbitrarily into several stages. As a bacterium approaches a surface, a number of specific and non-specific interactions will occur between the substratum and the cell, and these will determine whether successful attachment and colonisation will take place. Distinct stages in plaque formation are summarised below, and are shown schematically in Figure 5.2.

However, it should be remembered that biofilm formation is a dynamic process and the phases described below are only arbitrary and are for the benefit of discussion. The attachment, growth, removal and reattachment of bacteria are continuous processes, and a microbial biofilm such as plaque will undergo constant reorganisation.

ACQUIRED PELLICLE FORMATION

The earliest colonisers rarely come into contact with a 'naked' tooth surface. As soon as a tooth is cleaned, molecules from the environment, especially salivary

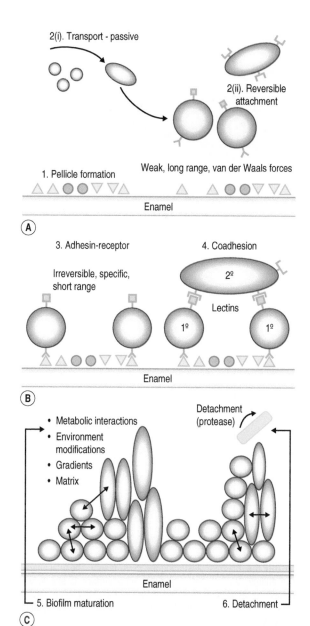

2(i). Transport - passive

2(ii). Reversible attachment

1. Pellicle formation

Weak, long range, van der Waals forces

Enamel

(A)

3. Adhesin-receptor

4. Coadhesion

Irreversible, specific, short range

2º

Lectins

1º   1º

Enamel

(B)

- Metabolic interactions
- Environment modifications
- Gradients
- Matrix

Detachment (protease)

Enamel

5. Biofilm maturation   6. Detachment

(C)

FIGURE 5.2 Schematic representation of the different stages in the formation of dental plaque: (**A**) 1. Pellicle forms on a clean tooth surface. 2(i) Bacteria are transported passively to the tooth surface where they 2(ii) may be held reversibly by weak electrostatic forces of attraction. (**B**) 3. Attachment becomes irreversible by specific stereochemical molecular interactions between adhesins on the bacterium and receptors in the acquired pellicle, and 4. secondary colonisers attach to primary colonisers, often by lectin-like interactions (coadhesion). (**C**) 5. Growth results in biofilm maturation, facilitating interbacterial interactions. 6. Eventually, detachment can occur, sometimes as a result of the degradation by bacteria of their adhesins.

proteins and glycoproteins, are adsorbed forming a surface-conditioning film, which is termed the acquired enamel pellicle. The major constituents of pellicle are salivary glycoproteins, phosphoproteins and lipids, and include statherin, proline-rich peptides (PRPs) and host defence components (see Chapter 2). Several enzymes of host and bacterial origin are immobilised in an active form in the pellicle. The enzymes include amylase, lysozyme, carbonic anhydrases, fructosyltransferases (FTFs) and glucosyltransferases (GTFs); glucans have also been detected in the pellicle, and play a significant role in bacterial attachment. Depending on the site, the pellicle can also contain components from gingival crevicular fluid (GCF).

Pellicle formation starts within seconds of a clean surface being exposed to the oral environment. An equilibrium between adsorption and desorption of salivary molecules occurs after 90 to 120 minutes. The thickness of the pellicle is influenced by the shear forces at the site of formation. After 2 hours, the pellicle on lingual surfaces is 20 to 80 nm thick, whereas buccal pellicles can be 200 to 700 nm deep. Depending on the site, further increases in pellicle depth can occur over time. Pellicle has an electron dense basal layer covered by a more loosely arranged globular surface (see Fig. 5.3). When salivary molecules bind to the tooth surface, they can undergo conformational changes. This can lead to exposure of new receptors for bacterial attachment (**cryptitopes**; see later) or, in the case of glucosyltransferases, an altered activity resulting in the synthesis of a glucan with a modified structure. Pellicle has several functions; it can act as a diffusion barrier and as a buffer and plays a critical role in determining the pattern of microbial colonisation.

TRANSPORT OF MICROORGANISMS AND REVERSIBLE ATTACHMENT

Microorganisms are generally transported passively to the tooth surface by the flow of saliva; only a few oral bacterial species are actively motile (e.g., possess flagella), and these are mainly located subgingivally.

Long-range but relatively weak physicochemical forces are generated as a microorganism approaches the pellicle-coated surface. Microorganisms are negatively-charged because of the molecules on their cell surface,

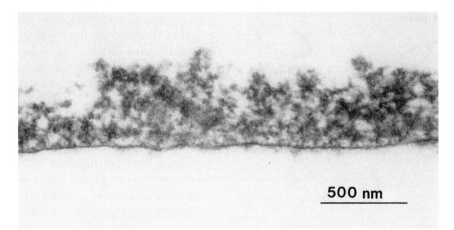

FIGURE 5.3 Transmission electron micrograph of the acquired pellicle on an enamel surface. (Reproduced with permission of Prof M Hannig.)

while many proteins present in the acquired pellicle also have a net negative charge. The Derjaguin and Landau and the Verwey and Overbeek (DLVO) theory has been used to describe the interaction between an inert particle (as a microorganism might be envisaged at large separation distances) and a substratum. This theory states that the total interactive energy, V_T, of two smooth particles is determined solely by the sum of the van der Waals attractive energy (V_A) and the usually repulsive, electrostatic energy (V_R). Particles in aqueous suspension and surfaces in contact with aqueous solutions can acquire a charge because of, for example, the preferential adsorption of ions from solution or the ionisation of certain groups attached to the particle or surface. The charge on a surface in solution is always exactly balanced by an equivalent number of counter ions; the size of this electrical double layer is inversely proportional to the ionic strength of the environment. As a particle approaches a surface, therefore, it experiences a weak van der Waals attraction induced by the fluctuating dipoles within the molecules of the two approaching surfaces. This attraction increases as the particle moves closer to the substratum. A repulsive force is encountered if the surfaces continue to approach each other, because of the overlap of the electrical double layers. Curves can be plotted to show the variation of the total interactive energy, V_T, of a particle and a surface with the separation distance, h (See Fig. 5.4). A net attraction can occur at two values of h; these are referred to as

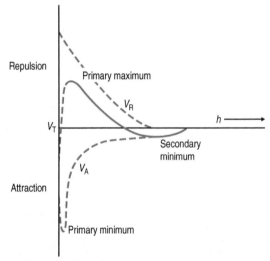

FIGURE 5.4 Diagram illustrating the DLVO theory. The total interactive energy, V_T, between a particle and a surface is shown with respect to the separation distance, h. The total interaction curve is obtained by the summation of an attraction curve, V_A, and a repulsion curve, V_R.

the primary minimum (h very small) and the secondary minimum (h = 10 to 20 nm) and are separated by a repulsive maximum. The primary minimum is not usually encountered, while the high ionic strength of saliva increases the likelihood that oral bacteria could be retained reversibly near a surface by a secondary minimum area of attraction (e.g., about 10 to 20 nm from the surface).

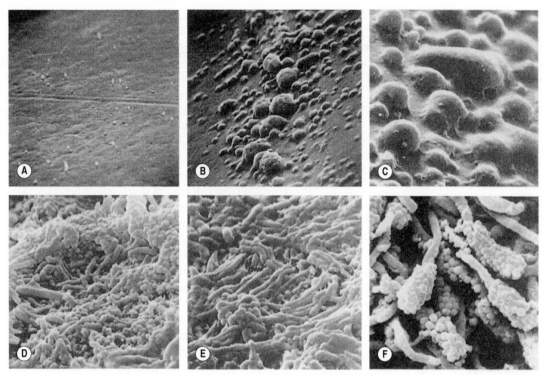

FIGURE 5.5 Development of dental plaque on a clean enamel surface. Coccal bacteria attach to the enamel pellicle as pioneer species (**A**) and multiply to form microcolonies (**B**), eventually resulting in confluent growth (biofilm formation) embedded in a matrix of extracellular polymers of bacterial and salivary origin (**C**). With time, the diversity of the microbiota increases, and rod and filament-shaped bacteria colonise (**D** and **E**). In the climax community, many unusual associations between different bacterial populations can be seen, including corn-cob formations (**F**). (Magnification approx. × 1150) (Published with permission of Dr A. Saxton.)

PIONEER MICROBIAL COLONISERS AND MORE PERMANENT ATTACHMENT (ADHESIN–RECEPTOR INTERACTIONS)

Within a short time, these weak physicochemical interactions may become stronger because of molecules (**adhesins**) on the microbial cell surface engaging in specific, short-range interactions with complementary **receptors** in the acquired pellicle. These interactions are highly specific, occur over short distances and make the attachment more permanent. For this to occur, water films must be removed from between the interacting surfaces. A major role of cell hydrophobicity and hydrophobic cell surface components is their dehydrating effect on this water film enabling the surfaces to get closer so that short-range interactions can occur. The specificity of these molecular interactions contributes to the often observed associations (**tropisms**) of certain microbes with a particular surface or habitat.

Irrespective of the type of tooth surface (enamel or cementum), the initial colonisers constitute a highly selected part of the oral microbiota. Within minutes, coccal bacteria appear on the surface (See Fig. 5.5, *A*), and these pioneer organisms are mainly streptococci, especially members of the mitis group of streptococci (e.g., *S. sanguinis, S. oralis* and *S. mitis* biovar 1) (Table 5.2). *Streptococcus sanguinis* and *S. oralis* produce an immunoglobulin A_1 (IgA_1) protease which may help them to survive and overcome a major component of the host defences during the early stages of biofilm formation. *Actinomyces* spp. are also commonly isolated after 2 hours, as are haemophili and *Neisseria*

TABLE 5.2   Proportions of cultivable bacteria in developing supragingival plaque

Bacterium	TIME OF PLAQUE DEVELOPMENT (h)		
	2	24	48
Streptococcus sanguinis	8	12	29
Streptococcus oralis	20	21	12
Mutans streptococci	3	2	4
Streptococcus salivarius	<1	<1	<1
Actinomyces naeslundii	6	7	5
Actinomyces odontolyticus	2	3	6
Haemophilus spp.	11	18	21
Capnocytophaga spp.	<1	<1	<1
Fusobacterium spp.	<1	<1	<1
Black-pigmented anaerobes	0	<0.01	<0.01

species, whereas obligately anaerobic species are detected only rarely at this stage and are usually in low numbers. Some aggregates of mixtures of cells may also attach.

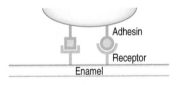

Many examples of the adhesion-receptor interactions have been characterised, and some are listed in Table 5.3. Bacteria are richly decorated with molecules that can interact with receptors in the pellicle or on the surface of already attached microbes. Some bacteria possess surface appendages (e.g., pili and fimbriae) that can penetrate mucus layers and the conditioning film; adhesins can be present along the length of these structures but, importantly, are also located on the tip. Adhesion often involves (bacterial) protein – (host) carbohydrate interactions, that is, lectin-like. There are a number of protein groups that can function as adhesins, and these include Antigen I/II, serine-rich repeat proteins, proteins binding glucan, collagen or immunoglobulins, etc. Among the carbohydrates that can act as receptors are glucose, galactose, sialic acid, fucose, N-acetyl glucosamine and N-acetyl galactosamine. Specific examples include: adhesins on *S. gordonii* that can bind to α-amylase, whereas *A. naeslundii* and *F. nucleatum* interact with statherin. *Streptococcus mutans*, *Porphyromonas gingivalis*, *Prevotella loescheii* and *Prevotella melaninogenica* adhere preferentially to surfaces coated with proline-rich peptides (PRPs), although different regions of the molecule bind to particular organisms. Colonisation by *S. sobrinus* is more dependent on sucrose-mediated mechanisms, including the interaction of glucans with receptors such as glucan-binding proteins. *Streptococcus sanguinis* can bind to terminal sialic acid residues in adsorbed salivary glycoproteins, whereas *S. oralis* expresses either a galactose-binding lectin or a lectin that interacts with a trisaccharide structure containing sialic acid, galactose and *N*-acetylgalactosamine. The large size of some bacterial cell wall proteins means that they may be involved in more than one function. For example, a protein of *S. gordonii* can interact both with salivary proteins and with *A. naeslundii* (coaggregation). Streptococci can use multiple adhesins to bind to saliva-coated surfaces; as an example, *S. sanguinis* can adhere via lectin-like, hydrophobic and/or specific protein (adhesin) interactions.

Actinomyces spp. have two antigenically and functionally distinct types of fimbriae; type 1 fimbriae mediate bacterial adherence to PRPs and to statherin (a protein-protein interaction), whereas type 2 fimbriae are associated with a lactose-sensitive mechanism (a lectin-like activity) involving the adherence of cells to already attached bacteria (**coadhesion**; see later in this section) or to buccal epithelial cells. Attempts are being made to interfere with bacterial attachment to prevent or reduce biofilm formation.

A critical factor in plaque formation concerns the site at which the specific interactions between

TABLE 5.3 Some examples of host-bacterial interactions involved in adhesion

Bacterium	Adhesin	Receptor
Streptococcus spp.	Antigen I/II	Salivary agglutinin
Streptococcus spp.	Lipoteichoic acid (LTA)	Blood group reactive glycoproteins
Mutans streptococci	Glucan binding protein	Glucan
Streptococcus parasanguinis	35 kDa lipoprotein	Fibrin, pellicle
Actinomyces naeslundii	Type 1 fimbriae	Proline-rich proteins
Porphyromonas gingivalis	150 kDa protein	Fibrinogen
Prevotella loescheii	70 kDa lectin	Galactose
Fusobacterium nucleatum	42 kDa protein	Coaggregation with *Porphyromonas gingivalis*

bacterial adhesins and host receptors take place. The host-derived receptors reside on molecules that are not only adsorbed to the tooth surface, but which are also freely accessible in solution in saliva. Some of these molecules are designed to aggregate bacteria in solution, thereby facilitating their removal from the mouth by swallowing. For plaque formation to proceed, however, it is implicit that not all bacteria are aggregated in saliva before they reach the tooth surface. A novel mechanism may function to overcome this problem. Although *A. naeslundii* could bind to acidic PRPs when the latter were bound to a surface, cells did not interact with these proteins in solution. It has been proposed that hidden molecular segments of PRPs become exposed only when the proteins are adsorbed to hydroxyapatite, as a result of conformational changes. Such hidden receptors for bacterial adhesins have been termed '**cryptitopes**'. In this way, a selective mechanism for facilitating natural plaque formation has evolved by which the host can promote the attachment of specific bacteria without compromising this process in the planktonic phase. Adhesins which recognise cryptitopes in surface-associated molecules would provide a strong selective advantage for any microorganism which colonises a mucosal or tooth surface. Another example of a cryptitope involving conformational change is the binding of members of the mitis group of streptococci to fibronectin when complexed to collagen, but not to fibronectin in solution. This might also be a mechanism enabling certain oral streptococci to colonise damaged

heart valves in infective endocarditis (see Chapter 11; Fig. 11.5).

A different type of cryptitope involves the recognition of galactosyl-binding lectins by oral bacteria. Epithelial cells and the acquired enamel pellicle have mucins with oligosaccharide side chains with a terminal sialic acid. Bacteria such as *A. naeslundii* synthesise neuraminidase which cleaves the sialic acid exposing the penultimate galactosyl sugar residue. Many oral bacteria possess galactosyl-binding lectins including *A. naeslundii, Leptotrichia buccalis, Fusobacterium nucleatum, Eikenella corrodens* and *P. intermedia*, and would benefit from the exposure of these cryptitopes. Similarly, the binding of *P. gingivalis* is greater to epithelial cells that have been mildly treated with trypsin. Some periodontal pathogens, including *P. gingivalis*, produce proteases with an arginine-x specificity (arg-gingipains) that may create appropriate cryptitopes for their colonisation.

Once attached, these pioneer populations start to divide and form microcolonies; these early colonisers synthesise extracellular polysaccharides, and salivary proteins and glycoproteins continue to be adsorbed (See Figures 5.5, B and C). The early streptococcal colonisers (mitis group of streptococci) possess a range of glycosidase activities that enable them to interact and use salivary glycoproteins as substrates (see Fig. 5.11 later). The fastest rates of multiplication occur during these early stages of biofilm formation; the mean doubling times of pure cultures of *S. mutans* and *A. naeslundii* were calculated to be 1.4 and 2.7 hours, respectively, in studies using rodents.

COAGGREGATION/COADHESION AND MICROBIAL SUCCESSION

Over time, the plaque microbiota becomes more diverse; there is a shift away from the initial preponderance of streptococci to a biofilm with increasing proportions of *Actinomyces* and other Gram-positive bacilli. Some organisms that were unable to colonise the pellicle-coated tooth surfaces are able to attach to already-adherent pioneer species by further adhesin–receptor interactions (coaggregation/coadhesion). In addition, the metabolism of the pioneer community alters the local environment and makes conditions more suited to the growth of some fastidious bacteria. Early colonisers are tolerant of a high redox potential; species such as *Neisseria* spp. can consume oxygen and produce carbon dioxide and more 'reduced' end products of metabolism. Gradually, conditions become more favourable for the growth of obligately anaerobic bacteria. Similarly, the metabolism of pioneer species produce end products of metabolism (e.g., peptides) and fermentation products (lactate, butyrate, acetate) that can be used by other organisms as primary nutrient sources (i.e., food chains develop; see later, Figs 5.12, 5.13 and 5.14). Thus, the composition of the plaque microbiota changes over time because of a series of complex interactions and becomes more diverse; the process is termed **microbial succession** (see Fig. 4.1).

Coaggregation or coadhesion (the term coadhesion is used by some to distinguish between the adhesive interaction of cells on a surface rather than those in suspension) is the cell-to-cell recognition of genetically distinct partner cell types, and is an important process in microbial succession and biofilm formation. Coaggregation occurs among most oral bacterial genera (see Fig. 5.6). Early plaque accumulation is facilitated by intrageneric coaggregation among streptococcal species and among *Actinomyces* spp., as well as by intergeneric coaggregation between streptococci and *Actinomyces*. The subsequent development of dental plaque will involve further intergeneric coaggregation between other genera and the primary colonisers.

Coaggregation often involves lectins; these proteins bind to the complementary carbohydrate-containing receptor on another cell. Thus, the lectin-mediated interaction between streptococci and *Actinomyces* can

be blocked by adding galactose or lactose, or by treating the receptor with a protease. Coaggregation can result in some unusual morphological formations, for example corn-cob structures (See Fig. 5.5, *F*). 'Corn-cobs' can be formed between streptococci and *Coryne-bacterium matruchotii*, and between *Eubacterium* and *Veillonella* species.

Fusobacteria have been found to coaggregate with the widest range of bacterial genera, although curiously, they do not coaggregate with each other. Early colonisers of plaque coaggregate extensively with *F. nucleatum*, whereas later colonisers such as *Selenomonas*, *Prevotella* or *Eubacterium* species do not coaggregate with early colonisers, but do coaggregate with *F. nucleatum*. It has been proposed that fusobacteria act as important 'bridges' between early and late colonising bacteria (see Fig. 5.6).

Coaggregation may also be an important mechanism in the functional organisation of microbial communities such as dental plaque. The persistence and survival of obligately anaerobic bacteria in an essentially aerobic habitat such as the mouth is enhanced if they are physically close to oxygen-consuming species such as *Neisseria* species; such interactions can be mediated by coaggregation, with fusobacteria facilitating the interaction of otherwise non-coaggregating species. The development of food chains, including those between streptococci and *Veillonella* species, might also be facilitated by coaggregation. Coaggregation could be a mechanism to increase the probability that species that need to interact and collaborate (to survive) will actually combine physically, especially during the earlier stages of biofilm development. Cell-cell signalling can occur between bacteria, such as streptococci and *Veillonella* species, to facilitate their involvement in a food chain (see later sections).

MATURATION OF THE BIOFILM AND MATRIX FORMATION

The microbial diversity of plaque biofilms increases over time because of successive waves of microbial succession and subsequent growth. The growth rate of individual bacteria within plaque slows as the biofilm matures, and the mean doubling times of 1 to 2 hours observed during the early stages of plaque formation rise to between 12 to 15 hours after several days of biofilm development. Confluent growth on the

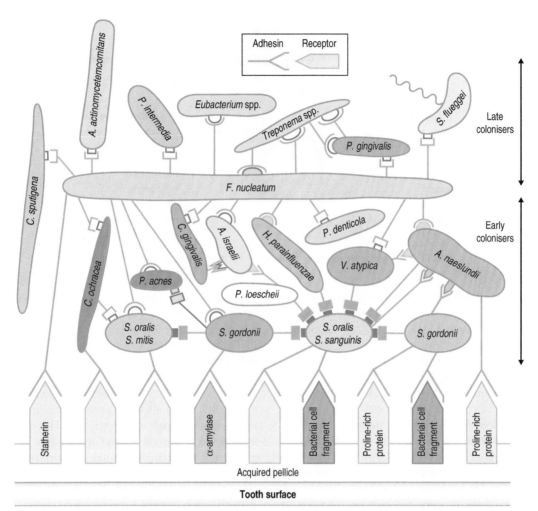

FIGURE 5.6 Schematic representation of the patterns of coaggregation (coadhesion) in human dental plaque. Early colonisers bind to receptors in the acquired pellicle; subsequently, other early and later colonisers bind to receptors on the surface of these already attached cells (coadhesion). Adhesins (symbols with stems) are cell components that are heat or protease sensitive; the receptor (complementary symbol) is insensitive to either treatment. Identical symbols do not imply identical molecules. The symbols with rectangular shapes represent lactose-inhibitable coaggregations. (Reproduced from Kolenbrander and London, J Bacteriol 1993 175:3247–3252; with permission from the American Society for Microbiology.)

tooth surface produces a biofilm with a 3-dimensional structure (See Fig. 5.5, *D* and *E*).

A key feature of the maturation of a biofilm is the development of an extracellular matrix of polymers; in dental plaque, the matrix includes soluble and insoluble glucans, fructans, proteins and extracellular deoxyribonucleic acid (eDNA). Glucans (see Fig. 4.11) are synthesised by glucosyltransferases; these enzymes can be secreted and adsorbed onto other bacteria or onto the tooth surface to form part of the

acquired pellicle, where they can remain functional and contribute further to matrix formation. In contrast, the fructans produced by fructosyltransferases (FTFs) are short-lived in plaque and act as extracellular nutrient storage compounds for use by other plaque bacteria (see Chapter 4). Recently, the importance of eDNA to the properties of the biofilm has become apparent. Extracellular DNA can be released from cells as a result of lysis, but in some situations it can also be actively secreted, for example, as a

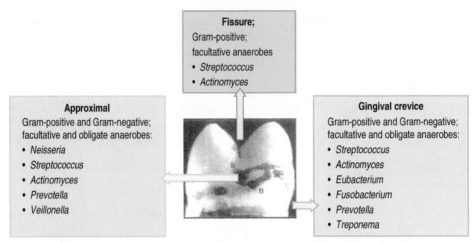

FIGURE 5.7 Predominant groups of bacteria found at distinct sites on the tooth surface.

consequence of cell-cell signalling (quorum sensing; see later), or via vesicles that bleb off the surface of Gram-negative bacteria (see Fig. 3.7, *B*). Enzymatic degradation of eDNA can weaken biofilm structure, and so it is believed that eDNA contributes to the structural integrity of the matrix as well as being involved in conventional gene transfer. Some bacteria produce DNases that can degrade eDNA, thereby generating nucleotides that can be used by organisms within the biofilm community.

A matrix is a common feature of all biofilms and is more than a chemical scaffold to maintain the structure of the biofilm. It makes a significant contribution to the structural integrity and general tolerance of biofilms to environmental factors (e.g., desiccation) and antimicrobial agents. The matrix can be biologically active and retain water, nutrients and enzymes within the biofilm. The chemistry of the matrix can also help exclude, or restrict, the penetration of other types of molecules including some charged antimicrobial agents.

As plaque matures, the microbiota becomes more diverse. A small sample of plaque may contain up to 100 distinct species, but the bacterial composition will vary at distinct anatomical sites because of the prevailing biological conditions (Fig. 5.7). Gradients continue to develop in factors that are critical to microbial growth so that sites close together may be vastly different in the concentration of essential nutrients and toxic products of metabolism, as well as in terms of pH and Eh, etc. These gradients are not necessarily linear; zones of quite different pH have been detected adjacent to each other in laboratory-generated plaque biofilms. Such **vertical and horizontal stratifications** will create local environmental heterogeneity resulting in a **mosaic of microhabitats or microenvironments**. Such heterogeneity can explain how organisms with apparently contradictory growth requirements in terms of nutritional, atmospheric or pH requirements are able to coexist in plaque at the same site. Each microhabitat potentially could support the growth of different populations and hence a distinct microbial community. Similarly, organisms residing in apparently the same general environment might be growing under quite dissimilar conditions and, therefore, exhibit a different phenotype. This is another reason why it is essential when studying plaque to take small samples from defined areas (see Chapter 4). The distribution of the main groups of microorganism at distinct sites on the tooth will be described later (see Fig. 5.7).

Multispecies biofilms create opportunities for numerous interactions among the constitutive species that are physically close to one another. These include examples of the conventional antagonistic and synergistic biochemical interactions, as well as gene transfer via plasmids and cell–cell signalling mediated by small diffusible molecules that enable similar bacteria to communicate with each other and coordinate their activities; these will be described later in this chapter.

Electron microscopy has been used extensively to view dental plaque, the structure of which appeared typically as compressed layers of diverse morphological types of cells that are densely packed together. However, contemporary studies now use FISH and confocal microscopy (see Chapter 4), and have demonstrated a more open biofilm architecture. Palisaded regions can be seen where filaments and cocci appear to be aligned in parallel at right angles to the enamel surface, while microcolonies, presumably of single cell populations, have also been observed. In addition, horizontal stratification has been described; examples of the ultrastructure of dental plaque are shown in Figures 5.8, 5.9 and 5.10. In mature plaque, organisms have been seen in direct contact with the enamel because of enzymatic attack on the pellicle. In the gingival crevice, plaque has a thin densely adherent layer on the root surface, with the bulk of the biofilm having a looser structure, especially where it comes into contact with the epithelial lining of the gingival crevice/periodontal pocket. *Synergistetes* spp. have been observed in the outer layer of subgingival biofilms, perhaps significantly, in close proximity to cells resembling neutrophils, implying that these organisms may play a direct role in host-biofilm interactions. Many bacterial associations have been observed subgingivally in these outer layers, in which cocci are arranged along the length of filamentous organisms, for example corn-cob, test tube brush or rosette formations (see Fig. 5.5, *F*); the identity of the bacteria involved in some of these associations has been confirmed using FISH. Corn-cob formations between streptococci and *Candida* have been observed in supragingival biofilms, whereas corn-cob and test-tube brush associations between *Tannerella*, *Prevotella* and *Synergistetes* organisms and between streptococci and fusiform bacteria have been detected in subgingival biofilms.

DETACHMENT FROM SURFACES

Shear forces can remove microorganisms from oral surfaces, but some bacteria can actively detach themselves from within the biofilm so as to be able to colonise elsewhere. *Streptococcus mutans* can synthesise an enzyme that cleaves proteins from its own cell surface and thereby detach itself from a mono-species biofilm. Similarly, a protease produced by *Prevotella loescheii* can

hydrolyse its own fimbrial-associated adhesin responsible for coaggregation with *S. oralis* as well as binding to fibrin. Bacteria may be able to sense adverse changes in environmental conditions, and these may act as cues to induce the genes involved in active detachment.

KEY POINTS

Adhesion of microorganisms to the conditioned tooth surface is a complex process involving, initially, weak long-range electrostatic attractive forces, followed by a variety of specific, strong and short-range molecular interactions between bacterial adhesins and receptors adsorbed to the surface (acquired pellicle). These latter processes together with the synthesis of extracellular polysaccharides from, for example, sucrose serve to increase the probability of permanent attachment. Extracellular polysaccharides contribute to the plaque matrix, along with proteins, lipids and eDNA. Pioneer species interact directly with the acquired pellicle whereas subsequent biofilm formation is dependent on intra- and intergeneric coadhesion between bacteria (involving lectin-mediated binding) and the subsequent growth of the attached microorganisms. Fusobacteria act as a bridge between early and late colonising bacteria. If conditions become unfavourable, some cells are able to actively detach, which creates an opportunity for them to colonise other sites.

CONSEQUENCES OF BIOFILM FORMATION
BIOCHEMICAL INTERACTIONS

The close proximity of microorganisms in biofilms facilitates a range of biochemical interactions which can be beneficial to one or more of the interacting populations, although others can be antagonistic (Table 5.4).

Synergistic interactions: Although competition for nutrients will be one of the primary ecological determinants in dictating the prevalence of a particular species in dental plaque, bacteria also have to collaborate to break down the complex host molecules that act as their primary substrates. Salivary proteins and glycoproteins are the major sources of nitrogen and carbon at healthy sites. Individual species of oral bacteria possess different but overlapping patterns of enzyme activity, so that the concerted action of several species is usually necessary for the complete degradation of host molecules (see Figs 5.11 and 5.14). For example, the growth of some organisms will be dependent on others for removing the terminal sugar

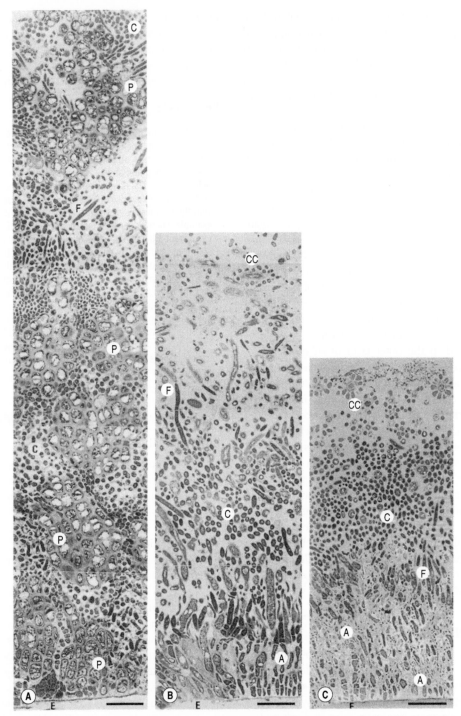

FIGURE 5.8 Ultrastructure of 2-week-old dental plaque from three individuals with different patterns of microbial colonisation (**A** to **C** labelling within the images). C, Gram-positive coccal bacteria; F, Gram-negative filamentous bacteria; CC, corn-cob formations; P, large, irregular-shaped bacteria. Bar, 5 μm. (Published with the permission of Professor B Nyvad, Professor O Fejerskov and Munksgaard.)

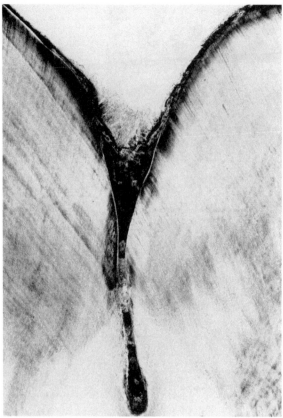

FIGURE 5.9 Dental plaque in a fissure on the occlusal surface of a molar. (Magnification approx. × 60.) (Published with permission of K. M. Pang.)

TABLE 5.4 Factors involved in beneficial and antagonistic microbial interactions in dental plaque

Beneficial (synergistic)	Antagonistic
Enzyme complementation	Bacteriocins
Food chains (food webs)	Hydrogen peroxide
Coadhesion	Organic acids
Cell-cell signalling	Low pH
Gene transfer	Nutrient competition
Environmental modification	Bacteriophage release

from the oligosaccharide side chain of the glycoprotein to expose a new sugar which they are able to utilise.

Microbial cooperation in the breakdown of host macromolecules has been noted when subgingival bacteria were grown on human serum (used to mimic GCF). Shifts in the microbial composition of the consortia were evident at different stages of glycoprotein breakdown. Initially, carbohydrate side-chains were removed by organisms with complementary glycosidase activities including, for example, *S. oralis, E. saburreum* and *Prevotella* spp. This was followed by the hydrolysis of the protein core by anaerobes (e.g., *P. intermedia, P. oralis, F. nucleatum*); some amino acid fermentation occurred and the remaining carbohydrate side-chains were metabolised leading to the emergence of *Veillonella* species. A final phase was characterised by progressive protein degradation and extensive amino acid fermentation; the predominant species included *Parvimonas micra* and *E. brachy*. Significantly, individual species grew only poorly in pure culture on serum. A consequence of these interactions is that different species avoid direct competition for individual nutrients, and hence are able to coexist.

Bacterial polymers are also targets for degradation. Extracellular polysaccharides synthesised by many plaque bacteria (see Table 4.8) can be metabolised by other organisms in the absence of exogenous (dietary) carbohydrates. The fructan of *S. salivarius* and other streptococci, and the glycogen-like polymer of *Neisseria*, are particularly labile, and only low levels of fructan can be detected in plaque *in vivo*. In addition, mutans streptococci, members of the mitis or salivarius groups of streptococci, *A. israelii, Capnocytophaga* spp., and *Fusobacterium* spp. possess exohydrolytic and/or endohydrolytic activity and metabolise streptococcal glucans.

An important nutritional interaction is when the products of metabolism of one organism (primary feeder) become the main source of nutrients for another (secondary feeder). For example, lactate produced from the metabolism of dietary carbohydrates by a range of other species, can be used by *Veillonella* spp. and converted to weaker acids. In this way, *Veillonella* spp. can reduce the cariogenic potential of other plaque bacteria; fewer carious lesions were obtained in rats inoculated with either *S. mutans* or *S. sanguinis* and *Veillonella* than in animals monoinfected

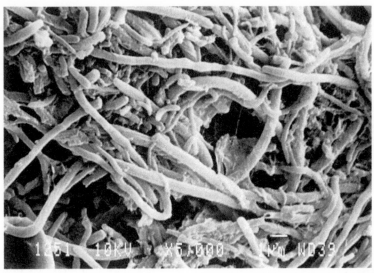

FIGURE 5.10 Scanning electron micrograph of subgingival plaque, showing rods, curved rods, filaments and spiral-shaped cells. (Magnification approx. × 5000.) (Published with permission of K. M. Pang.)

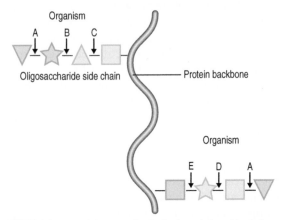

FIGURE 5.11 Bacterial cooperation in the degradation of host glyco-proteins (enzyme complementation). For example, organism A is able to cleave the terminal sugar of the oligosaccharide side-chain, which enables organism B or D to cleave the penultimate residue, etc.

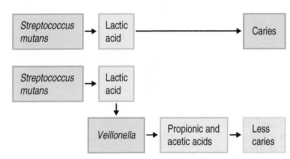

FIGURE 5.12 Establishment of a simple food-chain. Bacteria such as *Streptococcus mutans* produce lactate from fermentable sugars that can be metabolised to weaker acids by *Veillonella* species; in gnotobiotic animals, this food-chain can reduce the cariogenic potential of these streptococci.

with either of the streptococci (Fig. 5.12). Other bacteria (e.g., *Neisseria*, *Corynebacterium*, and *Eubacterium*) are also able to metabolise lactate. A range of other nutritional interactions between oral bacteria has been described (Fig. 5.13). A mutually beneficial interaction occurs between *S. sanguinis* and *Campylobacter rectus*; the anaerobe scavenges inhibitory oxygen, or possibly hydrogen peroxide produced by the streptococcus, whereas *S. sanguinis* provides

C. rectus with formate following the fermentation of glucose under carbohydrate-limiting conditions. *Campylobacter rectus* is also able to produce proto-haeme for the growth of black-pigmented anaerobes.

Numerous interbacterial nutritional interactions occur in plaque, with the growth of some species being dependent on the metabolism of other organisms. Indeed, our failed attempts to grow some species in pure culture are because of their dependence on the metabolism of other bacteria. The diversity of the plaque microbiota is caused, in part, by:

- the development of such food chains and food webs (Figs 5.12, 5.13 and 5.14), and to

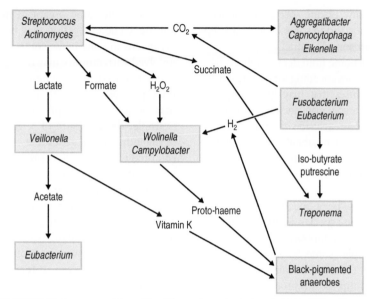

FIGURE 5.13 Some potential nutritional interactions (food chains) among plaque bacteria.

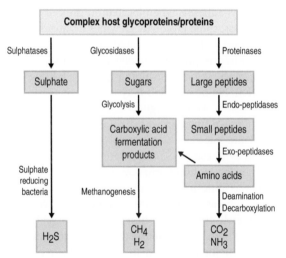

FIGURE 5.14 Illustration of the concerted and sequential breakdown of complex host substrates by communities of oral bacteria with complementary enzyme activities.

• the lack of a single nutrient limiting the growth of all bacterial species.

Antagonistic interactions: The production of antagonistic compounds (such as bacteriocins or bacteriocin-like substances) can give an organism a competitive advantage during colonisation and when interacting with other microbes (see Table 5.4). Bacteriocins are relatively high molecular weight proteins that can inhibit the growth of related bacteria whereas the producer strains are resistant to the action of the bacteriocins they produce. Bacteriocins are produced by most species of oral streptococci, and examples include mutacin by *S. mutans* and sanguicin by *S. sanguinis*; in contrast, *Actinomyces* species are not generally bacteriocinogenic. Although bacteriocins are usually limited in their spectrum of activity, many of the streptococcal bacteriocins are broad spectrum, inhibiting species belonging to Gram-positive (including *Actinomyces*) and Gram-negative genera.

Other inhibitory factors produced by plaque bacteria include organic acids, hydrogen peroxide, and enzymes. The production of hydrogen peroxide by members of the mitis group of streptococci has been proposed as a mechanism whereby the numbers of periodontal pathogens are reduced in plaque to levels at which they are incapable of initiating disease. The corollary of this, though, is that some periodontal pathogens (e.g., *A. actinomycetemcomitans*) produce factors inhibitory to oral streptococci, so that certain periodontal diseases (see Chapter 6) might result from an ecological imbalance between dynamically-interacting groups of bacteria. The low pH generated from carbohydrate metabolism is also inhibitory to many plaque species, particularly Gram-negative organisms and to some beneficial streptococci associated with sound enamel.

Studies of the metagenome from dental biofilms have shown the presence of genes encoding for bacteriophage. Phages are bacterial viruses that may lyse competing cells. The production of antagonistic factors will not necessarily lead to the complete exclusion of sensitive species as the presence of distinct microhabitats within a biofilm such as plaque enable bacteria to survive under conditions that would be incompatible to them in a homogeneous environment.

Antagonism will also be a mechanism whereby exogenous (allochthonous) species are prevented from colonising the oral cavity (colonisation resistance; see Chapter 4). For example, some *S. salivarius* strains produce an inhibitor (enocin or salivaricin) active against Lancefield Group A streptococci (such as *S. pyogenes*), which is an opportunistic pathogen. Bacteriocin-producing strains may prevent colonisation of the mouth by this pathogen in a manner similar to that proposed for streptococci in the pharynx. It has been claimed that *S. salivarius* is more frequently isolated from the throats of children who do not become colonised following exposure to Group A streptococci than from those who do become infected. In New Zealand, children can be deliberately implanted with bacteriocin-producing strains of *S. salivarius* to reduce infections by Group A streptococci; this process is termed **replacement therapy**. These, and other inhibitory bacteria such as lactobacilli and bifidobacteria from the dairy industry, are being considered for future use as oral **probiotics** (see Chapter 6). Probiotics are living bacteria that, when administered, deliver health benefits to the host. The regular intake of oral probiotics might alter colonisation by cariogenic bacteria, and there are claims that their use can reduce plaque formation and gingival inflammation, but more studies are needed. Thus, microbial interactions will play a major role in determining both the final composition and the pattern of development of the plaque microbiota.

IMPACT ON GENE EXPRESSION

Plaque maturation involves the growth of attached bacteria to produce a structurally and functionally organised biofilm. The phenotype of bacteria in a biofilm can differ markedly from that predicted from studies of the same organism in liquid (planktonic) culture. Gene expression may be altered when microorganisms initially make contact with a surface. Genes involved with motility may be repressed whereas other genes required for attachment, synthesis of extracellular polysaccharides or growth on new substrates may be induced or upregulated (see Table 5.1). For example, the exposure of *S. gordonii* to saliva results in the induction of genes that encode for adhesins that can bind to salivary glycoproteins and engage in coaggregation with *Actinomyces* species. Marked changes in protein profiles following attachment have been identified in *S. mutans* using a whole cell proteomic (protein analysis) approach. During the initial stages of biofilm formation by *S. mutans* (the first two hours following attachment), over 30 proteins were differentially expressed (most were upregulated but some were downregulated). There was an increase in the relative synthesis of enzymes involved in carbohydrate catabolism; these might be needed for energy generation, although these molecules are multifunctional and can also act as adhesins when located on the cell surface. In contrast, some glycolytic enzymes involved in acid production were downregulated in older (3 day) biofilms, whereas proteins involved in a range of biochemical functions, including protein folding and secretion, amino acid and fatty acid biosynthesis, and cell division, were upregulated. Novel proteins of as yet unknown function were expressed by biofilm but not planktonic cells. Genes involved with glucan and fructan synthesis in *S. mutans* are differentially regulated during biofilm formation. In laboratory models, there was little influence of surface growth on gene expression associated with exopolymer synthesis during early stages of biofilm formation (<48 hours), but *gtf* expression was markedly upregulated in older (7 day) biofilms whereas *ftf* activity was repressed. This was interpreted as an indirect effect of biofilm growth on gene expression, probably as a response to changes in local environmental conditions such as sugar concentration or pH as the biofilm matured, rather than because of initial attachment.

Subgingival bacteria also undertake substantial changes in gene expression during biofilm formation. *Porphyromonas gingivalis* differentially regulated nearly 20% of its genome during biofilm formation, with genes involved in adhesion upregulated during attachment. Later, there were increases in proteins associated with haemin transport and metabolism, which would be important for the growth of the organisms under nutrient-limited conditions. *Tannerella forsythia* also undergoes substantial adaptation during biofilm formation. Proteins associated with the outer membrane and with transport systems were upregulated, whereas the butyrate pathway was downregulated. Proteins involved with the oxidative stress response were also upregulated, and biofilm cells were 10- to 20-fold more tolerant of oxidative stress.

The situation can become complicated in multispecies consortia. In mixed culture biofilms of subgingival bacteria, the inclusion of *A. actinomycetemcomitans* resulted in an increase in proteins expressed by *P. intermedia* but substantial downregulation of proteins expressed by *C. rectus*, *S. anginosus* and *P. gingivalis*. Thus, the interactions among community members, and the response to local environmental conditions, will have profound consequences for the host.

CELL–CELL SIGNALLING

The close proximity of cells with each other in biofilms provides ideal conditions for cell-cell interactions. In addition to more conventional biochemical interactions, there is evidence from microbes in a number of habitats of cell density-dependent growth (quorum sensing), whereby individual cells are able to communicate with, and respond to, neighbouring cells by means of small, diffusible, effector molecules. These include acyl-homoserine lactones produced by Gram-negative bacteria and small peptides secreted by Gram-positive cells. The peptides are generally detected via two-component signal transduction systems. These cell–cell signalling strategies enable cells to sense and adapt to various environmental stresses, and regulate (and coordinate) the expression of genes that influence the ability of pathogens to cause disease.

Quorum sensing is mediated by a competence-stimulating peptide (CSP) in *S. mutans*. This peptide also induces genetic competence in *S. mutans* (i.e., the ability to take up DNA) so that the transformation efficiency of biofilm-grown *S. mutans* was 10- to 600-fold greater than for planktonic cells. Lysed cells in biofilms such as plaque could act as donors of DNA, thereby increasing the opportunity for horizontal gene transfer in oral biofilms. CSP is also directly involved

in biofilm formation since mutants in some of the genes involved in the CSP signalling system produce defective biofilms. This quorum sensing system also functions to regulate acid tolerance in *S. mutans* in biofilms. When cells are exposed to an acid shock, CSP is released which can initiate a coordinated protective biochemical response by more distant *S. mutans* cells, enabling them to survive a potentially lethal stress.

CSPs are specific for cells of the same species, but other communication systems may function between different genera. Surveys of Gram-negative periodontal bacteria suggest that these organisms do not possess the acyl-homoserine lactone signalling molecules detected in environmental bacteria. LuxS genes encode for autoinducer-2 (AI-2), and these have been detected in several genera of oral Gram-positive and Gram-negative bacteria, implying that AI-2 may be a universal language for interspecies communication in plaque bacteria. Several periodontal bacteria, including *F. nucleatum*, *P. intermedia*, *P. gingivalis* and *A. actinomycetemcomitans*, secrete a signal related to AI-2. AI-2 is involved in leukotoxin production and iron acquisition in *A. actinomycetemcomitans* and protease (arg-gingipain and lys-gingipain) and haemagglutinin activities in *P. gingivalis*. *Streptococcus gordonii* and *P. gingivalis* can respond to LuxS signals from each other (i.e., they can sense heterologous signals), but the pattern of genes that are regulated by LuxS differs in each species. In LuxS mutants, genes associated with carbohydrate metabolism such as glucosyltransferase and fructosidase were downregulated in the *Streptococcus* whereas genes relating to haemin acquisition and an arginine-specific protease were upregulated in *P. gingivalis*. These findings have led to a quest to understand and identify more of these communication networks. A possible practical outcome from such studies might be the development of synthetic analogues of specific signalling molecules that could be used as a novel therapeutic approach to manipulate the properties of oral biofilms.

Emerging evidence also suggests that members of the resident microbiota can also engage in 'cross-talk' with the host, for example, by downregulating the potential induction of proinflammatory cytokines, and upregulating beneficial pathways, thereby actively promoting a harmonious relationship between the normal microbiota and the host (see Chapter 4).

GENE TRANSFER

The close proximity of cells in biofilms provides ideal conditions for horizontal gene transfer. As described earlier, signalling molecules such as competence-stimulating peptide (CSP) markedly increase the ability of recipient cells to take up DNA. Extracellular DNA (eDNA) is present in biofilms, and CSPs increase the likelihood of it being take up by recipient cells. eDNA can be released during cell lysis, but it is also linked to the production of hydrogen peroxide by some oral streptococci. eDNA can also be found in vesicles released from the cell surface, especially by Gram-negative bacteria. Bacteriophage capable of delivering and integrating DNA into oral bacteria are also present in dental biofilms. In addition, the transfer of conjugative transposons encoding tetracycline resistance between streptococci has been demonstrated in laboratory biofilm models.

Evidence that horizontal gene transfer does occur in the mouth has come from the discovery that both resident (*S. mitis, S. oralis*) and pathogenic (*S. pneumoniae*) bacteria isolated from the nasopharyngeal area possess genes conferring penicillin resistance that display a common mosaic structure. Similar evidence suggests sharing of genes encoding penicillin-binding proteins among resident oral and pathogenic *Neisseria* species. These findings suggest that plaque can function as a genotypic reservoir by harbouring transferable mobile elements and genes. Such genetic exchange could have a wide clinical significance given the number of overtly pathogenic bacteria that can appear transiently in the mouth.

ANTIMICROBIAL TOLERANCE

Oral bacteria growing as a biofilm such as dental plaque display a markedly reduced sensitivity to antibiotics and antimicrobial agents (Table 5.5; see Fig. 5.15), including those used in toothpastes and mouthwashes. As discussed earlier, this is not genetic resistance, as the cells display normal sensitivity to the antimicrobial agent if the biofilm is dispersed; therefore, it is referred to a phenotypic tolerance. For example, the biofilm inhibitory concentration of chlorhexidine and amine fluoride was 300 and 75 times greater, respectively, when *S. sobrinus* was grown as a biofilm compared with the minimum bactericidal

TABLE 5.5   Increase in tolerance to antimicrobial agents when oral bacteria are grown as a biofilm

Bacterium	Antimicrobial agent	Biofilm effect*
Streptococcus sanguinis	Chlorhexidine	$10–50 \times$ MIC[†]
Streptococcus sobrinus	Amine fluoride	$75 \times$ MBC[‡]
	Chlorhexidine	$300 \times$ MBC
Porphyromonas gingivalis	Metronidazole	$2–8 \times$ MBC
	Doxycycline	$4–64 \times$ MBC
	Amoxicillin	$2–4 \times$ MBC

*Biofilm effect, change in sensitivity of cells growing as a biofilm compared to when cells were grown in liquid (planktonic) culture.
[†]MIC, minimum inhibitory concentration of planktonic cells.
[‡]MBC, minimum bactericidal concentration of planktonic cells.

concentration of planktonic cells. Similarly, antibiotics such as amoxicillin and doxycycline had no effect on the viability of biofilms of *S. sanguinis* when used at MIC levels, and laboratory biofilms of *P. gingivalis* displayed increased tolerance to doxycycline and metronidazole. Complete elimination of biofilms sometimes required exposure to levels that were 500-fold greater than the MIC for a particular antibiotic, although *S. sanguinis* biofilms were killed following exposure to 10 to 50 times the MIC of chlorhexidine.

The age of the biofilm can affect the sensitivity of cells to an antimicrobial agent. Older biofilms of *S. sanguinis* were less susceptible to chlorhexidine than younger biofilms; the biofilm killing concentration for the former being 200 μg/ml compared with 50 μg/ml for the latter. Similarly, being part of a microbial community can influence the sensitivity of cells to an antibiotic; susceptible organisms can appear 'resistant' if neighbouring cells secrete a neutralising or drug-degrading enzyme. Bacteria in subgingival plaque can produce sufficient β-lactamase to inactivate penicillin delivered to that site during therapy.

The mechanisms that cause the increased tolerance of biofilm cells to antimicrobial agents include:

(a) limited penetration (diffusion-reaction theory) (Fig. 5.15),
(b) inactivation (e.g., by neutralising enzymes),
(c) quenching,

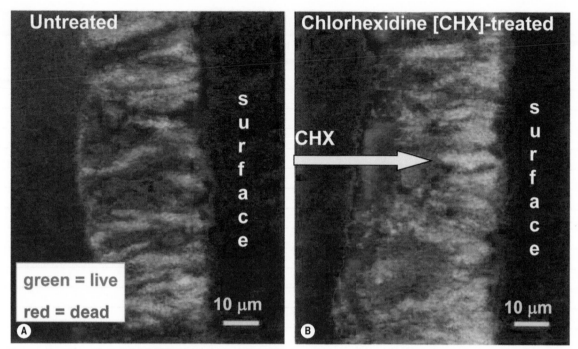

FIGURE 5.15 Penetration of chlorhexidine (CHX) into a dental plaque biofilm; an untreated biofilm is shown in (**A**), and the treated biofilm is shown in (**B**). The biofilm was visualised with a live/dead stain, in which viable bacteria stain green and dead cells are red. The chlorhexidine has an antimicrobial effect in the outermost layers of dental plaque, but failed to kill cells deeper in the biofilm. (Reproduced with permission of Dr. E. Zaura-Arite.)

(d) unfavourable environmental conditions for activity,

(e) slow microbial growth rates, and

(d) expression of a novel microbial phenotype (see Table 5.1).

KEY POINTS

A biofilm lifestyle has a direct and indirect impact on gene expression by oral bacteria, with many biofilm-specific genes being expressed. Cells in biofilms also display a decreased sensitivity to antimicrobial agents. Microorganisms in biofilms are in close proximity with one another which facilitates a range of biochemical (antagonistic and synergistic) interactions, as well as opportunities for gene transfer. In addition, attached cells can communicate with one another, and coordinate gene expression, via the production of small diffusible signaling molecules, such as competence-stimulating peptide by *S. mutans* and autoinducer-2 by a range of oral species. The final outcome is the development of spatially and functionally organised multispecies biofilms.

BACTERIAL COMPOSITION OF THE CLIMAX COMMUNITY OF DENTAL PLAQUE FROM DIFFERENT SITES

Environmental conditions on a tooth are not uniform. Differences exist in the prevalent nutrients, degree of protection from oral removal forces and in other biological and chemical factors that influence the growth of the resident microbiota. These differences are reflected in the composition of the microbial community, particularly at sites so obviously distinct as the gingival crevice, approximal regions, smooth surfaces, and pits and fissures. The predominant bacterial genera at these sites are shown in Figure 5.7, and a more detailed description of the microbiota at each site is given below. The application of culture-independent molecular techniques has increased our knowledge of the diversity of the microbiota from dental biofilms, and many new species are being described (see Chapters 3 and 4).

TABLE 5.6 The predominant cultivable microbiota of 10 occlusal fissures in adults			
Bacterium	Median percentage of total cultivable microbiota	Range (%)	Percentage isolation frequency
Streptococcus	45	8–86	100
Staphylococcus	9	0–23	80
Actinomyces	18	0–46	80
Propionibacterium	1	0–8	50
Eubacterium	0	0–27	10
Lactobacillus	0	0–29	20
Veillonella	3	0–44	60
Individual species:			
Mutans streptococci	25	0–86	70
Streptococcus mitis-group	1	0–15	50
Streptococcus anginosus-group	0	0–3	10
Actinomyces naeslundii	3	0–44	70
Lactobacillus casei	0	0–10	10
Lactobacillus plantarum	0	0–29	10

FISSURE PLAQUE

The microbiology of fissure plaque has been determined using either artificial fissures implanted in occlusal surfaces of preexisting restorations, or by sampling natural fissures. The cultivable microbiota is mainly Gram-positive and is dominated by streptococci, especially extracellular polysaccharide-producing species. In one study, no obligately anaerobic Gram-negative rods were found, although others have recovered anaerobes in low numbers such as *Veillonella* and *Propionibacterium* species (Table 5.6). Aerobic and facultatively anaerobic Gram-negative species, such as *Neisseria* spp. and *Haemophilus parainfluenzae*, have also been isolated on occasions. A striking feature of the microbiota is the wide range of numbers and types of bacteria in the different fissures. In one study, the total anaerobic microbiota ranged from 1×10^6 to 33×10^6 colony-forming units (CFU) per fissure. Saliva has a major influence on the biological properties of fissures, and diet may also be a significant factor because food can become impacted. The simpler community found in fissures compared with other enamel surfaces probably reflects a more severe environment. The distribution of bacteria within a fissure has not

been studied in detail, although it has been claimed that lactobacilli and mutans streptococci preferentially inhabit the lower depths of a fissure. It is clear from Figure 5.9 that environmental conditions at the base of the fissure will be very different in terms of nutrient availability, pH, and buffering effects of saliva than areas nearer the plaque surface.

APPROXIMAL PLAQUE

Streptococci are present in high numbers, but approximal sites are frequently dominated by Gram-positive rods, particularly *Actinomyces* species such as *A. naeslundii* and *A. israelii* (Table 5.7). The site has a lower redox potential than fissures, resulting in a higher recovery of obligately anaerobic organisms, although spirochaetes are not usually found.

The recovery and proportions of different groups of bacteria varies around the contact area. The isolation frequency of *S. mutans* and *S. sobrinus* was higher at subsites from below the contact area, and this is also the most caries-prone site. Similarly, *A. naeslundii* and *A. odontolyticus* were found more commonly below the contact area, whereas *Neisseria*, *S. sanguinis* and *S. mitis* biovar 1 were recovered more frequently at subsites

TABLE 5.7 **The predominant cultivable microbiota of approximal plaque**

Bacterium	Mean percentage of total cultivable microbiota	Range (%)	Percentage isolation frequency
Streptococcus	23	0.4–70	100
Gram-positive rods (predominantly *Actinomyces*)	42	4–81	100
Gram-negative rods (predominantly *Prevotella*)	8	0–66	93
Neisseria	2	0–44	76
Veillonella	13	0–59	93
Fusobacterium	0.4	0–5	55
Lactobacillus	0.5	0–2	24
Rothia	0.4	0–6	36
Some individual species:			
Mutans streptococci	2	0–23	66
Streptococcus sanguinis	6	0–64	86
Streptococcus salivarius	1	0–7	54
Streptococcus anginosus-group	0.5	0–33	45
Actinomyces israelii	17	0–78	72
Actinomyces naeslundii	19	0–74	97

away from, and to the side of, the contact area. Such variations again emphasise the need for accurate sampling of discrete sites when attempting to correlate the composition of plaque with disease.

GINGIVAL CREVICE PLAQUE

An obviously distinct ecological climate is found in the gingival crevice. This is reflected in the higher species diversity of the bacterial community at this site (Fig. 5.10) although the total numbers of cultivable bacteria can be low (10^3 to 10^6 CFU/crevice). Obligately anaerobic bacteria are cultured in high numbers from this site, many of which are Gram-negative or are *Eubacterium*-like (see Table 5.8 and Fig. 3.6), and spirochaetes and anaerobic streptococci are isolated almost exclusively from subgingival biofilms. The ecology of the crevice is influenced by the anatomy of the site and the flow and properties of gingival crevicular fluid (GCF; Chapter 2). Most of the organisms that inhabit this site are asaccharolytic and proteolytic, and derive their energy from the hydrolysis of host proteins and peptides and from the catabolism of

amino acids. In disease the gingival crevice enlarges to become a periodontal pocket (see Fig. 2.1), and the flow of GCF increases. The diversity of the microbiota increases still further in disease and will be described in more detail in Chapter 6.

Among the genera and species associated with the healthy gingival crevice are members of the mitis and anginosus groups of streptococci; in addition, Gram-positive rods such as *Actinomyces* spp. (*A. odontolyticus, A. naeslundii, A. georgiae*) and *Rothia dentocariosa* are also found. The most commonly isolated black-pigmented anaerobe in the healthy gingival crevice is *Prevotella melaninogenica* whereas *P. nigrescens* has also been recovered on occasions. Fusobacteria are among the commonest cultivable anaerobes found in the healthy gingival crevice, and capnophilic species such as *Capnocytophaga ochracea* can be isolated.

Molecular studies using culture-independent approaches (e.g., 16S rRNA gene amplification, FISH; Chapter 3) have shown that the subgingival microbiota is extremely diverse, even in health. Around 40% of the amplified clones represented novel phylotypes.

TABLE 5.8 The predominant cultivable microbiota of the healthy gingival crevice*

Bacterium	Mean percentage of total cultivable microbiota	Range (%)	Isolation frequency (%)
Gram-positive facultatively anaerobic cocci (predominantly *Streptococcus*)	40	2–73	100
Gram-positive obligately anaerobic cocci	1	0–6	14
Gram-positive facultatively anaerobic rods (predominantly *Actinomyces*)	35	10–63	100
Gram-positive obligately anaerobic rods	10	0–37	86
Gram-negative facultatively anaerobic cocci (predominantly *Neisseria*)	0.3	0–2	14
Gram-negative obligately anaerobic cocci (predominantly *Veillonella*)	2	0–5	57
Gram-negative facultatively anaerobic rods	ND	ND	ND
Gram-negative obligately anaerobic rods	13	8–20	100

*Samples were taken from the gingival crevice of seven adult humans.
ND, Not detected.

Human oral TM7 bacteria, of which no oral examples have been grown in pure culture, were detected frequently in samples and made up around 1% of the total bacteria in healthy subgingival sites (see Fig. 5.16). A number of spirochaetes have been detected, including *Treponema vincentii, T. denticola, T. maltophilum* and *T. lecithinolyticum*, as well as members of the genera *Selenomonas, Prevotella, Capnocytophaga* and *Campylobacter*.

KEY POINTS

The microbial composition of biofilms on teeth varies at distinct surfaces because of differences in the local environment.

Fissures are influenced by the properties of saliva, and the biofilms are dominated by streptococci; these bacteria have a saccharolytic style of metabolism.

The gingival crevice supports the growth of fastidious, obligately anaerobic bacteria, many of which are Gram-negative and proteolytic. GCF has a major influence on the biology of this site.

DENTURE PLAQUE

The microbiota of denture plaque from healthy sites (i.e., with no sign of denture stomatitis, Chapter 8) is highly variable as can be deduced from the wide ranges in viable counts obtained for individual bacteria as

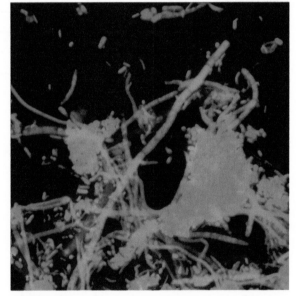

FIGURE 5.16 Unculturable bacteria belonging to the TM7 group (blue) in subgingival dental plaque. (Reproduced from Ouverney et al, Appl Environ Microbiol 2003 69:6294-6298; with permission from the American Society for Microbiology.)

illustrated in Table 5.9. Differences also occur between the fitting and the exposed surfaces of the denture. In the relatively stagnant area on the denture-fitting surface, plaque tends to be more acidogenic, thereby favouring streptococci (especially mutans streptococci)

TABLE 5.9 **The predominant cultivable microbiota of denture plaque**			
Microorganism	**Percentage viable count**		**Percentage isolation frequency**
	Median	Range	
Streptococcus	41	0–81	88
Mutans streptococci	<1	0–48	50
S. mitis group	2	0–30	75
S. anginosus group	2	0–51	63
S. salivarius group	0	0–41	38
Staphylococcus	8	1–13	100
S. aureus	6	0–13	88
S. epidermidis	0	0–7	13
Gram-positive rods	33	1–74	100
Actinomyces	21	0–54	88
A. israelii	3	0–47	63
A. naeslundii	3	0–48	63
A. odontolyticus	1	0–17	63
Lactobacillus	0	0–48	25
Propionibacterium	<1	0–5	50
Veillonella	8	3–20	100
Gram-negative rods	0	0–6	38
Yeasts	0.002	0–0.5	63

and sometimes *Candida* species. In edentulous subjects, dentures become the primary habitat for mutans streptococci and members of the mitis group of streptococci. Denture plaque can harbour obligate anaerobes including *A. israelii* and low proportions of Gram-negative rods. *Staphylococcus aureus* can be isolated from denture plaque, and this species is also found commonly in the mucosa of patients with denture stomatitis (see Chapter 8).

Culture-independent molecular techniques have detected periodontal pathogens such as *P. gingivalis, T. forsythia* and *A. actinomycetemcomitans* in the biofilms that develop on dentures in edentulous patients. High numbers of *Actinomyces* spp. and *Capnocytophaga* have also been detected.

DENTAL PLAQUE FROM ANIMALS

There is interest in the microbial composition of dental plaque from animals for two main reasons: (a) to study the influence of widely different diets and lifestyles on the microbiota, and (b) to determine the similarity between the microbiota of an animal with that of humans to ascertain their relevance as a model of human oral disease. At the genus level, the plaque microbiota is similar among animals representing such diverse dietary groups as insectivores, herbivores and carnivores. This is similar to recent data in humans which indicated that diet (omnivore, vegetarian or vegan) had no substantial effect on the oral microbiota. This emphasises the significance of endogenous nutrients in maintaining the stability and diversity of the resident microbiota.

CALCULUS

Calculus or tartar are the terms used to describe calcified dental plaque. Calculus consists of intra- and extracellular deposits of mineral, including apatite, brushite and whitlockite, as well as protein and carbohydrate. Mineral growth can occur around any bacteria; areas of mineral growth can then coalesce to form calculus which may become covered by an unmineralised layer of bacteria. Calculus occurs both supragingivally (especially near the salivary ducts) and subgingivally, where it may act as an additional retentive area for biofilm accumulation, thereby increasing the likelihood of gingivitis and other forms of periodontal disease. Calculus can be porous, leading to the retention of bacterial antigens and the stimulation of bone resorption by toxins from periodontal pathogens. Over 80% of adults have calculus, and its prevalence increases with age. An elevated calcium ion concentration in saliva may predispose some individuals to be high calculus formers. Once formed, huge removal forces are required to detach calculus; this removal takes up a disproportionate amount of clinical time during routine visits by patients to the dentist. Consequently, a number of dental products are now formulated to restrict calculus formation. These products contain pyrophosphates, zinc salts or polyphosphonates to inhibit mineralisation by slowing crystal growth and reducing coalescence.

DENTAL PLAQUE AS A MICROBIAL COMMUNITY

Oral bacteria do not behave randomly during the formation of dental plaque. Plaque forms in an organised manner via physicochemical and specific intermolecular, adhesin-receptor interactions, followed later by interbacterial coadhesion, metabolic interactions and cell–cell communication (see previous Sections). These interactions produce a spectrum of ecological niches (metabolic functions; Chapter 1), that offer a number of distinct benefits for the component microorganisms enabling the survival and growth of fastidious species by:

- efficient nutrient and energy cycling via cross-feeding and food webs.
- the synergistic catabolism of complex host macromolecules so that substrates can be utilised that would be recalcitrant to degradation by individual species,
- modulation of local environmental conditions (pH, oxygen tension, redox potential). For example, this enables the growth of (a) obligate anaerobes in an overtly aerobic habitat, and (b) pH-sensitive bacteria during periods of low pH, and
- increased protection from the host defences, antimicrobial agents, and from environmental stresses.

Great metabolic diversity exists within the plaque microbiota, ranging from organisms that can catalyse the initial splitting of complex host polymers into smaller units, to those such as sulphate-reducing bacteria and methanogens that gain energy from the utilisation of simple end products of metabolism (Fig. 5.14). The presence of these organisms in plaque confirms that this biofilm acts as a true microbial community because it is capable of fully exploiting the total energetic potential of the available nutrients. In such a microbial community, the metabolic efficiency of the whole is greater than that of the sum of the individual species since substrate use involves both the concerted and sequential catabolism of these complex molecules. Growth of such a community as a biofilm confers additional benefits since cells are protected from the host defences, antimicrobial agents and from other hostile factors; for example, a sensitive

organism can be protected by neighbouring cells expressing enzymes such as β-lactamase, IgA-protease or catalase that can inactivate or neutralise inhibitors or antimicrobial agents. In addition, the closely coupled physical and metabolic interactions leave few niches unfilled thereby reducing the likelihood of colonisation by exogenous microbes, and contributing to the natural microbial stability of the microbiota of plaque (microbial homeostasis; see next section).

For some groups of interacting consortia of organisms, the community lifestyle also increases their pathogenic potential (**pathogenic synergism**; see Fig. 6.18). Groups of weakly pathogenic organisms are able to cause disease that would be unable to do so in pure culture; examples include most periodontal diseases (Chapter 6) as well as abscesses (Chapter 7). In these polymicrobial infections, organisms that are not involved directly in tissue destruction can play vital roles in the disease process. Some organisms can support those with a more obvious pathogenic role by, for example, providing protection from host defences (e.g., by the production of IgA proteases), modifying the local environment (e.g., consuming oxygen and lowering the redox potential), providing key nutrients (e.g., via food chains or by contributing to the catabolism of complex host molecules), and by inactivating inhibitors (e.g., β-lactamase production to neutralise penicillins), and have been termed **accessory pathogens**.

An overview of some of the potential interactions in a microbial community such as dental plaque is shown in Figure 5.17.

KEY POINTS

> The overall benefits of a microbial community lifestyle to the component species are an increased:
> - Habitat range,
> - Ability to use complex host substrates,
> - Metabolic efficiency,
> - Protection from host defences and environmental stresses, and
> - Pathogenic potential.

MICROBIAL HOMEOSTASIS IN DENTAL PLAQUE

Despite its microbial diversity, the composition of dental plaque at any site is characterised by a remarkable

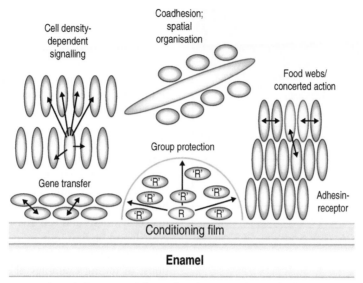

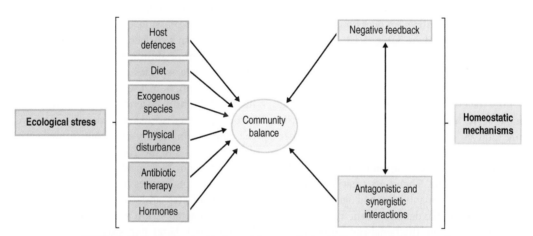

FIGURE 5.17 Schematic representation of the types of interaction that occur in a microbial community, such as dental plaque, growing as a biofilm. R, resistant organism to an antimicrobial agent; 'R', sensitive cell that is protected by the activity of its resistant neighbour.

FIGURE 5.18 Factors involved in the maintenance of microbial homeostasis in the mouth.

degree of stability or balance among the component species. This stability is maintained despite the host defences and the regular exposure of the plaque community to a variety of modest environmental stresses. These stresses include diet, the regular challenge by exogenous species, the use of dentifrices and mouthwashes containing antimicrobial agents and changes in saliva flow and hormone levels (Fig. 5.18). The ability to maintain community stability in a variable environment has been termed **microbial homeostasis**. This

stability stems not from any metabolic indifference among the components of the microbiota but results rather from a balance of dynamic microbial interactions, including both synergism and antagonism (see earlier sections). When the environment is perturbed, self-regulatory mechanisms (homeostatic reactions) come into force to restore the original balance. An essential component of such mechanisms is negative feedback, whereby a change in one or more organisms results in a response by others to oppose or neutralise

TABLE 5.10 **Factors responsible for the breakdown of microbial homeostasis in dental plaque**	
Immunological factors	**Non-immunological factors**
sIgA-deficiency	Xerostomia
Neutrophil dysfunction	Antibiotics
Chemotherapy-induced myelosuppression	Dietary carbohydrates/low pH
Infection-induced myelosuppression (e.g., AIDS)	Increased GCF flow
	Oral contraceptives

AIDS, Acquired immune deficiency syndrome; *GCF*, gingival crevicular fluid; *sIgA*, secretory immunoglobulin A.

such a change. There is a tendency for homeostasis to be greater in microbial communities with a higher species diversity.

Despite the microbial diversity of dental plaque, homeostasis does break down on occasions. The main causes for this are listed in Table 5.10 and can be divided into either:

- deficiencies in the immune response, or
- other (non-immune) factors.

The host defences, together with the resident microbiota, serve to maintain microbial homeostasis in plaque (and on other oral surfaces), and together they act synergistically to prevent colonisation by exogenous species and the invasion of host tissues by opportunistic pathogens. Therefore, treatment strategies, including the use of antimicrobial agents, should avoid causing irreversible damage to the resident oral microbiota so as to retain the beneficial properties of dental plaque and the microbiota of other oral sites.

The remainder of this book will be devoted to describing the consequences of the breakdown of microbial homeostasis in the mouth and the aetiology of the major oral diseases.

CHAPTER SUMMARY

Dental plaque is a microbial biofilm with a high species diversity found on the tooth surface, embedded in polymers of salivary and bacterial origin. The development of dental plaque is an example of autogenic succession where microbial factors influence the pattern of the development of the microbiota.

The formation of dental plaque can be divided arbitrarily into a number of distinct stages. These include the adsorption of host and bacterial molecules to form the acquired pellicle, passive transport of bacteria to the pellicle-coated tooth surface, a weak and reversible phase of adherence involving van der Waals attractive forces and electrostatic repulsion, a more permanent phase of attachment involving specific, short range and strong intermolecular interactions between bacterial adhesins and host receptors, coadhesion of bacteria to already attached organisms, matrix synthesis and cell division leading to confluent growth and biofilm formation. The close proximity of different bacterial species results in extensive interactions, including examples of synergism and antagonism. Some organisms produce signalling molecules enabling cells to communicate with one another and coordinate their activity. The properties of bacteria in a biofilm are different to those of planktonically grown cells. Gene expression can be altered when microorganisms are on a surface, whereas cells in biofilms are more tolerant of antimicrobial agents.

The pioneer species that form the plaque biofilm include members of the mitis group of streptococci, haemophili and *Neisseria* species; many of the streptococci produce an IgA protease. The composition of the climax community of plaque shows variations at different sites on the tooth surface reflecting differences in their biological properties. The microbial community of fissures is less diverse than that of approximal sites and the gingival crevice. Obligate anaerobic bacteria form a significant part of the microbiota at these latter two sites, so special precautions are necessary when sampling and processing plaque from these areas to maintain the viability of the resident microorganisms.

The balance of the microbiota at a site remains reasonably stable unless severely perturbed by an environmental stress. Such a stable microbiota is also able to prevent exogenous species from colonising. This stability (termed microbial homeostasis) is due, in part, to a dynamic balance of synergistic (e.g., coadhesion, the development of food chains, and metabolic cooperation) and antagonistic (e.g., production of bacteriocins, hydrogen peroxide, organic acids and a low pH) microbial interactions. Disease can occur when homeostasis breaks down.

The spatial heterogeneity within a biofilm such as plaque can lead to the coexistence of species that would be incompatible with one another in a homogeneous environment. Dental plaque functions as a true microbial community; the interactions of the component species result in a metabolic efficiency and diversity that is greater than the sum of its constituent species.

Dental plaque must never be regarded as a constant, static ecosystem: a consideration of the points raised throughout this chapter serve to emphasise its dynamic nature.

FURTHER READING

Aas JA, Paster BJ, Stokes LN, et al. Defining the normal bacterial flora of the oral cavity. *J Clin Microbiol.* 2005;43:5721-5732.

Carlsson J. Growth and nutrition as ecological factors. In: Kuramitsu HK, Ellen RP, eds. *Oral bacterial ecology. The molecular basis.* Wymondham: Horizon Scientific Press; 2000:67-130.

Cook LC, Federle MJ. Peptide pheromone signaling in *Streptococcus* and *Enterococcus. FEMS Microbiol Rev.* 2014;38:473-492.

Duran-Pinedo AE, Frias-Lopez J. Beyond microbial community composition: functional activities of the oral microbiome in health and disease. *Microbes Infect.* 2015;17:505-516.

Flemming HC, Wingender J. The biofilm matrix. *Nat Rev Microbiol.* 2010;8:623-633.

Gungor OE, Kirzioglu Z, Kivanc M. Probiotics: can they be used to improve oral health? *Benef Microbes.* 2015;6:647-656.

Hannig M, Joiner A. The structure, function and properties of the acquired pellicle. *Monogr Oral Sci.* 2006;19:29-64.

Höiby N, Bjarnsholt T, Givskov M, et al. Antibiotic resistance of bacterial biofilms. *Int J Antimicrob Agents.* 2010;35:322-332.

Jakubovics NS. Talk of the town: interspecies communication in oral biofilms. *Mol Oral Microbiol.* 2010;25:4-14.

Jakubovics NS, Shields RC, Rajarajan N, et al. Life after death: the critical role of extracellular DNA in microbial biofilms. *Lett Appl Microbiol.* 2013;57:467-475.

Jakubovics NS, Yassin SA, Rickard AH. Community interactions of oral streptococci. *Adv Appl Microbiol.* 2014;87:43-110.

Jolivet-Gougeon A, Bonnaure-Mallet M. Biofilms as a mechanisms of bacterial resistance. *Drug Discov Today Technol.* 2014;11:49-56.

Kolenbrander PE, ed. *Oral Microbial Communities. Genomic enquiry and interspecies communication.* Washington DC: American Society for Microbiology Press; 2011.

Koo H, Falsetta ML, Klein MI. The exopolysaccharide matrix. A virulence determinant of cariogenic biofilm. *J Dent Res.* 2013;92:1065-1073.

Kuboniwa M, Lamont RJ. Subgingival biofilm formation. *Periodontol 2000.* 2010;52:38-52.

Lindh L, Aroonsang W, Sotres J, et al. Salivary pellicles. *Monogr Oral Sci.* 2014;24:30-39.

Marsh PD, Takahashi N, Nyvad B. Biofilms in caries development. In: Fejerskov O, Nyvad B, Kidd EAM, eds. *Dental caries. The disease and its clinical management.* 3rd ed. Oxford: Blackwell Munksgaard; 2015:107-131.

Nikikova AE, Haase EM, Scannapieco FA. Taking the starch out of oral biofilm formation: Molecular basis and functional significance of salivary α-amylase binding to oral streptococci. *Appl Environ Microbiol.* 2013;79:416-423.

Nobbs AH, Jenkinson HF, Jakubovics NS. Stick to your gums: mechanisms of oral microbial adherence. *J Dent Res.* 2011;90: 1271-1278.

Nobbs AH, Lamont RJ, Jenkinson HF. Streptococcus adherence and colonization. *Microbiol Mol Biol Rev.* 2009;73:407-450.

Okshevsky M, Meyer RL. The role of extracellular DNA in the establishment, maintenance and perpetuation of bacterial biofilms. *Crit Rev Microbiol.* 2015;41:341-352.

Pereira CS, Thompson JA, Xavier KB. AI-2-mediated signaling in bacteria. *FEMS Microbiol Rev.* 2013;37:156-181.

Roberts AP, Kreth J. The impact of horizontal gene transfer on the adaptive ability of the human oral microbiome. *Cell Infect Microbiol.* 2014;4:article 124.

Socransky SS, Haffajee AD. Dental biofilms: difficult therapeutic targets. *Periodontol 2000.* 2002;28:12-55.

Wickstrom C, Nerzberg MC, Beighton D, et al. Proteolytic degradation of human salivary MUC5B by dental biofilms. *Microbiology.* 2009;155:2866-2872.

Wilson M, Devine D, eds. *Medical implications of biofilms.* Cambridge: Cambridge University Press; 2003.

Wright CJ, Burns LH, Jack AA, et al. Microbial interactions in building of communities. *Mol Oral Microbiol.* 2013;28:83-101.

Zijnge V, Ammann T, Thurnheer T, et al. Subgingival biofilm structure. *Front Oral Biol.* 2012;15:1-16.

Zijnge V, van Leeuwen MBM, Degener JE, et al. Oral biofilm architecture on natural teeth. *PLoS ONE.* 2010;5:e9321.

MULTIPLE CHOICE QUESTIONS

Answers on p. 249

1 *Which of the following is a major property of dental biofilms and is of clinical significance?*
   a. Allows many fastidious bacteria to survive and grow
   b. Increased sensitivity to antibiotics
   c. Increased tolerance of antimicrobial agents
   d. Enhanced development of halitosis

2 *Which of the following are the weak, long-range forces that promote the attachment of an oral microorganism to the tooth surface?*
   a. van der Waals forces
   b. Electromagnetic energy
   c. Adhesin-receptor interactions
   d. Proton-motive force

3 *Which of the following terms describes hidden receptors in the pellicle for bacterial attachment?*
a. Glucan
b. Fimbriae
c. Amylase
d. Cryptitope

4 *Which of the following is not a consequence of biofilm formation?*
a. Upregulation of genes associated with bacterial motility
b. Enhanced cell-cell signalling
c. Enhanced horizontal gene transfer
d. Reduced sensitivity to antimicrobial agents

5 *Early bacteria colonisers of a tooth surface are able to do which of the following to provide more favourable conditions for the growth of later colonising species that are obligately anaerobic?*
a. Synthesise proline-rich peptides
b. Catabolise exopolymers
c. Remove sialic acid from host glycoproteins
d. Consume oxygen and release carbon dioxide

6 *What is the product of a food chain between* Streptococcus mutans and Veillonella *species, when the former is metabolising fermentable sugars:*
a. More lactic acid
b. Propionic and acetic acids, and more caries
c. Propionic and acetic acids, and less caries
d. Ammonia production

7 *Which of the following is not an example of a synergistic microbial interaction?*
a. Enzyme complementation
b. Coadhesion
c. Bacteriocin production
d. Food web formation

8 *Which of the following is not an example of an antagonistic microbial interaction?*
a. Cell-cell signalling
b. Hydrogen peroxide production
c. Nutrient competition
d. Organic acid/low pH formation

9 *Which of the following is not a property of the matrix of a microbial biofilm?*
a. Restricts the penetration of charged antimicrobial agents
b. Contributes to the structural integrity of the biofilm
c. Increases desiccation
d. Retain nutrients and enzymes within the biofilm

10 *Which of the following is the predominant group of bacteria isolated from occlusal fissures?*
a. *Streptococcus*
b. *Actinomyces*
c. *Prevotella*
d. *Treponema*

11 *Which of the following is the predominant group of bacteria found in approximal plaque?*
a. *Streptococcus*
b. *Actinomyces*
c. *Prevotella*
d. *Treponema*

12 *The gingival crevice is the sole habitat on the teeth for which of the following groups of bacteria?*
a. *Streptococcus*
b. *Actinomyces*
c. *Prevotella*
d. *Treponema*

13 *Which of the following is the mean doubling time of bacteria during the early stages of biofilm formation on teeth?*
a. 20 minutes
b. 1 to 2 hours
c. 6 to 7 hours
d. 12 to 15 hours

14 *Individual species of oral bacteria possess different but complementary patterns of which of the following to obtain nutrients from salivary mucins?*
  a. Glycosidases
  b. Glucosyltransferases
  c. Glucose phosphotransferases
  d. Fructosyltransferases

15 *Which of the following is* not *a 'non-immunological' factor responsible for the breakdown of microbial homeostasis in dental plaque?*
  a. Xerostomia
  b. Broad spectrum antibiotic treatment.
  c. Infection-induced myelosuppression
  d. Dietary sugars

CHAPTER 6

Plaque-mediated diseases: Dental caries and periodontal diseases

RELATIONSHIP OF PLAQUE BACTERIA TO DISEASE: PREVIOUS AND CONTEMPORARY PERSPECTIVES

Most classical infectious diseases satisfy Koch's postulates, for example, the microorganism is found in all cases of the disease and with a distribution corresponding to the observed lesions. Evidence will be presented in this chapter that plaque-mediated diseases do not satisfy these postulates. The contemporary view is that disease is a consequence of the activity of multiple bacterial species, often working in combination, as a result of a disruption (**dysbiosis**) to the normally beneficial resident oral microbiota.

There have been two main schools of thought on the role of plaque bacteria in the aetiology of caries and periodontal diseases. Originally, the **specific plaque hypothesis** was put forward. This proposed that only a few species out of the diverse collection of organisms comprising the resident plaque microbiota are actively involved in disease. This proposal has been valuable because it focused

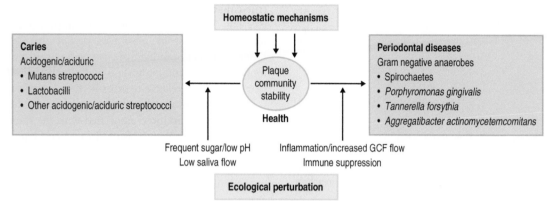

FIGURE 6.1 Ecological shifts in the dental plaque microbiota in health and disease.

efforts on controlling disease by targeting preventative measures and treatment against a limited number of organisms. Over time, however, it became apparent that disease could occur in the apparent absence of these putative pathogens, whereas these organisms were also recovered on occasions from healthy sites, and that many species had the potential to cause disease. This led to the **non-specific plaque hypothesis** being proposed, in which disease was considered to be the outcome of the overall activity of the total plaque microbiota. In this way, a diverse mixture of interacting microorganisms (a microbial community) could play a role in disease. The microbial composition of these communities could vary at different sites and subjects while still resulting in a similar clinical outcome. In some respects, the arguments about the relative merits of these hypotheses may be about semantics, because plaque-mediated diseases are essentially mixed culture (**polymicrobial**) infections, but in which only certain (perhaps relatively specific) species actively participate. The arguments then centre on the definitions of the terms specific and non-specific. If not actually specific, then the diseases certainly show evidence of specificity, especially in terms of function if not in microbial name.

These arguments led to an alternative hypothesis being proposed (the **ecological plaque hypothesis**), that reconciled the key elements of the earlier two hypotheses, but highlighted the importance of the oral environment. In brief, the ecological plaque hypothesis proposes that the organisms associated with disease may also be present at sound sites, but at levels too low to be clinically relevant. Disease is a result of

a shift in the balance of the resident microbiota because of a response to a change in local environmental conditions (**dysbiosis**) (Fig. 6.1). For example, repeated conditions of low pH in plaque following frequent sugar intake favours the growth of acid-producing and acid-tolerating species that will increase the risk of dental caries. In periodontal disease, the inflammatory response to dental plaque accumulation around the gums results in an increased flow in gingival crevicular fluid that not only delivers the host defences but also provides molecules that favour the growth of the proteolytic and obligately anaerobic bacteria that predominate in disease. Tissue damage is mainly because of an inappropriate and exaggerated host response to the biofilm rather than to the direct action of the microorganisms themselves. Importantly, therefore, prevention can be achieved not only by the direct inhibition of the causative bacteria but also by the 'removal' or 'neutralisation' of the factors that drive the selection of these organisms. Additional theories and models have been proposed (e.g., the **extended caries ecological hypothesis**, and the **polymicrobial synergy and dysbiosis** model for periodontal disease); all of these theories will be discussed later in more detail.

RELATIONSHIP OF PLAQUE BACTERIA TO DISEASE: IMPLICATIONS FOR STUDY DESIGN

Two types of epidemiological surveys have been designed to determine the role of plaque bacteria in human disease (Fig. 6.2). In **cross-sectional surveys**, predetermined surfaces in a population are sampled

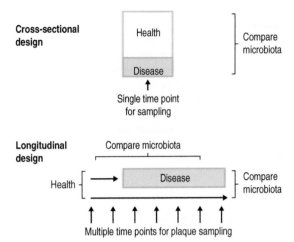

FIGURE 6.2 Distinction between cross-sectional and longitudinal study designs to investigate the role of dental plaque bacteria in caries or periodontal diseases.

at a single time point, and the plaque microbiota is related to the caries or periodontal status of the site at that time. However, with this type of study, it cannot be determined with certainty whether the species that were isolated at the time when disease was diagnosed caused the decay or inflammation, or arose because of it. Only associations can be derived from this study design, but they have the advantage that large numbers of sites/people can be analysed, and different patient groups, age groups, tooth surfaces, diets, intervention strategies, and so on can be compared. Likewise, it cannot be determined whether the site, at the time of sampling, was progressing, arrested, or healing, nor whether each phase may have a different microbiota. To overcome these difficulties, **longitudinal studies** can be performed in which initially clinically healthy sites are sampled at regular intervals over a set time period (see Fig. 6.2). Sites are selected on the basis of previous epidemiological surveys from which it can be predicted that a statistically relevant number of sites should suffer disease within the time span of the study. The microbiota can then be compared: (a) before and after the diagnosis of disease, and (b) between those sites that became diseased and those that remained healthy throughout the study, so that

true **cause-and-effect** relationships can be established (see Fig. 6.2). A consequence of this approach is that, for practical reasons, resources permit that only a limited number of individuals can be followed for prolonged periods, and far fewer longitudinal studies have been performed relative to cross-sectional surveys.

Superimposed on the challenges of study designs outlined above are those associated with the sampling and microbiological analysis of plaque (see Chapter 4). Biofilms are difficult to remove, and the oral microbiota is diverse. Disease is not because of colonisation by exogenous (non-oral) species (such events might be easier to recognise), but to changes in the relative proportions of members of the resident microbiota. Traditional culture techniques can presently recover only about 50–70% of the microbiota (see Chapter 3), and so the role of potentially significant organisms could be underestimated or missed using these approaches. Furthermore, irrespective of the methods used, there are wide intersubject variations in the composition of the plaque microbiota (see Chapter 5), so that when data are averaged from numerous individuals, clear associations between bacteria and disease can be obscured. Similarly, the composition of dental plaque can vary over relatively small distances. This can pose difficulties during longitudinal studies because, ideally, the same location should be resampled on each occasion. In addition, there is the possibility that regular sampling could distort the subsequent reestablishment of plaque.

In some studies, only a small number of predetermined bacteria are monitored, so a complete picture of the role of other bacteria in disease would not be apparent. For example, in several early studies of dental caries, only viable counts of mutans streptococci (with and without lactobacilli or *S. sanguinis*) were determined. It is possible that clearer relationships might emerge if biofilm communities were analysed on the basis of 'function' rather than merely the name of the component species. It is probable that several species could perform the same biochemical or physiologic function in biofilms from different individuals. Despite these problems of study design and methodology, much progress has been made, and the major findings will now be discussed in the following sections.

DENTAL CARIES

In 2010, untreated caries in permanent teeth was reported to be the most prevalent condition globally, affecting 2.4 billion people, whereas untreated caries in deciduous teeth was the tenth most prevalent condition, affecting 621 million children. Caries of enamel surfaces is particularly common up to the mid-twenties, whereas, in later life, root-surface caries is an increasing problem caused by gingival recession exposing the vulnerable cementum to microbial colonisation. Evidence is emerging that there are three peaks of caries prevalence, at ages 6, 25 and 70.

Dental caries can be defined as the localised destruction of the tissues of the tooth by bacterial fermentation of dietary carbohydrates. Cavities begin as small demineralised areas below the surface of the enamel (Fig. 6.3); once the enamel has been affected, caries can progress through the dentine and into the pulp (Fig. 6.4). Demineralisation of the enamel is caused by acids, particularly lactic acid, produced from the microbial fermentation of dietary carbohydrates. Lesion formation involves dissolution of the enamel and the transport of the calcium and phosphate ions away into the surrounding environment. The initial stages of caries are reversible and remineralisation can occur, particularly in the presence of fluoride.

EVIDENCE FOR THE ROLE OF MICROORGANISMS IN THE AETIOLOGY OF DENTAL CARIES

In his famous Chemico-Parasitic Theory, Miller (1890) proposed that oral bacteria converted dietary carbohydrates into acid, which solubilised the calcium phosphate of the enamel to produce a caries lesion. Although Clarke isolated an organism (which he called *Streptococcus mutans*) from a human caries lesion in 1924, definitive proof for the causative role of bacteria in caries came only in the 1950s and 1960s following experiments with germ-free (or gnotobiotic) animals. Pioneering experiments showed that germ-free rats developed caries when infected with bacteria, which were described as enterococci. Evidence for the transmissibility of caries came from studies on hamsters. Caries-inactive animals had no caries even when fed a highly cariogenic (i.e., sucrose-rich) diet. Caries only developed in these animals when they were caged with, or ate the faecal pellets of a group of caries-active hamsters. Further proof came when streptococci, isolated from caries lesions in rodents, caused rampant decay when inoculated into the oral cavity of previously caries-inactive hamsters, whereas

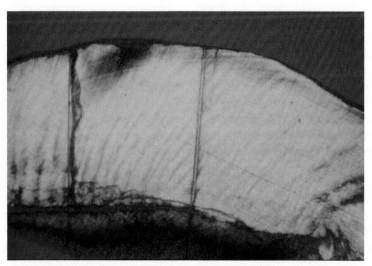

FIGURE 6.3 Subsurface demineralisation of enamel (viewed in cross-section).

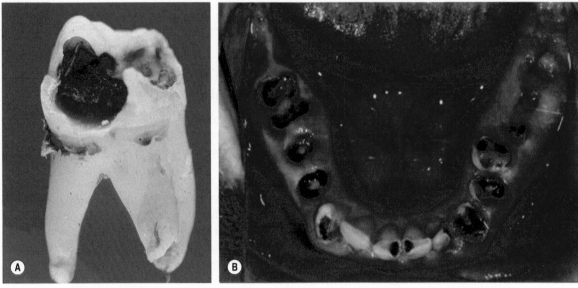

FIGURE 6.4 Photograph showing (**A**) extensive cavitation of a tooth, and (**B**) cavitation of teeth in the mouth.

animals treated with appropriate antibiotics did not develop caries. The importance of diet became apparent when caries development was found to occur only in the presence of fermentable sugars such as sucrose. This is an important finding because it confirms that the mere presence of a potentially cariogenic bacterium is insufficient for disease to occur.

Mutans streptococci can cause caries of smooth surfaces, as well as in pits and fissures, in hamsters, gerbils, rats and monkeys fed on cariogenic diets, and these are the most cariogenic group of bacteria found. Other bacteria, including members of the mitis-, anginosus-, and salivarius-groups of streptococci, *Enterococcus faecalis*, *Actinomyces naeslundii*, *A. viscosus* and lactobacilli, can also produce caries under conducive conditions in some animals, although the lesions are usually restricted to fissures. The ability of mutans streptococci to cause dental caries has also been confirmed during vaccination studies. Immunisation of rodents or primates fed a cariogenic (high sugar) diet with whole cells or specific antigens of *S. mutans* and *S. sobrinus* led to a reduction in the number of these organisms in plaque and a decrease in the number of caries lesions when compared with control animals. Subsequent experiments using defined mutants helped to confirm the importance

of traits such as the production of intracellular and extracellular polysaccharides from sucrose to the cariogenic potential of mutans streptococci (see later; Table 6.5).

Unlike animal studies, any relationship between particular oral bacteria and caries in humans must be derived by indirect means in epidemiological surveys. Patients on long-term, broad-spectrum antibiotic therapy frequently exhibit a reduced caries experience.

AETIOLOGY OF HUMAN ENAMEL CARIES

Cavitation is the final stage of enamel caries (see Fig. 6.4); it is preceded by a clinically-detectable small lesion, known as a white spot, and before that by subsurface demineralisation, which can only be detected by histological techniques (see Fig. 6.3). Not all white-spot lesions progress to cavitation; in some studies only about half of these early lesions penetrated the dentine after 3 to 4 years. White spot lesions do not just arrest, but can even remineralise, a process that is enhanced by fluoride. Enamel caries often occurs in teeth shortly after eruption (hence, its historical association with young people), and some teeth and surfaces are more vulnerable than others. The prevalence of caries is highest on the occlusal surfaces of first and second molars, and lowest on the lingual surfaces of mandibular teeth. The risk to approximal surfaces is intermediate to those described above. With the reduction in the incidence of dental caries in the young, it is predicted that the caries risk for some surfaces will now extend over the life-time of an individual, and this has important implications for caries prevention strategies. Some individuals are more caries prone than others, and this may be related to their diet (e.g., frequency of sugar intake), lack of optimum saliva flow (e.g., flow is severely reduced in xerostomia patients), or a low exposure to fluoride. Most caries is now concentrated in a minority of the population, especially in the most marginalised and disadvantaged groups.

MICROBIOLOGY OF ENAMEL CARIES

Buccal and lingual **smooth surfaces** are easy to clean and generally only rarely suffer from decay. However, they are easy to study for experimental purposes, both in terms of clinical diagnosis and in plaque sampling. Higher proportions (10- to 100-fold) of mutans streptococci have been cultured from white-spot lesions on smooth surfaces compared with adjacent sound enamel. As stated earlier, such an association does not prove a causal relationship and the actual proportions of mutans streptococci are often low. Suspensions of plaque from white-spot lesions produce a lower pH minimum and a faster rate of pH-fall than plaque from sound enamel. Molecular studies have found an association between *S. mutans*, *Atopobium parvulum*, *Dialister invisus* and species of *Prevotella* and *Scardovia* with white-spot lesions, whereas a number of Gram-negative taxa have been linked to sound enamel (*Fusobacterium*, *Campylobacter*, *Kingella*, *Capnocytophaga*). Similar associations were found in a study of white-spot lesions associated with orthodontic bands in adolescent patients. This study, using a microarray approach (human oral microbe identification microarray [HOMIM], see Chapter 3) found correlations between lesions and the presence of *Granulicatella elegans*, *Veillonella* species, bifidobacteria, mutans streptococci and *Scardovia wiggsiae*.

Fissures on occlusal surfaces (see Figs. 2.2 and 5.9) are the most caries-prone sites. Caries can develop rapidly on these surfaces, and it is at these sites that the strongest association between mutans streptococci and dental decay has been found. In one cross-sectional study, 71% of carious fissures had viable counts of mutans streptococci that were more than 10% of the total cultivable plaque microbiota, whereas 70% of the fissures that were caries free at the time of sampling had no detectable mutans streptococci. However, this also meant that mutans streptococci were present in 30% of caries-free fissures. An inverse relationship between mutans streptococci and *S. sanguinis* is frequently observed. In a longitudinal study of North American children, the proportions of mutans streptococci, *S. sanguinis* and lactobacilli were monitored before and at the time of caries development in occlusal fissures. The subjects were divided into several groups according to their previous caries experience and to their caries activity during the study. The proportions of mutans streptococci increased significantly at the time of diagnosis of most lesions. However, mutans streptococci were only a minor component of the plaque from five fissures which became carious. Counts of lactobacilli were significantly higher at these sites and, it was concluded, that these were probably responsible for lesion formation. A subsequent longitudinal study confirmed these findings, and demonstrated an even stronger relationship between mutans streptococci and caries initiation (see Table 6.1), whereas lactobacilli, when present, were

TABLE 6.1 **Mean proportions of mutans streptococci and lactobacilli teeth in schoolchildren (7–8 years old) who remained caries free or who developed a caries lesion during a longitudinal study**

Time (months) before caries diagnosis	MEAN BACTERIAL PROPORTIONS IN FISSURE PLAQUE					
	CARIES SITES		FILLED SITES		CARIES FREE SITES	
	MS	L	MS	L	MS	L
0	29	8	–	–	9	2
6	25	8	15	3	17	1
12	16	1	20	2	9	3
18	9	<1	16	1	11	1

Data taken from: Loesche WJ, Eklund S, Earnest R, Burt B. Longitudinal investigation of bacteriology of human fissure decay: epidemiological studies in molars shortly after eruption. Infect Immun 1984 46: 765–772.

L, Lactobacilli; *MS*, mutans streptococci.

associated with sites requiring restoration. Although there was a correlation between mutans streptococci and fissure decay, lesions could also develop at some sites in the apparent absence of this group of bacteria, and there were also surfaces where mutans streptococci persisted in moderately high numbers without any evidence of detectable caries.

A major prospective study of young Swiss children (7 to 8 years) specifically examined whether or not colonisation by mutans streptococci was a risk factor for caries in fissures (and on smooth surfaces). Both fissures and smooth surfaces of first permanent premolars that suffered demineralisation without cavitation were heavily colonised with mutans streptococci (10^4 to 10^5 colony forming units [CFU]/ml of sample) around 12 to 18 months before the clinical diagnosis of the lesion. The proportion of mutans streptococci appeared to increase markedly 6 to 9 months before lesion detection to reach 11% to 18% and 10% to 12% of the total streptococcal microbiota of fissures and smooth surfaces, respectively. This study demonstrated that colonisation and an increase in proportion of mutans streptococci preceded lesion formation by about six months. As with other studies of caries, however, several sites had high counts of mutans streptococci (>20% of the total streptococcal count) but no evidence of caries. Larger lesions (with cavitation) were found only at a relatively few sites. In five out of six carious fissures, the median count of mutans streptococci rose from 10^2 to more than 10^4 CFU/ml around 12 months before lesion detection; this represented a final mean proportion of 18% of the total streptococcal count. The remaining carious fissure had no detectable mutans streptococci at any time during the study, again illustrating that species other than mutans streptococci can play a role in lesion formation on occasions. An additional feature of the design of this study was that some sites were diagnosed with a lesion, which subsequently remineralised. Some of these sites had levels of mutans streptococci greater than 20% of the streptococcal microbiota, and yet the lesion remineralised within 12 months. During this period, the levels of mutans streptococci fell markedly between 6 and 9 months before the diagnosis of the reversal.

More recent studies have expanded the spectrum of bacteria being evaluated for their role in caries. When appropriate isolation media were used, a number of bifidobacteria were isolated from occlusal lesions in children and adults; these included *Bifidobacterium dentium*, *B. longum*, *B. breve*, *Parascardovia denticolens* and *Scardovia inopicata*. The architecture of biofilms from sites with occlusal caries has been studied using fluorescence in situ hybridisation (FISH) combined with confocal microscopy. *Actinomyces* organised in palisades formed an inner layer at the fissure entrance, and bacteria within the fissure appeared to be less metabolically active, perhaps reflecting difficulties of penetration of substrates. Bacterial invasion of dentinal tubules by lactobacilli and bifidobacteria was observed in advanced lesions.

A challenge for studies of **approximal** surfaces lies with the difficulty in accurately diagnosing early lesions, and with the fact that plaque samples are inevitably removed from the whole interproximal area, including that overlying sound enamel as well as carious enamel. The microbiota can vary markedly at different sites around the contact area between teeth, irrespective of whether or not a lesion is developing, so that specific associations can sometimes be obscured. Early cross-sectional studies found a positive correlation between elevated levels of mutans streptococci and lesion development. Many of these studies, however, were limited in scope, and only monitored a few types of microorganism. A limited number of longitudinal studies have been performed; in a survey of English schoolchildren, aged 11 to 15 years, mutans streptococci could be found in high numbers before demineralisation at a number of sites, but lesions also appeared to develop on occasions in the apparent absence of these bacteria. Mutans streptococci were also present at other sites in equally high numbers for the duration of the study without any diagnosis of caries. There was evidence that the isolation frequency and proportions of mutans streptococci increased after, rather than before, the first radiographic detection of some lesions, especially in those that progressed deeper into the enamel, suggesting that the composition of the microbiota changes as the lesion progresses through the tooth (microbial succession; see Chapter 4).

Similar findings were found in a study of Dutch army recruits, aged 18 to 20 years. Mutans streptococci were isolated from 40% and 86% of sites from caries-free and caries-active recruits, respectively

TABLE 6.2   Prevalence of mutans streptococci at approximal tooth surfaces with and without caries progression

	TOTAL NUMBER OF TOOTH SURFACES	THE NUMBER OF SITES WITH MUTANS STREPTOCOCCI AT PROPORTIONS OF*:	
		0%	0–5%	>5%
Caries progression	14	1†	3	10
No caries progression	41	21	17	3

*The number of sites in which mutans streptococci were detected at a particular percentage of the total cultivable microbiota.
†Number of tooth surfaces.

(Table 6.2). Marked differences in the distribution of individual species were found; *S. mutans* (serotype *c*) strains were isolated from both groups whereas *S. sobrinus* (serotype *d*) was recovered almost exclusively from caries-active recruits. The prevalence of both species of mutans streptococci also showed a direct but not unique correlation with the progression of a lesion into the dentine. Again, relatively high proportions of mutans streptococci persisted at some tooth surfaces without caries progression although on occasion caries could develop in their apparent absence.

A major limitation of traditional culture approaches is that nearly a third of the oral microbiota cannot as yet be grown in the laboratory, and so, more recently, molecular methods have been applied to characterise the complex microbial communities associated with caries. A more diverse microbiota was found when these methods were applied to sites with caries, and novel taxa have been described. One study confirmed the relationship of *S. sanguinis* with sound enamel and *S. mutans* and lactobacilli with caries lesions, but additionally found *Actinomyces gerencseriae* and other *Actinomyces* spp. to be implicated in caries initiation and *Bifidobacterium* spp. with advanced lesions. Another study used molecular approaches to investigate the microbial diversity of plaque from teeth with lesions at different stages of disease. They found 10% of subjects with rampant caries in the secondary dentition did not have detectable levels of *S. mutans*; these lesions had high levels of lactobacilli, low pH tolerating non-mutans streptococci and *Bifidobacterium* species. High levels of *Actinomyces* species and non-mutans streptococci were found in early (white spot) lesions, whereas mutans streptococci and lactobacilli, together with *Propionibacterium* and *Bifidobacterium* spp. dominated advanced (deep dentine) lesions. The data support the ecological plaque hypothesis in that shifts in the bacterial composition of plaque were seen between healthy sites and those with lesions of increasing severity, and the organisms associated with caries were all acid producing species.

Rampant caries can occur in particular subgroups of people who are especially prone to decay, such as xerostomic patients (who have a markedly reduced salivary flow rate because of radiation treatment for head and neck cancer), those with Sjögren's syndrome, or as a side-effect of medication. These patients also generally consume soft diets, with high sucrose content, and may often suck candies to relieve their symptoms of dry mouth. Longitudinal studies of patients undergoing radiation treatment showed large increases in the numbers and proportions of mutans streptococci and lactobacilli in plaque and saliva. Other species associated with sound enamel, such as *S. sanguinis, Neisseria* spp. and Gram-negative anaerobes, decreased during this period.

Early childhood caries (ECC) and **severe early childhood caries** (S-ECC) are increasing public health problems. The clinical definition of these conditions varies in different regions, and relates to the age profile of the children. Their prevalence in Europe ranges between 16% and 86% of children depending on the country, whereas S-ECC affects about 3% to 12% of infants. The prevalence of early caries is higher in those from lower socioeconomic groups and in the poor; it also tends to be more common in immigrants within a country. Apart from the impact on the primary dentition, ECC and S-ECC reduce the quality of life of an infant by impacting on their sleep and affecting their ability to eat so that they can be underweight, and they are risk factors for caries in permanent teeth. These conditions include caries covered by the previous term 'nursing-bottle caries', which described the extensive and rapid decay of the maxillary anterior teeth associated with the prolonged and frequent feeding of young infants with bottles or pacifiers containing formulas with a high concentration of fermentable carbohydrate. Plaque bacteria receive an almost continuous provision of substrates from which they can make acid. Such prolonged conditions of low pH are conducive, and indeed selective, for mutans streptococci and lactobacilli, and proportions of mutans streptococci in plaque can reach more than 50% of the cultivable microbiota. Other studies have reported elevated levels of *S. mutans, Actinomyces israelii,* lactobacilli, *Veillonella* spp. (presumably reflecting high concentrations of lactate; see Chapter 5), and *C. albicans* (which also tolerates acidic conditions) in ECC and S-ECC. In a study of ECC using molecular approaches, *S. sanguinis* was associated with sound surfaces whereas, in order of decreasing cell numbers, *A. gerencseriae, Bifidobacterium, S. mutans, Veillonella,* other streptococci, and *Lactobacillus fermentum* were linked with caries. Other studies reported that particular bifidobacteria, namely *Scardovia wiggsiae* and *Slackia exigua,* were associated with lesions in children with S-ECC. A similar, but less diverse, microbiota was found in infected pulp from primary teeth in children with S-ECC. In particular, *S. mutans, Parascardovia denticolens, B. longum, V. dispar* and several *Lactobacillus* and *Actinomyces* species were preferentially isolated from cariously-exposed pulps.

Caries can reoccur beneath and around previous restorations (**recurrent or secondary caries**), and treatment of this accounts for a large proportion of the restorative needs of the adult population. Secondary dentinal involvement is of particular concern because it can be difficult to diagnose non-invasively, and it poses the threat of pulpal inflammation and infection (see later). Mutans streptococci and lactobacilli have been isolated in high numbers from recurrent caries whereas a more diverse microbiota has been isolated when dentine is affected (see later).

Numerous studies have shown mutans streptococci to be important cariogenic bacteria; they generally appear in the mouth once teeth have erupted, although mutans streptococci have been detected in pre-dentate infants. The mother is the main source of these bacteria; additional factors that correlate with *S. mutans* colonisation are sweetened drinks taken by infants to bed, frequent exposure to sugar, snacking, and sharing of foods with adults, whereas non-colonisation is associated with toothbrushing and multiple courses of

antibiotics. This information can play an important part in developing appropriate caries control strategies.

KEY POINTS

> Enamel caries is associated with a shift in the balance of the microbiota of dental plaque. The isolation frequency and proportions of acid-producing and acid-tolerating species, especially mutans streptococci, bifidobacteria and lactobacilli, are higher at sites with caries. No single species is uniquely associated with dental caries, so that caries can occur on occasions in the apparent absence of mutans streptococci, whereas these organisms can persist at some sites without evidence of demineralisation.

MICROBIOLOGY OF ROOT-SURFACE CARIES AND INFECTED DENTINE

The reduction in enamel caries in industrialised societies has resulted in large proportions of the public retaining their teeth into later life. Gingival recession occurs in old age exposing the susceptible cementum surface of the root to microbial colonisation; root surfaces can also become exposed because of mechanical injury or to periodontal surgery (e.g., following scaling and root planing). These cementum surfaces are even more vulnerable than enamel to demineralisation by plaque acids, although the flow of saliva is lower in older age groups. The prevalence of root surface caries increases with age; approximately 60% of individuals aged 60 years or older now have root caries or fillings.

Direct evidence for the role of oral microorganisms in root-surface caries came from early studies with animals in which filamentous bacteria were observed invading the root surfaces of hamsters and causing caries. Human isolates of *Actinomyces naeslundii* were then shown to cause root surface caries in germ-free rats and hamsters, as were pure cultures of mutans streptococci and representatives of the mitis- and anginosus-groups of streptococci.

Early studies were designed around the findings from the first animal experiments, and focused on the role of Gram-positive filamentous bacteria, especially *Actinomyces* spp., in root surface caries. Among the organisms isolated from lesions were *Rothia dentocariosa, Actinomyces naeslundii* and *A. odontolyticus;* in some studies, mutans streptococci were also associated with root surface caries.

TABLE 6.3 Mean percentage viable counts (and percentage isolation frequencies in parentheses) of some plaque bacteria from root surfaces, with and without caries

Bacterium	Sound root surface	Root surface caries	
		Initial (soft)	Advanced (hard)
Mutans streptococci	2 (84)	29 (92)	8 (92)
Streptococcus sanguinis	19 (96)	11 (97)	22 (85)
Actinomyces naeslundii	12 (90)	11 (85)	13 (96)

Subsequent studies have tended to confirm a stronger association between mutans streptococci and lactobacilli with root surface caries. In a major longitudinal survey in Canada, although no direct correlation between specific bacteria and root caries was found, the presence of mutans streptococci and lactobacilli on root surfaces was predictive for the subsequent development of a lesion. Other studies have attempted to subdivide the lesions into initial (or soft) and advanced (or hard). Several groups reported higher proportions (often around 30% of the total cultivable microbiota) of mutans streptococci at the initial lesion (Table 6.3), sometimes in association with lactobacilli. Lactobacilli have occasionally been found at arrested (hard, black-coloured) lesions. Following improvements to the classification of *Actinomyces* spp., the predominant species isolated from infected dentine of active root caries lesions were *A. israelii* > *A. gerencseriae* > *A. naeslundii* > *A. odontolyticus* > *A. georgiae*.

In situ devices have been worn by volunteers to study the microbiota of actively-progressing root surface caries lesions. In one study, elderly subjects (mean age: 70 years) carried root surface specimens from human molars on their partial dentures for 3 months. After this period, the predominant plaque microbiota was determined and the integrity of the experimental root surface was measured by highly sensitive techniques (quantitative microradiography).

Although the composition of the microbiota showed distinct individual differences, plaque samples from surfaces showing the highest loss of mineral were dominated either by (a) *A. naeslundii*, or (b) a combination of mutans streptococci and lactobacilli. Plaque from root surfaces with less pronounced mineral loss harboured a more complex microbiota including *Actinomyces* spp., mutans streptococci, *S. mitis* biovar 1, *Veillonella* spp., Gram-negative rods, and low numbers of lactobacilli.

The recent application of more sophisticated approaches to sampling plaque has given new insights into the relationship between the composition of the microbiota and lesion development. One study used a specially designed device to lift plaque from discrete areas directly into reduced transport fluid to preserve the viability of obligately anaerobic bacteria. The caries status of these precise sampling sites was then assessed by a variety of sensitive techniques including contact microradiography, and light and electron microscopy. In this way, the surface directly beneath the plaque that had been sampled could be reliably classified as being sound, active or an arrested carious root lesion. Regardless of the degree of mineralisation, the cultivable microbiota from these root surfaces was more diverse than had previously been reported, and resembled that associated with gingivitis (see later). On all surfaces, *Actinomyces* were the predominant group of bacteria, especially *A. naeslundii*, *A. odontolyticus* and *A. gerencseriae*. Arrested lesions had significantly lower numbers of bacteria than either sound surfaces or active lesions. Gram-negative species formed around 50% of the microbiota on sound and active carious surfaces, with *Prevotella* spp. (particularly *P. nigrescens*) being highly prevalent. Other Gram-negative bacteria, including *Capnocytophaga* spp., *Campylobacter* spp. and *Leptotrichia buccalis*, were preferentially isolated from plaque overlying active lesions. This may be because a number of these species are sufficiently saccharolytic to demineralise cementum and dentine, whereas others are proteolytic, and could hydrolyse the dentine collagen matrix. A metagenomics approach compared the microbiota from supragingival biofilms from healthy and carious sites in elderly patients with root caries. *Propionibacterium acidifaciens*, *S. mutans*, *Olsenella profusa*, *Prevotella multisaccharivorax* and *L. crispatus* were most associated with root caries.

Collectively, these data suggest that (a) caries initiation on root surfaces has a polymicrobial aetiology, and (b) bacterial succession occurs during the development of root surface lesions. There is a diversity of bacterial species recovered from root surface lesions, but most probably there is a consistency in the properties of the predominant species in that they are generally acidogenic and acid-tolerating. Dentine can be invaded: (a) by direct progression of an enamel caries lesion; (b) from caries of the root surface (see above); (c) from a periodontal pocket via lateral or accessory canals (Fig. 6.5); (d) as a result of fracture or trauma during operative procedures, or (e) as a result of secondary or recurrent caries (see above). The microbial community from the advancing front of a dentinal lesion is diverse and contains many facultatively- and obligately-anaerobic Gram-positive bacteria belonging to the genera *Actinomyces, Bifidobacterium, Eubacterium, Lactobacillus, Parvimonas, Propionibacterium* and *Rothia*. Streptococci are recovered less frequently, but when mutans streptococci have been isolated they can be one of the predominant members of the community. Gram-negative bacteria such as *Prevotella, Porphyromonas*, and *Fusobacterium* spp. can also be isolated but they are generally present only in low numbers.

The microbiota found in the dentine and pulp of periodontally-diseased human teeth is also diverse and may be derived predominantly from the subgingival area. Numerous Gram-positive and Gram-negative species have been identified; some are more prevalent in the dentine (e.g., *A. odontolyticus, Bifidobacterium* spp.), some predominate in the pulp (e.g., black-pigmented anaerobes), whereas others are found equally at both sites (e.g., *A. naeslundii, Veillonella* spp., *F. nucleatum*). Dentine collagen is denatured and modified during the caries process, and becomes more susceptible to breakdown by non-specific proteases, and this explains the presence of both acidogenic and proteolytic bacteria.

Bacteria in the dentine tubules obtain their nutrients from dentinal fluid, which contains glycoproteins such as IgG, albumin and fibrinogen. When streptococci come into contact with exposed type I collagen there is upregulation of specific genes that enhances cell adhesion and growth. For example, *S. gordonii* increases expression of the adhesin, antigen I/II, and long chains of streptococci develop along collagen fibrils.

Once bacteria are in the pulp, inflammation can occur which may result eventually in necrosis of the root canal. A further consequence is that microorganisms can invade and destroy tissue surrounding the apex of the root, producing a spreading or localised infection (see Fig. 6.5). Diverse consortia of bacteria

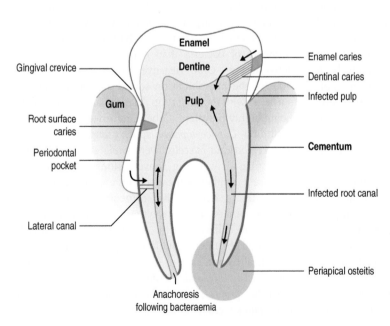

Enamel
Dentine
Pulp
Gum

Gingival crevice

Root surface caries

Periodontal pocket

Lateral canal

Anachoresis following bacteraemia

Enamel caries
Dentinal caries
Infected pulp

Cementum

Infected root canal

Periapical osteitis

FIGURE 6.5 Progression of infections affecting the tooth and its supporting structures.

are cultured, including black-pigmented anaerobes (*Prevotella intermedia*, *Prevotella melaninogenica*, *Porphyromonas endodontalis*, *P. gingivalis*), and *Prevotella dentalis*, *Campylobacter sputorum*, *Eubacterium* spp. and *Parvimonas* species. Some of these species (*P. endodontalis*, *P. dentalis*) are found almost exclusively in infected root canals and abscesses of endodontal origin. Another study of necrotic pulps found *Propionibacterium*, *Eubacterium* and *Fusobacterium* spp. to be the predominant bacteria, with *Bifidobacterium*, *Lactobacillus*, *Actinomyces* and *Veillonella* spp. as minor components. *Enterococcus faecalis* is also commonly associated with infected root canals.

More recently, combinations of culture and molecular approaches have been used to characterise the microbial community of carious dentine. In one study, the predominant cultivable bacteria included a novel *Propionibacterium* spp., *Olsenella profusa* and *Lactobacillus rhamnosus*, but even more taxa were detected when deoxyribonucleic acid (DNA) was extracted directly from the lesions, amplified by polymerase chain reaction, and bacterial identification was based on 16S ribosomal ribonucleic acid (rRNA) gene sequence analysis (see Chapters 3 and 4). The predominant taxa included *S. mutans*, lactobacilli and *Rothia dentocariosa* along with many taxa that had never been described previously (although they were generally close relatives of cultivable species). Other studies of infected dentine also detected diverse microbial consortia dominated by *Prevotella*, *Lactobacillus*, *Selenomonas* and *Streptococcus* species. Some samples were dominated by lactobacilli, whereas those with low levels of lactobacilli had high numbers of *Prevotella* species. The pH can vary within the dentinal lesion, and this can influence the composition of the microbiota. Although some species were unaffected by the pH, acidic areas were often dominated by lactobacilli (e.g., *L. fermentum*, *L. rhamnosus*, *L. crispatus*) whereas regions where the pH was nearer neutrality had a more diverse microbiota which included *Alloprevotella* and *Streptococcus* species.

The treatment of infections of the root canal (endodontics) involves the removal of infected and dead tissue both mechanically and by irrigation, sometimes accompanied by treatment with antimicrobial agents to reduce the microbial community to a level where the cavity can be restored effectively.

KEY POINTS

Root surface caries is common in older age groups when the cementum is exposed and becomes susceptible to microbial colonisation, and saliva flow is reduced. Although mutans streptococci and lactobacilli are common at sites with root surface caries, the microbiota can be complex from deeper lesions. Infected dentine has high proportions of *Actinomyces* spp. and lactobacilli, as well as a diverse range of proteolytic and obligately anaerobic species that may be involved in the degradation of dentine. There is no absolute specificity in terms of the microbiota isolated from root caries lesions or from infected dentine, but the predominant species are probably acidogenic and acid-tolerating, combined with some proteolytic organisms.

PATHOGENIC DETERMINANTS OF CARIOGENIC BACTERIA

Determinants of cariogenicity are often linked to sugar metabolism (Table 6.4). Mutants defective in various aspects of sucrose metabolism have been compared in

TABLE 6.4 **Characteristics of mutans streptococci that contribute to their cariogenicity**

Property	Comment
Sugar transport	High and low affinity transport systems operating over a wide range of conditions to ensure substrate uptake, even under extreme environments; for example, low pH.
Acid production	An efficient glycolytic pathway rapidly producing low terminal pH values in plaque.
Aciduricity	Cells have specific biochemical attributes enabling them to survive, metabolise and grow at low pH values.
Extracellular polysaccharide (EPS) production	EPS contributes to the plaque matrix, consolidates attachment of cells, and may localise acidic fermentation products.
Intracellular polysaccharide (IPS) production	IPS use allows acid production to continue in the absence of dietary sugars.

TABLE 6.5 The use of mutants of mutans streptococci to determine traits linked to cariogenicity

Trait	Property of mutant	Effect on cariogenicity*
glucosyltransferase[†]	decreased colonisation and plaque formation	reduced
fructosyltransferase	loss of extracellular fructans	none
fructanase	no breakdown of extracellular fructans	none
intracellular polysaccharide (IPS) production	no intracellular glycogen	reduced
antigen 1/11	decreased ability to adhere	none
enzyme II (PTS)	decreased sucrose transport	none
lactic dehydrogenase	no lactic acid production	reduced
aciduricity[‡]	reduced tolerance of low pH	reduced

*If a mutation did not lead to a reduction in caries, it does not necessarily mean that the trait is not important in cariogenicity. It may reflect the fact that the particular trait is not essential for caries in an animal model; also, mutans streptococci often have more than one mechanism for a particular function, for example, adherence.
[†]Mutations in *gtfB* and *gtfC*, but not in *gtfD*, led to a reduction in cariogenicity.
[‡]This mutant was not fully characterised.

terms of their relative cariogenicity in animal models (Table 6.5). Strains of *S. mutans* defective in insoluble glucan synthesis were unable to colonise teeth as effectively as the parent strains, and caused fewer smooth surface caries lesions in an animal model. The synthesis of intracellular storage compounds enables *S. mutans* to continue making acid even in the absence of dietary carbohydrates. Mutants defective in intracellular polysaccharide (IPS) synthesis produced fewer caries lesions than parent strains when inoculated in pure cultures in gnotobiotic rodents. Mutants of *S. mutans* defective in either lactic dehydrogenase or fructosyltransferase (see Chapter 4) activity are also markedly less cariogenic in rat caries models whereas, in contrast, fructanase was shown not to be essential for virulence.

Distinctive characteristics of cariogenic bacteria are:
- the ability to rapidly transport sugars when in competition with other plaque bacteria;
- the rapid conversion of such sugars to acid; and
- the ability to maintain these activities and grow at a low pH.

Few oral bacteria are able to tolerate acidic conditions for prolonged periods, but most strains of mutans streptococci and lactobacilli are not only able to remain viable (survive) at a low pH, but are able to continue to metabolise and multiply, that is, they are **acidogenic** (strongly acid producing) and **aciduric** (acid-loving). Microbial survival in acidic environments depends on the cell maintaining a favourable intracellular pH despite sharp fluctuations in external pH (see Chapter 4), and *S. mutans* achieves this by a number of specific mechanisms (see Table 4.7). Some strains of the anginosus-, mitis- and salivarius-groups of streptococci can also display an acid tolerant phenotype, whereas there can be variation in acid tolerance even among strains of *S. mutans*. Some bacteria can adapt to frequent conditions of sugar exposure and acid production, which eventually increases their acidogenic potential.

CONTEMPORARY PERSPECTIVES ON THE MICROBIAL AETIOLOGY OF DENTAL CARIES

Although many studies have shown an association between mutans streptococci, lactobacilli and dental caries, a consistent feature of most of the clinical studies already described has been the occasional but consistent finding of carious sites from which neither of these two groups of bacteria can be isolated. This suggests that organisms other than mutans streptococci can make a contribution to the demineralisation process, although their mere presence does not inevitably result in disease. Mutans streptococci generally display faster rates of acid production at low environmental pH values, but other streptococci might have greater rates at pH 7.0 and pH 6.0. Such findings reinforce the view that although mutans streptococci are clearly well-equipped biochemically to play a key role in enamel caries, other bacteria can contribute to, and modulate, the strength of the cariogenic challenge at a site. The converse situation is also not uncommon, where mutans streptococci are found in high numbers but in the apparent absence of any demineralisation of the underlying enamel. This may be because of the presence of lactate-consuming species (e.g., *Veillonella*), or to the production of alkali at low pH (e.g., ammonia production by urease or arginine deiminase activities of bacteria such as *S. salivarius* and *S. sanguinis*, respectively).

These findings allow a model to be constructed to explain the changes in the ecology of dental plaque that lead to the development of a caries lesion. Potentially cariogenic bacteria may be found naturally in dental plaque but, at neutral pH, these organisms are weakly competitive and are present only as a small proportion of the total plaque community. In this situation, with a conventional diet, the levels of such potentially cariogenic bacteria are clinically insignificant, and the processes of demineralisation and remineralisation are in equilibrium. If the frequency

of fermentable carbohydrate intake increases, then plaque spends more time below the critical pH for enamel demineralisation (approximately pH 5.5; see Fig. 2.3). The effect of this on the microbial ecology of plaque is twofold. Conditions of low pH favour the proliferation of mutans streptococci and lactobacilli, and tip the balance towards demineralisation. Greater numbers of mutans streptococci and lactobacilli in plaque result in more acid being produced at even faster rates, thereby enhancing demineralisation still further. Bacteria could also adapt to these repeated conditions of low pH, and become even more actively involved in the caries process by producing acid over a wider pH range. Other bacteria could also make acid under similar conditions, albeit at a slower rate, but would contribute to the initial stages of demineralisation, or could cause lesions in the absence of other (more overt) cariogenic species in a susceptible host. This sequence of events would account for the lack of total specificity in the microbial aetiology of caries and explain the pattern of bacterial succession observed in many clinical studies. This model forms the basis of the **ecological plaque hypothesis** (Fig. 6.6). In this hypothesis, caries is a consequence of changes in the natural balance of the resident plaque microbiota brought about by an alteration in local environmental conditions (e.g., repeated conditions of high sugar and low plaque pH). The hypothesis also acknowledges the dynamic relationship that exists between the

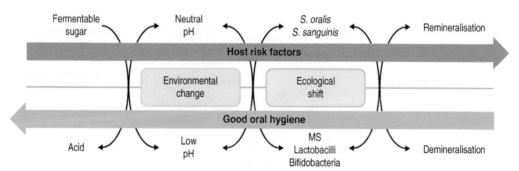

FIGURE 6.6 A schematic representation of the ecological plaque hypothesis in relation to the aetiology of dental caries. Frequent metabolism of fermentable sugars in dental plaque produces regular and prolonged conditions of low pH; this environmental change in plaque favours the growth of acid-tolerating bacteria (such as mutans streptococci [MS], lactobacilli and bifidobacteria) at the expense of species associated with sound enamel. Such a change in the microbiota predisposes a surface to demineralisation. Caries is promoted in individuals who regularly consume fermentable carbohydrates and/or have an impaired saliva flow, whereas good oral hygiene and exposure to optimum levels of fluoride would reduce the risk of demineralisation. Disease could be prevented by not only targeting the putative pathogens, but also by interfering with the factors driving their selection.

microbiota and the host, so that the impact of alterations in key host factors (such as saliva flow) on plaque composition is taken into account. This is of great significance for caries prevention because implicit in the hypothesis is the concept that disease can be controlled not only by targeting directly the putative pathogens (e.g., by inhibition of mutans streptococci by antimicrobial agents) but also by interfering with the factors that are driving the deleterious shifts in the balance of the microbiota (e.g., lowering the acid challenge by reducing the frequency of sugar intake, or by promoting the use of snacks containing sugar substitutes). These, and other caries preventive strategies, will be discussed in a later section.

The concepts behind the original ecological plaque hypothesis have been extended for dental caries to take into account the ability of some bacteria to adapt to acid stress. In this **extended caries ecological hypothesis**, the caries process is divided into three reversible stages (Fig. 6.7). In early biofilms, when acid is produced mainly during main meals (see Fig. 2.3), the acids can be readily neutralised by saliva or by any alkali production in the biofilm, and demineralisation and remineralisation are in equilibrium (the dynamic stability stage). If sugar intake becomes more frequent, then the regular conditions of low pH encourage acid adaptation in some bacteria, which can result in increased acid production. Such conditions start to favour the growth of acidogenic and acid-tolerating strains of streptococci and *Actinomyces*, and the mineral equilibrium is shifted towards demineralisation (the acidogenic stage). If these conditions persist, and the biofilm spends even more time at a low pH, then the most efficient of the acidogenic and aciduric bacterial populations will be selected; these can also adapt to the new conditions and increase their acidogenicity. This aciduric stage further disturbs the mineral balance, and accelerates the progression of caries. In the extended ecological caries hypothesis, environmental acidification acts as the main driving

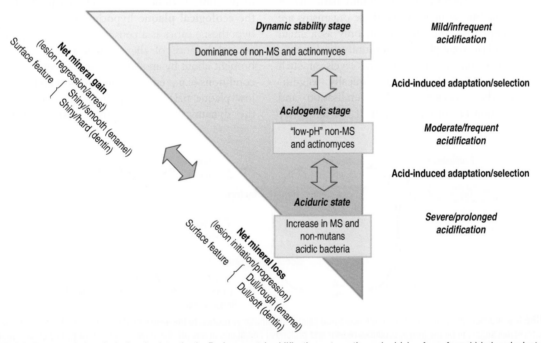

FIGURE 6.7 The extended ecological caries hypothesis. Environmental acidification acts as the main driving force for acid-induced adaptation and acid-induced selection of the microbial community as it passes from the dynamic stability stage via the acidogenic stage to the aciduric stage. Concurrently, caries lesion dynamics shift towards net mineral loss. The reactions can be reversed by elimination of the acid stress. (Reproduced with permission from Marsh PD, Takahashi N, Nyvad B. Biofilms in caries development. In: *Dental caries. The disease and its clinical management.* 3rd Ed. Fejerskov O, Nyvad B, Kidd E eds, 2015;108–131, Oxford: Wiley Blackwell.)

force for both adaptation and enrichment of an acid-tolerating bacterial community.

The ecological plaque hypotheses also define aetiological agents for caries in a different way. Rather than just focusing on the association of particular named organisms in disease, the ecological plaque hypotheses attempt to **define the involvement of microbes on the basis of their properties or functions**. Thus cariogenic bacteria are acidogenic and aciduric, and some species also produce extracellular and intracellular polysaccharides. Such properties will not be unique to a single species in the same way that toxin production can be specific to a medical pathogen such as *Clostridium tetani* (the aetiological agent of tetanus), and could vary among strains of a particular species. Indeed, there will be a spectrum of pathogenic potential among many species of plaque bacteria and even among strains within a species, and bacteria are able to adapt to a low pH environment within the biofilm. In general, however, the organisms that are optimally equipped biochemically to be acidogenic and aciduric belong to the mutans streptococci (these

strains also produce glucans that contribute to the plaque matrix, and they store fermentable intracellular polysaccharides [IPS] produced from sucrose) and lactobacilli, and these organisms are consistently isolated in elevated numbers from caries lesions, but other bacteria (e.g., bifidobacteria) will contribute to a degree that is proportional to their acidogenic/aciduric phenotype.

KEY POINTS

Dental caries is associated with a disruption to the normally beneficial relationship between the microbiota in supragingival plaque biofilms and the host. This disruption (dysbiosis) is driven by an increased frequency of exposure to fermentable dietary sugars, and/or a reduction in saliva flow. This disruption is described by the 'Ecological plaque hypothesis' and the 'Extended caries ecological hypothesis'. Caries can be prevented not only by targeting the putative pathogens but also by modifying the factors driving their selection.

PERIODONTAL DISEASES

The term periodontal diseases embraces a number of conditions in which the supporting tissues of the teeth are attacked. Periodontal diseases are common in developed countries, and are a leading cause of tooth loss (see Chapter 1), and are emerging as risk factors for some systemic diseases (see Chapter 11). In periodontal diseases, the junctional epithelium at the base of the gingival crevice migrates down the root of the tooth to form a periodontal pocket (see Fig. 6.5). This is partly as a result of direct action by the microorganisms themselves, but mainly because of the side-effects of a damaging deregulated inflammatory response mounted by the host in response to plaque accumulation. Thus the aetiology of periodontal diseases does not behave like a classical infectious disease. It is both more subtle and complex in its nature in that it is an exaggerated inflammatory response to an altered resident microbiota driven by changes in the local environment and the lifestyle of the individual.

ECOLOGY OF THE PERIODONTAL POCKET: IMPLICATIONS FOR PLAQUE SAMPLING

As discussed in Chapters 2 and 5, the ecology of the gingival crevice is different to that of other sites in the mouth; it is more anaerobic and the site is bathed in gingival crevicular fluid (GCF). In disease, the crevice becomes a pocket, and the Eh (oxidation-reduction potential; see Chapter 2) falls to low levels (i.e., it is highly anaerobic), whereas the flow of GCF increases significantly in gingivitis and by many fold in periodontitis as part of the host inflammatory response. GCF delivers humoral and cellular defence factors to combat the microbial insult, but it also provides a number of proteins and glycoproteins that can serve as novel substrates for bacterial metabolism, for example iron and haeme-containing molecules such as transferrin and haemoglobin. In contrast to dental caries, many of the bacteria associated with periodontal diseases are asaccharolytic (i.e., cannot metabolise carbohydrates for energy) but are proteolytic. A consequence of proteolysis is that the pH in the pocket during disease becomes slightly alkaline (pH 7.4 to 7.8) compared with near neutral values in health (c. pH 6.9). Likewise, the temperature of the periodontal pocket can increase slightly during inflammation. These changes in environment affect gene expression and alter the competitiveness of periodontal pathogens, thereby changing the natural balance (homeostasis) of the subgingival microbiota to favour the growth of proteolytic and, obligately anaerobic species, many of which are Gram-negative, which leads to dysbiosis (see Fig. 6.1).

The flow of GCF can remove microorganisms not attached firmly to a surface. The cementum surface of the tooth is colonised by Gram-positive bacteria belonging to the genera *Streptococcus* and *Actinomyces*. Many putative periodontal pathogens (*Prevotella, Porphyromonas, Fusobacterium* spp.) can attach to this layer of cells by coaggregation/coadhesion (see Chapter 5). Likewise, black-pigmented anaerobes and *Parvimonas micra* may persist in the pocket because of their ability to adhere to crevicular epithelial cells. Indeed, their attachment to these cells is markedly enhanced when the epithelium has been treated with proteases of bacterial or host origin.

When attempting to determine the microbiota of a periodontal pocket, care has to be taken to preserve the viability of the obligately anaerobic species during the taking, dispersing, diluting and cultivation of the sample (see Chapter 4). Ideally, the sample should be taken from the base of the pocket, near the advancing front of the lesion to avoid removing organisms that are not associated with tissue destruction, and which might obscure any association between specific bacteria and disease activity. Also, it is often difficult to diagnose periodontal diseases accurately, so not all studies are comparing identical pathological conditions. Furthermore, it is not clear whether chronic periodontitis progresses at (a) a continuous slow rate, or (b) by distinct periods of disease activity over relatively short periods of time, followed by phases of quiescence or even repair. This would have implications for sampling strategies, because it would be necessary to remove plaque only during periods of disease activity. The use of rigorous plaque recovery approaches, together with the application of molecular techniques has led to the discovery of organisms never before described. As discussed in Chapter 4, irrespective of whether culture or non-culture-based approaches are used to determine the microbiota, the validity of the data generated will be totally dependent on the quality and relevance of the sample that is taken.

EVIDENCE FOR MICROBIAL INVOLVEMENT IN PERIODONTAL DISEASES

Classical experiments have demonstrated that the accumulation of plaque around the gingival margin in human volunteers reproducibly induces an inflammatory response in the tissues in 10 to 20 days (the experimental gingivitis model). Removal of plaque results in resolution of the inflammatory response. Similarly, plaque control and antibiotic treatment studies have confirmed the essential role of microorganisms in human disease. These latter types of studies, however, can give no information as to whether disease results from the activity of (a) a single, or only a limited number of species (the **specific plaque hypothesis**); or (b) any combination of a wider range of plaque bacteria (the **non-specific plaque hypothesis**) (see earlier). Studies with animals have shown that bacteria, alone or as part of a consortium, can induce bone loss, though sometimes these models require a ligature to be tied around teeth to initiate inflammation.

To test these hypotheses, a large number of cross-sectional epidemiological studies have been performed on patients with particular forms of periodontal disease (see Fig. 6.2). As with dental caries, a disadvantage of this type of study is that true cause-and-effect relationships can never be determined. Microorganisms that appear to predominate at diseased sites might be present as a result of the disease, rather than having actually initiated it. With the exception of gingivitis, longitudinal studies (which do not suffer from this drawback) are not usually possible because of the lengthy natural history of most forms of periodontal disease and the difficulties in predicting subjects and sites likely to be affected. Recently, as with dental caries, the **ecological plaque hypothesis** has been applied to explain the aetiology of periodontal disease. This hypothesis proposes that changes in local environmental conditions in the subgingival region (e.g., the increased flow of GCF that occurs during inflammation, and the resultant increases in pH and temperature) favour the growth of the proteolytic and obligately anaerobic species (many of which are Gram-negative) at the expense of those bacteria seen in health. This results in a shift in the overall balance of the subgingival microbiota (dysbiosis), thereby predisposing a site to disease. A similar set of concepts are developed in the **polymicrobial synergy and dysbiosis** model.

Both hypotheses have been augmented by the **keystone pathogen hypothesis** that proposes that certain bacteria (e.g., *P. gingivalis*) can be present in relatively low numbers but have a disproportionate impact on tissue destruction, by orchestrating changes in the relationship between the host defences and the subgingival microbial community. These hypotheses will be described in relation to periodontal diseases in more detail later in this chapter.

MICROBIOLOGY OF PERIODONTAL DISEASES

The main types of periodontal disease are: (a) gingival diseases; (b) chronic periodontitis; (c) necrotising forms of periodontal diseases; and (d) aggressive periodontitis. Chronic and aggressive periodontitis can be localised or generalised, and there can be modifiers of chronic periodontitis such as diabetes, smoking, certain medications and human immunodeficiency virus (HIV) infection. Periodontitis can also occur as a manifestation of systemic diseases, for example, as a result of haematological disorders (e.g., neutropaenia and leukaemia) or genetic disorders, many of which affect neutrophil function (e.g., Papillon–Lefèvre syndrome, Chediak–Higashi syndrome). There are other rare forms of periodontal diseases that will not be covered in this chapter that are caused by developmental and acquired deformities and conditions, or to endodontic lesions.

In periodontal diseases, there is a shift in the balance of the normal subgingival microbiota (see Fig. 6.1). The healthy gingival crevice has substantial proportions of Gram-positive, facultatively anaerobic bacteria such as *Streptococcus* and *Actinomyces* species together with some obligately anaerobic bacteria (see Table 5.8). The most commonly isolated black-pigmented anaerobe

in the healthy gingival crevice is *Prevotella melaninogenica* although *P. nigrescens* has also been recovered on occasions; *Porphyromonas gingivalis* is rarely isolated from healthy sites. Molecular studies using culture-independent approaches (e.g., 16S rRNA amplification; FISH) have shown that the subgingival microbiota is extremely diverse, even in health, but becomes much richer and more diverse in disease.

GINGIVITIS

Chronic marginal gingivitis is a non-specific, reversible inflammatory response to biofilm accumulation around the gingival margin (Fig. 6.8). If good oral hygiene is restored, then gingivitis is usually eradicated and the tissues becomes clinically normal again (Fig. 6.9). Estimates of the incidence of gingivitis are difficult to determine but probably the whole dentate population is affected by this condition at some stage. Generally, gingivitis is regarded as resulting from a non-specific proliferation of the normal gingival crevice microbiota caused by poor oral hygiene. Gingival diseases can also be modified by systemic factors. The clinical signs are exaggerated and the gingivae are more oedematous and inflamed in individuals undergoing hormonal disturbances (e.g., during puberty or pregnancy), while certain drug therapies (e.g., immunosuppressive drugs) can also result in gingivitis.

The observation in the 1960s that gingivitis develops in a predictable and reproducible manner in volunteers who refrain from oral hygiene permitted the design of longitudinal studies (see Fig. 6.2)

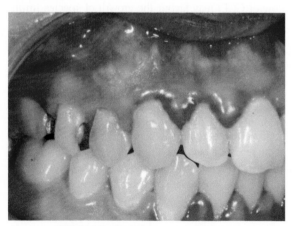

FIGURE 6.8 Clinical image of gingivitis.

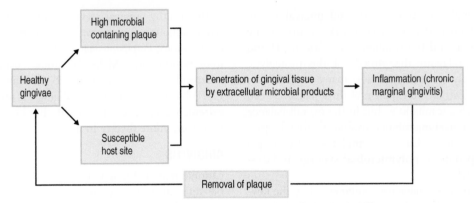

FIGURE 6.9 Schematic diagram of the aetiology of chronic gingivitis.

to determine the bacteriologic events that lead to disease. The microbiota associated with gingivitis is more diverse and differs in overall composition from that found in health. There is an increase (10- to 20-fold) in plaque mass, and there is a shift from the streptococci-dominated plaque of gingival health (see Chapter 5) to one in which *Actinomyces* spp., capnophilic (especially *Capnocytophaga* spp.) and obligately anaerobic Gram-negative bacteria predominate.

Not all sites with gingivitis progress to more serious forms of periodontal disease, but it is accepted that gingivitis must precede periodontitis. Certainly, some species that predominate in periodontitis, but which are not detectable in the healthy gingiva, have been found as a small percentage of the microbiota in gingivitis. This suggests that environmental conditions which develop during gingivitis (e.g., bleeding, increased flow of GCF) may favour the growth of species implicated in periodontitis.

CHRONIC PERIODONTITIS

This is the most common form of advanced periodontal disease affecting the general population, and is a major cause of tooth loss after the age of 25 years (see Chapter 1). It differs from chronic gingivitis in that in addition to the gingivae being involved, there is loss of attachment between the root surface, the gingivae and the alveolar bone, and bone loss itself may occur (Fig. 6.10), giving an increased depth on probi ng (Fig. 6.11), and bleeding. In contrast to gingivitis, these pathologic changes are irreversible. Factors that enhance plaque retention or impede plaque removal,

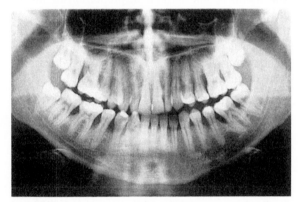

FIGURE 6.10 Radiograph of chronic periodontitis showing extensive bone loss.

such as subgingival calculus, overhanging restorations or crowded teeth, can predispose towards chronic periodontitis.

Early studies of plaque associated with chronic periodontitis relied on microscopy which showed that many of the bacteria in plaque from patients with deep pockets were motile (probably *Campylobacter rectus* and *Selenomonas sputigena*) and spiral-shaped (e.g., *Treponema* spp.). Attempts have been made to use the presence of these morphotypes as the basis of a cheap and rapid test for use in the clinic to monitor the status of a pocket or effectiveness of treatment. Numerous cross-sectional microbiologic culture studies have been performed on different patient groups with pockets of varying depths from numerous geographic regions. Studies agree that the cultivable microbiota is diverse and is composed of large numbers of

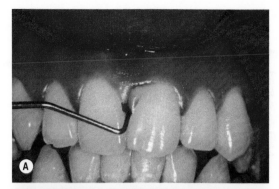

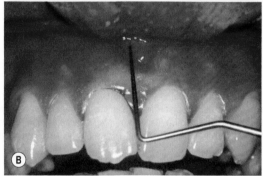

FIGURE 6.11 Use of a periodontal probe to determine the depth of a pocket: (**A**) the probe in situ; (**B**) the probe removed and overlain on the tissues to show the extent of the loss of attachment.

TABLE 6.6 Some of the predominant bacteria that have been commonly cultured from sites with chronic periodontitis in adults

Gram-positive	Gram-negative
Eubacterium brachy	Tannerella forsythia
Eubacterium nodatum	Fusobacterium nucleatum
Mogibacterium timidium	Porphyromonas gingivalis
Parvimonas micra	Prevotella intermedia
Peptostreptococcus stomatis	Prevotella loescheii
	Dialister pneumosintes
	Campylobacter rectus
	Treponema spp.

obligately anaerobic and proteolytic bacteria, many of which are also Gram-negative. Some of the bacteria that have been implicated from cultural studies are listed in Table 6.6.

Studies have implicated certain clusters or complexes of bacteria with disease. In a series of studies, over 13,000 subgingival plaque samples from nearly 200 subjects were screened for the presence of 40 preselected target bacterial species using a molecular approach (a DNA–DNA checkerboard hybridisation technique). Five clusters were identified (Fig. 6.12); the red complex was found most frequently in deeper periodontal pockets, and consisted of *Tannerella forsythia*, *Porphyromonas gingivalis* and *Treponema denticola*, and their presence was often preceded by members of the orange complex, which was also often found in deeper pockets, but was more diverse in membership. In contrast, species of the yellow, green and purple complexes, together with *A. naeslundii*, were considered to be host compatible, and were

generally associated with healthy sites. *Aggregatibacter* (formerly *Actinobacillus*) *actinomycetemcomitans* serotype *b* did not fall within a complex, and is associated more with aggressive periodontitis (see later). Thus, chronic periodontitis appears to result from the activity of mixtures of interacting bacteria, and therefore has a polymicrobial aetiology. There is a progressive change in the composition of the microbiota from health and gingivitis to periodontitis. This change involves not only the emergence of apparently previously undetected species, but also modifications to the numbers, or proportions, of a variety of species already present.

Two theories have been proposed to explain the emergence of previously undetected species. It may be because of the selective growth (enrichment) of a microorganism that is present in health in only very low numbers, caused by a change in the environment during disease. Alternatively, it might be because of the exogenous acquisition of periodontal pathogens from other diseased sites or subjects. The recent application of sensitive molecular approaches has identified low levels of many of the putative pathogens at healthy sites, whereas evidence of transmission of organisms such as *P. gingivalis* and *A. actinomycetemcomitans* between spouses has been obtained. However, in either situation, a major change to the ecology of the habitat has to occur to enable low levels of an

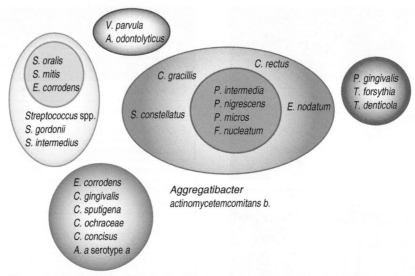

FIGURE 6.12 The grouping of bacteria into complexes to reflect their relationship with the host in health and periodontal disease. The red complex is found most frequently in deep periodontal pockets, and their presence was usually preceded by members of the orange complex. Members of the yellow, green and purple complexes were generally associated with gingivally healthy sites. *Aa, Aggregatibacter actinomycetem-comitans.* (Adapted from Socransky SS, Haffajee AD, Cugini MA, Smith C, Kent RL Jr. Microbial complexes in subgingival plaque. J Clin Periodontol 1998;25:134-144. Published with permission.)

organism to outcompete the existing members of the resident microbiota and reach clinically significant proportions within the subgingival biofilm. The most likely environmental changes capable of causing such a shift in the microbiota are associated with the host inflammatory response (Fig. 6.13). The increased flow of gingival crevicular fluid (GCF) not only introduces components of the host defences but also a range of molecules with the potential to act as novel nutrients for some of the proteolytic bacteria that reside subgingivally. This proteolytic metabolism also leads to a rise in local pH, and so the combination of altered nutrient status and change in environment (in terms of pH, temperature and Eh) would favour the growth of many of the bacteria that have been found to predominate in periodontitis.

The application of molecular methods to characterise the subgingival microbiota of sites with chronic periodontitis has further emphasised the diversity of bacteria found in these sites (Table 6.7). A large proportion of clones identified by 16S rRNA gene sequencing belong to novel phylotypes, some of which have no cultivable representatives. Some studies have detected unculturable examples of *Treponema* spp.

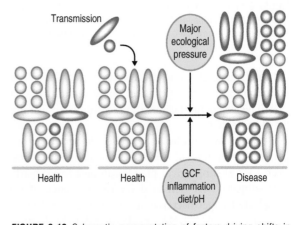

FIGURE 6.13 Schematic representation of factors driving shifts in the balance of the microbiota in health and periodontal diseases. The microbiota of dental plaque is distinct in health and disease. Potential pathogens (shown in red) may be present in low numbers in plaque at healthy sites or transmitted in low numbers from other sites. A major ecological pressure is necessary for such pathogens to outcompete other members of the resident microbiota (green) and achieve the numerical dominance needed for disease to occur.

TABLE 6.7 Bacteria detected directly in subgingival plaque by 16S rRNA sequencing, and implicated in chronic and necrotising periodontal diseases

Named species	Novel phylotype
Fusobacterium animalis	TM7 (clone I025)
Atopobium parvulum	Deferribacteres clones
Atopobium rimae	Selenomonas clone
Cantonella morbid	Desulfobulbus clone
Dialister pneumosintes	Megasphaera clone
Treponema socranskii, T. lecithinolyticum, T. vincentii	Treponema clones
Eubacterium saphenum	Eubacterium clone
Eubacterium nodatum	Desulfobulbus oral taxon
Slackia exigua	Fretibacterium oral taxon
Abiotrophia adiacens	
Filifactor alocis	
Gemella haemolysans	
Streptococcus constellatus	
Campylobacter gracilis	
Campylobacter rectus	
Haemophilus parainfluenzae	
Tannerella forsythia	
Porphyromonas gingivalis	
Porphyromonas endodontalis	
Peptostreptococcus stomatis	
Anaeroglobus germinatus	
Selenomonas sputigena	
Fretibacterium fastidiuosum	

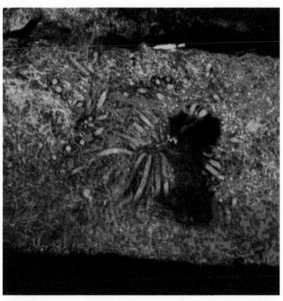

FIGURE 6.14 Unculturable *Treponema* species detected in subgingival plaque by fluorescent in situ hybridization (FISH). Red, *Treponema* spp; green, other bacteria. (Courtesy of Dr Annette Moter and produced with permission (see text on Fig. 3.3, *A*).)

A systematic review of the data from over 40 recent studies of periodontitis, in which culture-independent methods were used, has highlighted an association between 17 species or phylotypes and disease, and some are also listed in Table 6.7. These types of culture-independent studies are changing our views on the role of bacteria in disease. Such studies have confirmed that complex consortia are associated with sites with advanced disease, and that poorly classified organisms that are currently difficult or impossible to grow in the laboratory can predominate in deep pockets. It has yet to be determined whether these organisms are playing an active role in disease or are there as a consequence of tissue destruction (the causal versus casual argument). It is also now accepted that tissue destruction is a consequence of a subverted host inflammatory response to this dysbiotic microbiota. Many bacteria, therefore, might play an indirect role in periodontitis by being part of a microbial community that provokes the host and induces inflammation. In the future it may be possible to routinely screen for the presence of these disease-associated complexes using molecular-based tests, and facilitate improved diagnosis and treatment monitoring.

(Fig. 6.14) or unnamed members of the Obsidian Pool, OB11, and TM7 phylotypes (see Fig. 3.3). Other bacteria that have been recovered almost exclusively from diseased sites include *Treponema socranskii, Filifactor alocis, Dialister pneumosintes, Porphyromonas gingivalis* and *Porphyromonas endodontalis* (Table 6.7).

KEY POINTS

Gingivitis is a reversible condition associated with an increase in plaque mass. There is little evidence to implicate specific bacteria with the onset of inflammation, although the complexity of the microbiota increases, and there is a shift away from a Gram-positive-dominated community to one with larger numbers of Gram-negative obligate anaerobes. Some sites progress to chronic periodontitis in which the gingival crevice deepens to become a periodontal pocket, and there is loss of attachment and bone loss; tissue destruction is irreversible. The microbiota becomes even more diverse; culture-based studies have confirmed the shift to a Gram-negative, obligately anaerobic microbiota, with complexes containing mixtures of species such as *Porphyromonas gingivalis*, *Tannerella forsythia* and a range of spirochaetes being commonly isolated from deep pockets. Culture-independent approaches have found associations between disease and a larger number of novel phylotypes including *Filifactor alocis*, *Synergistetes* (e.g., *Fretibacterium* spp.), *Dialister pneumosintes*, as well as taxa that cannot yet be cultivated (unculturables), such as the TM7 group. Tissue destruction in periodontitis is mainly a consequence of a damaging and subverted host response to these inflammatory consortia.

NECROTISING PERIODONTAL DISEASES

Both necrotising ulcerative gingivitis and necrotising ulcerative periodontitis are included in this category. It is not clear whether these are separate diseases or are part of a single disease process. Both conditions can be manifestations of underlying systemic problems such as HIV infection, and they can be linked to emotional stress and tobacco smoking.

Necrotising ulcerative gingivitis (NUG), also described as Vincent disease, trench mouth, or acute necrotising gingivitis, is a severe form of necrotising inflammation of the interdental papillae, accompanied by spontaneous gingival bleeding and intense pain. It is characterised clinically by the formation of a grey pseudomembrane on the gingivae, which easily sloughs off revealing a bleeding area beneath. NUG can often be diagnosed by the characteristic halitosis (malodorous breath) it produces. Microorganisms can be seen invading the host gingival tissues, and spirochaetes and fusiform bacteria can be observed in smears of the affected tissues (fusospirochaetal complex; Fig. 6.15). Early electron microscopic investigations showed that the invading microorganisms consisted primarily of large and intermediate-sized spirochaetes that were present in the lesions in high numbers and in advance of other microorganisms. A heterogeneous collection of microorganisms has been isolated from ulcerated sites. Various spirochaetes (*Treponema* spp.) were found in high numbers (approximately 40% of the total cell count), but in view of the fusospirochaetal pattern characteristically observed by microscopy, the most unusual finding was the relatively low numbers of *Fusobacterium* spp. and the high

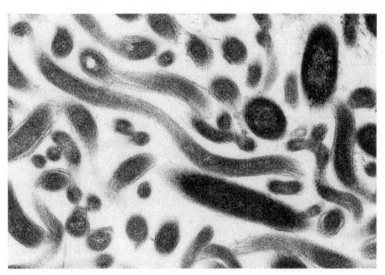

FIGURE 6.15 Electron micrograph of a sample from necrotising ulcerative gingivitis (NUG) showing spirochaetes.

proportions of *Prevotella intermedia*, which averaged 3% and 24% of the total cultivable microbiota, respectively. More recent studies using culture independent approaches (16S rRNA gene sequencing; FISH), have confirmed the predominance of a diverse range of *Treponema* species in lesions, many of which cannot be cultivated, but showed that the fusiform bacteria could belong to a broader range of genera including *Leptotrichia, Capnocytophaga* and *Tannerella* in addition to *Fusobacterium* species. Other non-culturable phylotypes have also been detected, including *Deferribacteres*, and some *Synergistete* taxa. One study also detected increased levels of *Porphyromonas gingivalis, Selenomonas sputigena* and *Actinomyces gerencseriae* in NUG. Metronidazole is effective in eliminating the fusospirochaetal complex from infected sites and this is associated with rapid clinical improvement.

Necrotizing ulcerative periodontitis is a painful condition that affects a small proportion of HIV-positive subjects. Molecular approaches detected a wide range of bacteria including *Bulleida, Dialister, Fusobacterium, Selenomonas, Veillonella*, members of the TM7 phylum, and anaerobic streptococci, although intriguingly some of the more common organisms isolated from periodontal diseases in HIV-negative patients (e.g., *P. gingivalis*) were not recovered.

KEY POINTS

> Necrotising ulcerative gingivitis is a painful, condition, which has a fusospirochaetal aetiology. Culture and molecular studies have detected a range of *Treponema* spp. and fusiform bacteria invading gingival tissues.

AGGRESSIVE PERIODONTITIS

Patients that were diagnosed previously as having localised juvenile periodontitis (LJP), generalised juvenile periodontitis or early onset periodontitis are now described as suffering from aggressive periodontitis (the age-related terminologies have been discarded) that can either be localised or generalised.

Aggressive periodontitis is a rare condition (affecting only around 0.1% of the susceptible age group) which usually occurs in adolescents. The disease appears to start around puberty, is more common in girls, cases often cluster in families, and loss of attachment is rapid. Aggressive periodontitis also shows some

genetic predispositions, being slightly more common in people of West African and Asian origin. Two forms of the disease have been described. In localised aggressive periodontitis there is a distinct pattern of alveolar bone loss that is characteristically localised, for as yet unknown reasons, to the first permanent molars and the incisor teeth (Fig. 6.16). In contrast, a generalised form has been described in which many teeth are affected. The majority of patients with aggressive periodontitis have a variety of functional abnormalities of neutrophils. These abnormalities have been associated with signal transduction pathways, and there is reduced chemotaxis and phagocytosis, but increased superoxide radical production. This deficiency is coupled with, or is a direct cause of, the presence of relatively high numbers of *Aggregatibacter* (formerly *Actinobacillus*) *actinomycetemcomitans*. The microbiota of plaque from patients with aggressive periodontitis is relatively sparse, considering the severity and rapidity of the tissue destruction and bone loss. There are relatively few microorganisms present (approximately 10^6 CFU/pocket) belonging to only a limited number of species, and the majority of these are capnophilic (CO_2-loving) Gram-negative rods. In some culture studies, *A. actinomycetemcomitans* could be recovered from 97% of affected sites and comprise up to 70% of the cultivable microbiota. However, *A. actinomycetemcomitans* can be detected using molecular techniques in low numbers quite commonly at healthy sites in some communities, e.g., 13% in Finland and 20% to 25% in urban U.S.A. This again emphasises the important role of the need for a susceptible host. Affected individuals tend to have elevated serum antibody titres to this microorganism, although its reduction or elimination results in a resolution of disease activity; recurrence of the disease is usually related to the reappearance of *A. actinomycetemcomitans*. These findings have important implications in treatment design because tetracycline is effective in eliminating *A. actinomycetemcomitans* from infected pockets, and resolving the clinical condition. This is in contrast to other forms of chronic inflammatory periodontal disease when metronidazole might be chosen because of its specific action against obligately anaerobic bacteria. Tetracycline does not always lead to complete elimination of *A. actinomycetemcomitans* from the pocket, and the combination of metronidazole and amoxicillin has

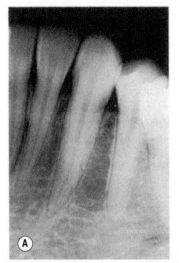

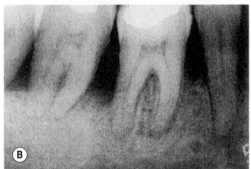

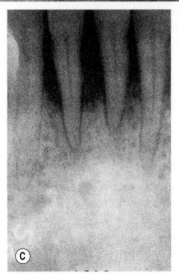

FIGURE 6.16 Radiograph of (**A**) normal periodontium, and (**B**) and (**C**) localised aggressive periodontitis, showing bone loss.

been found to be particularly effective in these situations, particularly when combined with scaling and root planing.

Five serotypes (*a–e*) of *A. actinomycetemcomitans* have been described, and more than one serotype can be found in the mouth of an individual. Strains of *A. actinomycetemcomitans* produce a range of virulence factors, including a powerful leukotoxin (i.e., a protein toxic for neutrophils), lipopolysaccharide (LPS; endotoxin, which can stimulate bone resorption), and cell surface associated material which induces bone resorption. In addition, *A. actinomycetemcomitans* produces enzymes with the ability to degrade collagen, as well as other, less well-defined factors, that modulate the activity of the host defences. *A. actinomycetemcomitans* can also invade gingival connective tissues, and intrafamily transmission of strains may occur.

Molecular studies have provided evidence for the existence of virulent clones. The JP2 clone overproduces the leukotoxin and is found endemically in people from Morocco and other parts of North West Africa. The presence of this JP2 clone in plaque significantly raises the risk of adolescents suffering from aggressive periodontitis (the risk increases 18-fold compared with subjects without *A. actinomycetemcomitans*, although this risk is reduced if sites harbour both JP2 and non-JP2 clones).

In contrast to most other forms of periodontal disease, therefore, localised aggressive periodontitis appears to result from the activity of a relatively specific microbiota dominated by a single species. As stated above, sites have been found in which *A. actinomycetemcomitans* is not necessarily the predominant microorganism, which is analogous to other dental diseases. In these pockets, small spirochaetes, *Eikenella corrodens*, *Wolinella* sp. and *Fusobacterium nucleatum* are often numerous.

In a study of generalised aggressive periodontitis, *Treponema* species were closely associated with disease (including morphotypes that could not be cultured but which could be distinguished by microscopy), as were *F. nucleatum*, lactobacilli, several species of *Eubacterium*, *Parvimonas* spp., *Prevotella intermedia* and *Selenomonas* species. The role, and therefore the significance, of most of these bacteria in disease has yet to be determined.

KEY POINTS

> Aggressive periodontitis is rare, and is associated with functional abnormalities of neutrophils. Plaque from affected sites is sparse but, in the localised form of the disease, often contains *Aggregatibacter actinomycetemcomitans*, strains of which produce a powerful leukotoxin. The presence of the JP2 clone is a major risk factor for subsequent disease, and is found in adolescents originating from North West Africa.

OTHER PERIODONTAL DISEASES

Acute, or exaggerated, forms of gingivitis can arise because of a variety of predisposing factors or circumstances including HIV infection, diabetes, pregnancy, puberty, menstruation, stress, or the use of oral contraceptives.

Pregnancy gingivitis. The exaggerated gingivitis seen in pregnancy is linked to an increase in the proportions of the black-pigmented anaerobe, *P. intermedia*, during the second trimester, possibly caused by the increased levels of steroid hormones in GCF.

Acute streptococcal gingivitis. This condition affects the gingivae which can result in severe illness. The gingivae become red, swollen and full of fluid (oedematous), the temperature is raised and the regional lymph nodes are also enlarged. Lancefield group A streptococci (*S. pyogenes*) can be isolated from the affected gingivae. This disease is usually preceded by a sore throat and hence it is possible that there is a direct spread of *S. pyogenes* from throat to gingivae.

Acute herpetic gingivitis. The majority of infectious cases of gingivitis are bacterial in origin but occasionally viral gingivitis is seen, predominantly in young people. The commonest form is acute herpetic gingivitis, the causative agent of which is herpes simplex type 1 (HSV-1). Acute herpetic gingivitis is seen usually in children and appears as ulcerated swellings of the gingivae which are acutely painful. The symptoms may persist for 7 to 21 days and herpetic lesions may concomitantly be present on lips or any area of the oral mucosa. The diagnosis is usually made on clinical criteria although cytological smears and cytopathic effects following culture have been used for confirmation; direct immunofluorescence is also used for diagnosis. Antiviral agents (e.g., acyclovir and penciclovir) can be effective treatments.

Diabetes mellitus-associated gingivitis. The relationship between diabetes and periodontal disease may be bi-directional (see Chapter 11). Both conditions stimulate the release of proinflammatory cytokines that have a direct effect on the periodontal tissues. In general, patients with diabetes have more severe episodes of gingivitis compared with healthy controls, especially in younger subjects whose condition is poorly controlled. Many of the host response traits that confer susceptibility in periodontal disease in otherwise healthy individuals are exaggerated in diabetics. Susceptibility traits include neutrophil dysfunction, altered cross-linking and glycosylation of collagen, defective secretion of growth factors and subsequent impaired healing. Diseased sites have higher proportions of *Capnocytophaga*, and other periodontal pathogens including *P. gingivalis* and spirochaetes. Sometimes, non-oral bacteria (e.g., staphylococci) have been isolated. These changes in microbiota may reflect a compromised host defence. Periodontal disease may increase insulin resistance in diabetic patients. Periodontal pathogens may raise pro-inflammatory mediators that result in insulin resistance and an increase in blood glucose, thereby predisposing individuals to develop type 2 diabetes. Mechanical treatment of periodontitis, when combined with antimicrobial agents, can improve glycaemic control.

HIV-associated periodontal disease. The impaired immune response in HIV patients can result in colonisation of subgingival sites by opportunistic oral pathogens, such as *Gemella, Dialister, Streptococcus* and *Candida* species. Classical periodontal pathogens, such as *P. gingivalis, T. forsythia* and spirochaetes are not necessarily prevalent.

Noma (cancrum oris). Noma is a severe gangrenous disease that causes a rapid necrotising destruction of soft and hard tissue of the face, including bone. Noma was often fatal before the use of antibiotics such as metronidazole. The classic form of the disease affects young children, although immunocompromised adults can also be affected; the disease is characterised by a strong putrid odour. Noma is most common in Africa, but is also reported in parts of Latin America and Asia. The World Health Organization (WHO) estimated that about 200,000 children under 6 years of age contract noma each year; consequently, noma has been declared a priority by WHO. Risk factors include malnutrition, poor oral hygiene and a compromised immune system caused by, for example, infection with measles, malaria or HIV. The disease process may involve three stages: (a) a staging period, where infection, for example measles, results in a lowered host resistance, and the appearance of oral lesions; (b) an infection period, where some trigger activates a polymicrobial infection; and (c) a tissue invasion and destruction phase, during which an acute ulcerative condition progresses to orofacial gangrene, which is life-threatening. *Fusobacterium necrophorum*, which can be acquired from domesticated livestock, has been isolated from some advanced noma lesions, and has been proposed as the trigger organism for the development of Cancrum oris; infected children are often in regular close contact with animals. Evidence of oral herpes virus, especially cytomegalovirus, has been found in noma patients, and it has been suggested that such an infection could lower local immunity leading to overgrowth by bacterial pathogens. Culture-based studies have recovered *P. intermedia*, streptococci and *Actinomyces* species from lesions, as well as opportunistic pathogens such as staphylococci and pseudomonads. A culture-independent study detected a diverse range of bacteria including 25 phylotypes that had never previously been grown in the laboratory. Bacteria that were unique to noma lesions included members of the genera *Eubacterium, Porphyromonas* and *Treponema*; species more commonly isolated from soil were also detected, and this might reflect the fact that advanced noma lesions are open to the environment. Treatment focuses on improving overall health (e.g., nutritional rehabilitation), administration of broad-spectrum antibiotics and, when possible, introduction of oral hygiene; reconstructive surgery is often necessary once healing is complete.

KEY POINTS

A number of distinct forms of periodontal disease may arise because of a range of predisposing factors, which include: viral infections (HIV, HSV-1), diabetes, and bacterial infection (group A streptococci). Noma is a severe gangrenous disease that often affects young children in the developing world. Risk factors include malnutrition, poor oral hygiene and a compromised immune system.

PATHOGENIC MECHANISMS IN PERIODONTAL DISEASES

Tissue damage can result from the direct action of bacterial enzymes and cytotoxic products of bacterial metabolism but mainly, indirectly, as a consequence of the inevitable side effect of a subverted and exaggerated host inflammatory response to plaque antigens (Fig. 6.17).

INDIRECT PATHOGENICITY

Any subgingival plaque bacterium could be considered to be playing a role in tissue destruction via the indirect pathogenicity route if they contribute to an inflammatory host response. Bacterial antigens can penetrate the crevicular epithelium and stimulate either humoral or cell mediated immunity. Humoral immunity results in the synthesis of immunoglobulins, which are involved in opsonisation and which activate the complement cascade that leads to inflammation and the generation of prostaglandins, which can stimulate bone resorption. Cellular immunity leads to the release of cytokines from activated T-lymphocytes, and these modulate macrophage activity. Activated macrophages release cytokines such as tumour necrosis factor-alpha (TNF-α) and interleukin-1 (IL-1). Both IL-1 and TNF-α can induce collagenase release from a variety of connective tissue cells, including fibroblasts, and cause bone resorption and tissue damage.

Important host tissue cells in the gingival crevice include the pocket epithelium and the periodontal ligament, and these are richly endowed with collagen and glycosaminoglycan (GAG) molecules linked to a protein core. The main proteoglycans of the gingivae and periodontal ligament are hyaluronic acid, heparin sulphate, dermatan sulphate and chondroitin sulphate 4. These proteoglycans can be degraded by elastase and cathepsin B; both enzymes are present in the inflamed gingival crevice, and are probably derived from neutrophils, macrophages and fibroblasts. Mast cells can be found migrating through the junctional epithelium and into the pocket, and can release histamine and other vasoactive molecules, as well as a range of proteases.

Many host cells in the gingival crevice also contain proteinase inhibitors such as α-1-proteinase inhibitor

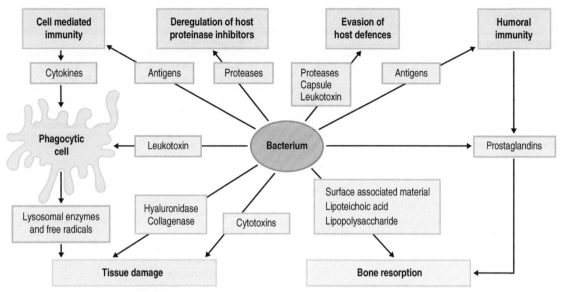

FIGURE 6.17 Diagram to illustrate the mechanisms by which dental plaque can cause damage to host tissues by indirect and indirect routes of pathogenicity.

and α-2-macroglobulin, which are responsible for inactivating proteases in host tissues, thereby theoretically enabling the host to control the potentially destructive forces of the inflammatory response. As will be discussed in the next section, bacterial proteases can degrade these important control molecules, leading to further damage to tissues. Tissue damage in active periodontal disease is due, therefore, to a deregulated and subverted immune response.

DIRECT PATHOGENICITY

The putative pathogens produce a range of potential virulence factors that enable them to:

 (a) colonise and multiply at subgingival sites;
 (b) evade or inactivate the host defences;
 (c) induce tissue damage; and on occasions,
 (d) invade host tissues.

These virulence factors are listed in Table 6.8.

Periodontal pathogens are able to attach to and colonise the subgingival surfaces via bacterial adhesins that interact with specific receptors (see Chapter 5). These receptors may be located either on the root surface or on gingival epithelial cells, or the pathogens may coadhere to already-attached Gram-positive bacteria such as streptococci and *Actinomyces* species. Many of the bacteria that colonise subgingivally are

proteolytic, and produce an array of proteases and glycosidases to obtain nutrients from the catabolism of host molecules; often several species with complementary enzyme profiles combine to break down these complex molecules (see Chapter 5). Bacteria such as *P. gingivalis* also possess haemagglutination and haemolytic activities, which may be a means of targeting appropriate substrates for the release of essential cofactors for growth, such as haemin, from host molecules. Lys-gingipain of *P. gingivalis* plays an essential role in nutrition by obtaining haemin from haemoglobin.

Phagocytic cells form the main defence strategy by the host against periodontal pathogens. Many strains of *A. actinomycetemcomitans* produce a powerful leukotoxin able to lyse human neutrophils, monocytes and a subpopulation of lymphocytes, whereas other cell types (e.g., epithelial and endothelial cells, fibroblasts, erythrocytes) are resistant. *Campylobacter rectus* also produces a leukotoxin. The JP2 clone of *A. actinomycetemcomitans* serotype *b* overproduces the leukotoxin by up to 20 times that seen in other strains, and its presence is a significant risk factor for localised aggressive periodontitis.

Periodontal pathogens express a range of molecules that cause tissue damage by inducing host cells to produce pro-inflammatory cytokines. These molecules

TABLE 6.8   Bacterial factors implicated in the aetiology of periodontal diseases

Stage of disease		Bacterial factor
Attachment to host tissues		Surface components, for example, adhesins Surface structures, for example, fimbriae
Multiplication at a susceptible site		Protease production to obtain nutrients Development of food chains Inhibitor production, for example, bacteriocins
Evasion of host defences		Capsules and slimes Neutrophil-receptor blockers Leukotoxin Immunoglobulin-specific proteases Complement-degrading proteases Suppresser T cell induction
Tissue damage	(a) direct	**Enzymes** 'Arginine-specific' proteases (gingipain) Collagenase Hyaluronidase Chondroitin sulfatase **Bone resorbing factors** Lipoteichoic acid Lipopolysaccharide (LPS) Capsule Surface-associated material. **Cytotoxins** Butyric and propionic acids Indole Amines Ammonia Volatile sulphur compounds
	(b) indirect	Inflammatory response to plaque antigens (see text).

include lipopolysaccharides and other less well-defined cell wall components. Other bacterial components can inhibit the chemotaxis of neutrophils, and interfere with their ability to kill bacteria or phagocytose cells. Bacteria, including *A. actinomycetemcomitans*, also exert an immunosuppressive effect, perhaps mediated by cell surface proteins, whereas *P. gingivalis* possesses a capsule, which protects cells against phagocytosis. *Aggregatibacter actinomycetemcomitans, T. forsythia, P. gingivalis*, and other pathogens may also evade the host defences by invading epithelial cells (see Chapter 4; Fig. 4.7).

The proteases of *P. gingivalis* play a critical role in deregulating the host control of the inflammatory response, and in evading the action of other components of the immune system. Arg-gingipain can inactivate both complement (e.g., by degrading C3 and C5) and antimicrobial peptides (see Chapter 2); a range of proteases can also degrade immunoglobulins (IgA, IgG and IgM) and interfere with the respiratory burst of neutrophils, reducing the likelihood of opsonisation. The maintenance of tissue homeostasis, and the coordination of the innate and adaptive immune response, is dependent on a complex intercellular signalling network mediated by cytokines. Arg-gingipain can also inactivate the two major plasma protease inhibitors, α_1-antitrypsin and α_2-macroglobulin, thereby reducing the ability of the host to regulate the scale and ferocity of the inflammatory response. Expression and activity of these enzymes is upregulated by environmental changes (e.g., by increases in local pH and haemin concentration) that occur during the transition from a normal gingival crevice to a periodontal pocket.

The subgingival microbiota also produces enzymes that may directly damage host tissues in the periodontal pocket. *Porphyromonas gingivalis* produces collagenases, although the majority of the collagen-degrading activity in GCF is host-derived. Once denatured, collagen may be broken down by bacterial proteases with a broader specificity. Other enzymes produced by subgingival bacteria that may damage tissue matrix molecules directly include hyaluronidase, chondroitin sulfatase, and glycylprolyl peptidase. These enzymes can also be detected on outer membrane vesicles of Gram-negative bacteria such as *P. gingivalis* (see Fig. 3.7, *B*); these vesicles can be shed from the bacterial cell surface during growth, enhancing the likelihood of tissue penetration by these enzymes. Once the integrity of the epithelium is impaired, the increased penetration of cytotoxic bacterial metabolites such as indole, amines, ammonia, volatile sulphur compounds (e.g., methyl mercaptan, H_2S), and butyric and propionic acids can induce further damage. Bone loss is a feature of advanced forms of periodontal disease (see Fig. 6.10); bone resorption can be induced by molecules from periodontal pathogens (e.g., LPS, lipoteichoic acid and cell surface-associated proteins).

Microbial invasion of host tissues occurs in periodontal diseases, and is a classic feature of NUG, where there is superficial invasion of the gingival connective tissues by spirochaetes. The persistence of putative pathogens such as *P. gingivalis* in health may be linked to their ability to invade host cells and survive in this privileged site, out of the reach of the host defences.

The invasion of gingival tissue by *A. actinomycetemcomitans* shows some similarities to other intracellular pathogens, such as *Shigella flexneri* and *Listeria monocytogenes*, but there are also unique features, especially with respect to cell-to-cell spread. Contact between *A. actinomycetemcomitans* and a host cell triggers effacement of the microvilli, formation of 'craters' on the host cell surface, and rearrangement of host cell actin at the site of entry. Bacteria appear to enter the host cell through ruffled apertures on the cell surface, and entry occurs in a host-derived, membrane-bound vacuole. The host-derived vacuolar membrane that initially surrounds the internalised bacterial cells soon disappears and cells of *A. actinomycetemcomitans* grow rapidly intracellularly, and spread to neighbouring cells by using host cell microtubules. These protrusions contain cells of *A. actinomycetemcomitans*, and interconnect with other host cells, enabling cell-to-cell spread of the bacteria to occur.

KEY POINTS

> The interaction between the developing subgingival microbiota and the host's immune and inflammatory response is a critical determinant in the balance between health/tissue homeostasis and destructive periodontal disease. Bacterial enzymes, including lys-gingipain, play a key role in sustaining microbial growth by acquiring essential nutrients and cofactors (e.g., haemin) from host molecules such as haemoglobin. Tissue damage can arise via direct (e.g., the action of bacterial enzymes such as collagenase and hyaluronidase, and cytotoxic metabolites such as butyrate and ammonia) but more probably by indirect routes, as an unintended consequence of a subverted and exaggerated host inflammatory response. Bacterial proteases can degrade components of the host defences (immunoglobulins and complement), as well as inhibitors produced by the host to regulate host proteases involved in inflammation. Some periodontal pathogens also evade the host defences by capsule production, or by invading epithelial cells. In this way, the balance can shift in favour of accelerated microbial growth, thereby invoking a further frustrated response by the host when trying to control the microbial assault on the subgingival tissues.

PATHOGENIC SYNERGISM AND PERIODONTAL DISEASE

One of the most consistent features of the microbiology of periodontal diseases is the isolation of complex consortia (complexes) of bacteria from diseased sites (see Fig. 6.12). In particular, in chronic periodontitis, the composition of these mixtures can differ considerably both between and within studies of patients presenting with apparently similar clinical features. This further emphasises that periodontal diseases should not be viewed in the same way as most classical infectious diseases.

For the establishment of disease, organisms must gain access to and adhere at a susceptible site, multiply, overcome or evade the host defences, and then produce or induce tissue damage (see previous section). A large number of virulence traits are needed for each stage in the disease process (Table 6.8), and it is unlikely that any single microorganism will produce all of these factors optimally or in every situation. Thus, tissue destruction is probably a result of consortia of interacting bacteria. In this way, periodontal diseases are a particularly striking example of a **polymicrobial infection,** whereby microorganisms that are individually unable to satisfy all of the requirements necessary to cause disease, combine forces to do so (**pathogenic synergism**). Thus, although a few species (e.g., *Porphyromonas gingivalis, Treponema* spp.) produce enzymes that cause tissue damage directly, the persistence of these 'primary pathogens' in the pocket may be dependent on other organisms to provide means of attachment (e.g., receptors for coaggregation on *Streptococcus* and *Actinomyces* spp.), or essential nutrients for growth (e.g., vitamin K, protohaeme, succinate) via food webs and food chains (see Chapter 5). Similarly, the bacteria that support the growth of the primary pathogens may also require other organisms to suppress or inactivate the host defences, or to inhibit competing organisms (e.g., by bacteriocin production) to ensure their survival. These microorganisms have been termed **accessory pathogens**. Bacteria could also have more than one function in the aetiology of periodontal disease and a schematic diagram illustrating this pathogenic synergism is shown in Fig. 6.18. Our ability to interpret results from future microbiologic studies of periodontal disease would be greatly enhanced if we knew more about the role (or niche; see Chapter 1) of particular species in the disease process. In a polymicrobial infection such as periodontal disease, a microorganism could still be highly significant without necessarily having the potential to cause tissue destruction directly (in other pockets, different bacteria could fill identical roles.

KEY POINTS

Subgingival bacteria may function as a community during the development of periodontal disease. Weakly pathogenic species may pool their metabolic resources to overcome the host defences, obtain nutrients, and persist at a site, and in so doing they create an environment that allows more virulent organisms to flourish (pathogenic synergism).

AETIOLOGY OF PERIODONTAL DISEASE: CONTEMPORARY PERSPECTIVES

Current theories are uniting in recognition that, although microorganisms are necessary for periodontal disease, tissue destruction is an unintended consequence of a dysregulated host response to the growth of a multispecies biofilm composed of a large

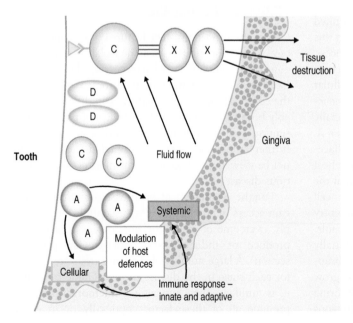

FIGURE 6.18 Pathogenic synergy in the aetiology of periodontal diseases. Bacteria capable of causing tissue damage directly (e.g., species X) may be dependent on the presence of other cells (e.g., organisms C and D) for essential nutrients or attachment sites so that they can grow and resist the removal forces provided by the increased flow of gingival crevicular fluid. Similarly, both of these groups of bacteria may be reliant for their survival on other organisms (e.g., A and C) to modulate the host defences. Individual bacteria may have more than one role (e.g., organism C) in the aetiology of disease. Bacteria that support the growth of the primary pathogens have been termed accessory pathogens.

number of bacteria that are adapted to, and selected by, the inflamed subgingival environment. There is agreement that there is a reciprocal relationship between the local subgingival environment and the microbiota and vice versa, and disease is a consequence when this dynamic relationship is subverted. In simple terms, biofilm accumulation can invoke and deregulate a host inflammatory response, which will change the subgingival microenvironment, which in turn can drive a reorganisation of the composition and activity of the microbiota, resulting in a more aggressive host response, leading to further changes in the environment, and subsequently the selection of communities of microorganisms that are even more suited to the prevailing conditions (the **ecological plaque hypothesis** (Fig. 6.19) and the **polymicrobial synergy and dysbiosis** model). What follows is a continuous sequence of positive feedback loops that drives a vicious circle of an ever increasingly damaging and locally uncontrolled immune response to an adapting microbiota. In different patients, and even at distinct sites in the same patient, the same pathologic processes may be driven by different combinations of bacteria. Thus, the current paradigm is moving away from disease being caused by a specific organism, or even a group of a limited number of species (i.e., beyond just the red complex; see Fig. 6.12),

to a situation in which combinations of interacting bacteria respond to and drive tissue damage by disrupting the host-microbe equilibrium and subverting the normally protective host response. Implicit in the ecological plaque hypothesis is that disease can be prevented not only by targeting the putative pathogens, but also by interfering with the environmental factors that drive the changes in the balance in the microbiota, for example by reducing the severity of the inflammatory response, or by altering the redox potential of the pocket to prevent the growth of the obligate anaerobes (see Fig. 6.19).

Innate immunity is the first line of defence in the clinically healthy gingival crevice, and the tissues are under constant immune surveillance (see Chapter 2). Host cells in the periodontium express toll-like receptors (TLRs) which are pattern-recognition receptors enabling the host to detect and respond to conserved molecules on microorganisms, termed PAMPs (pathogen-associated molecular patterns) or MAMPS (microbe-associated molecular patterns). MAMPs include molecules such as lipopolysaccharides and lipoteichoic acid in Gram-negative and Gram-positive bacterial cell walls, respectively. TLRs continually interact with the subgingival biofilm, and are able to activate innate immune cells via complex intracellular signalling pathways. TLR signalling upregulates the production of host defence

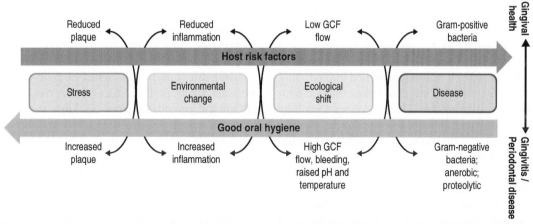

FIGURE 6.19 A schematic representation of the ecological plaque hypothesis in relation to periodontal disease. Plaque accumulation produces an inflammatory host response; this causes changes in the local environmental conditions which favour the growth of proteolytic and anaerobic bacteria, many of which are Gram-negative. The risk of disease is increased if the host has abnormalities in their host defences, or they have other risk factors such as tobacco smoking, whereas effective oral hygiene will reduce the likelihood of disease. Disease could be prevented by not only targeting the putative pathogens, but also by interfering with the factors driving their selection.

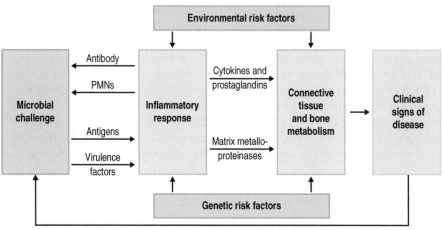

FIGURE 6.20 A schematic representation of the interrelationships between the host and dental plaque in periodontal disease. PMNs, polymorphonuclear leukocytes (mainly neutrophils).

peptides such as β-defensins, cathelicidin and calprotectin (see Chapter 2), as well as interleukin-8 (IL-8), which is now regarded as a chemokine (CXCL8) as it can induce chemotaxis. These defences are highly coordinated and tightly regulated, and there is only a low level expression of inflammatory mediators in healthy tissue. The expression of E-selectin on the vascular endothelium of the periodontium facilitates neutrophil exit into the surrounding tissues. The clinically healthy junctional epithelium expresses high levels of CXCL8 (IL-8), which is a potent neutrophil chemoattractant, and other chemokines such as intracellular adhesion molecule-1 (ICAM-1). ICAM-1 and CXCL8 (IL-8) expression increases from the basal cells toward the surface of the junctional epithelium and guide neutrophils towards areas exposed to potential bacterial challenges. It has been calculated that in health, approximately 30,000 neutrophils transit through periodontal tissue every minute. These processes contribute to the maintenance of a local host-microbe equilibrium and to the limitation of possible neutrophil-associated tissue damage. Some commensal bacteria engage in cross-talk with host cells to downregulate proinflammatory tendencies (see Chapter 4). Periodontal health, therefore, is a dynamic state in which proinflammatory and antimicrobial activities are balanced by antiinflammatory mechanisms to prevent unwarranted inflammation.

This highly ordered and tightly regulated situation can break down if biofilm continues to accumulate, and this can lead to periodontal disease (Fig. 6.20). A failure of the innate host defences to control biofilm development, perhaps coupled with other host-related factors (e.g., smoking, or immunocompromised patients/individuals with an impaired immune response) and ineffective plaque control, leads to an increased expression of inflammatory mediators that are normally present only in small amounts (such as Toll-like receptor-2), whereas different inflammatory molecules (such as Toll-like receptor-4) can be switched on.

The epithelial cells that line the gingival crevice are the first to respond to MAMPs. They express ICAM-1 and CXCL8 (IL-8) to enhance the migration of neutrophils. However, they also produce matrix metalloproteinases (MMPs) and reactive oxygen species in response to MAMPs, and these can cause tissue damage by degrading matrix and basement membrane components. Neutrophils produce reactive oxygen species (ROS) and proinflammatory cytokines such as IL-1, IL-6 and tumour necrosis factor (TNF-α) when stimulated by interaction of TLRs with MAMPs, and these cytokines can promote bone resorption and induce tissue degrading proteinases. The bacterial community can continue to provoke the host via surface antigens, soluble antigens and cytotoxins; antigenic molecules are also released extracellularly on membrane vesicles. Some subgingival bacteria are able to invade or damage the gingival epithelial barrier. This leads to activation of TLRs on other host cells, including macrophages, fibroblasts, dendritic cells, osteoblasts and osteoclasts.

Further cytokines are induced that activate T-lymphocytes to produce a Th-1 or Th-2 or Th-17 immune response, resulting in the production of specific antibodies and the release of a greater range of proinflammatory cytokines, chemokines, and biologic mediators such as prostaglandins and MMPs. Thus, there is an escalation in the host response with an increasing risk of self-induced tissue damage.

If these destructive processes continue, there is further reorganisation of the biofilm with the selection of a community that is even more subversive. Connective tissue attachment to the tooth is lost, and epithelial cells migrate apically along the root surface creating an ever deepening periodontal pocket that, if left untreated, can lead to the eventual loss of the tooth. The shift from a symbiotic microbiota to a dysbiotic, pathogenic community triggers the potent host inflammatory response that drives the tissue destruction and alveolar bone loss that is characteristic of periodontitis.

The response of the host to biofilm accumulation leads to an increased flow of gingival crevicular fluid (GCF) which delivers more components of the innate and adaptive host response, including complement (see Fig. 6.21). Complement is a cascade system involving a network of proteins and receptors that play a fundamental role in immunity. Complement is essential for opsonisation and phagocytosis, and direct lysis of targeted microorganisms. Some periodontal pathogens, for example P. gingivalis, are resistant to complement by means of the action of their gingipains and the synthesis of an alternative LPS. Crucially, however, GCF also delivers an array of other molecules that, coincidentally (and unintentionally), can also act as a source of nutrients for some normally minor components of the subgingival microbiota. In general, the putative periodontal pathogens are non-competitive with other members of the resident subgingival microbiota at healthy sites, but GCF provides molecules, such as transferrin and haemoglobin, that are a potential source of nutrients and essential growth cofactors for many of the proteolytic Gram-negative anaerobes that predominate in advanced periodontal lesions. This metabolism also leads to an increase in local pH and a fall in the redox potential (i.e., the pocket becomes slightly alkaline and more anaerobic), and there is a small rise in temperature as a result of the inflammatory response, which will favour their growth still further.

These changes in the local environment (increased pH, temperature and availability of essential cofactors such as haemin) can upregulate expression of some of the virulence factors associated with these putative pathogens (e.g., gingipain activity by P. gingivalis), and favour their growth at the expense of the species associated with gingival health (i.e., increase the competitiveness of the potential pathogens). For example, even the small rise in temperature associated with the host inflammatory response, together with the increased presence of haemin, can result in P. gingivalis altering the structure of its cell wall and the production of an LPS with an atypical structure. This modified LPS antagonises activation of TLR-4-dependent antimicrobial pathways, and helps to protect not just this organism but also the whole microbial community from the host response.

The role of P. gingivalis within a subgingival community has attracted a great deal of attention. Although this species can be found in health on occasions, it is present in very low numbers, but its growth is favoured by the changes in the biology of the inflamed pocket. Factors that are associated with its virulence are upregulated and it is argued that P. gingivalis can then play a significant part in the subversion of the host defences, and in manipulating the composition of the biofilm. For these reasons, P. gingivalis has been described as a **keystone pathogen**. A keystone pathogen plays a disproportionately important role in disease relative to its numbers within a microbial community. Its presence at a site may also be dependent on the properties of other bacteria, for example, factors that facilitate colonisation, help to inactivate the host defences, and contribute to the nutritional needs of P. gingivalis. These bacteria are termed **accessory pathogens**, and the enhanced virulence of the microbial community is referred to as **pathogenic synergism** (see Fig. 6.18). Bacteria other than P. gingivalis may also function as keystone pathogens.

Porphyromonas gingivalis can manipulate host immunity enabling overgrowth by other bacteria, thereby helping to tip the balance towards dysbiosis. Amongst other damaging attributes, P. gingivalis can:

- invade gingival epithelial cells and prevent production of CXCL8 (IL-8) by means of its serine phosphatase (a process termed 'local chemokine paralysis');

- transiently inhibit upregulation of E-selectin thereby interfering with neutrophil adhesion and migration;
- interfere with complement activation, by gingipain-mediated degradation of the central complement component, C3, thereby benefitting other subgingival pathogens, and resist complement-mediated lysis by expression of a novel form of LPS;
- degrade key host regulatory components, such as host protease inhibitors, and host defence peptides;
- subvert TLR2 and TLR4 responses; and
- produce cytotoxins.

The overall dynamics of the interactions between the host and subgingival biofilms in periodontal diseases are summarised in Figure 6.21.

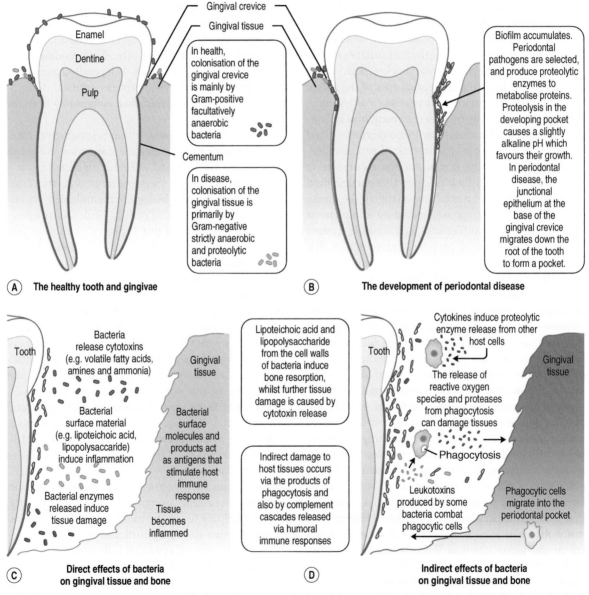

FIGURE 6.21 A schematic representation of the interactions between the host defences and the adapting subgingival biofilm during the development of a periodontal pocket.

KEY POINTS

> Periodontal diseases are a consequence of a deleterious shift in the balance of the subgingival microbiota (dysbiosis) in response to changes in local environmental conditions due to the host inflammatory response. The microbiota becomes more diverse, but some low abundance species may play a pivotal role in orchestrating disease (keystone pathogens). Tissue damage is mainly a consequence of a subverted and exaggerated host response to the dysbiotic biofilm.

PERIODONTAL DISEASES AND SYSTEMIC DISEASE

The periodontium is highly vascular, and this means that many of the bacteria and proinflammatory molecules described above can enter the circulatory system and potentially affect sites and systems elsewhere in the body. In this way, periodontal diseases have been reported as risk factors for atherosclerosis, rheumatoid arthritis, diabetes and chronic obstructive pulmonary disease. Periodontal diseases have also been associated with pregnancy complications and aspiration pneumonia. The possible association between periodontal and systemic diseases will be described in Chapter 11.

In this important clinical area, there is a need for further large, well-controlled investigations in diverse but homogeneous population groups, in which the statistical analyses are adequately adjusted for other lifestyle confounding risk factors (smoking, alcohol consumption, maternal education, etc.). Longitudinal, prospective studies are also needed to determine whether the observed periodontal disease is causal for these medical sequelae. The outcome of intervention studies, in which the impact of periodontal treatment on the subsequent development of systemic disease is monitored, will be crucial in confirming the impact of oral disease on general health.

APPROACHES FOR CONTROLLING PLAQUE-MEDIATED DISEASES

Mechanical removal of plaque by efficient oral hygiene procedures can almost completely prevent plaque-mediated diseases. Plaque control can be achieved by conventional oral hygiene measures such as toothbrushing and flossing, which can be augmented by professional prophylaxis during routine visits to the dentist. Plaque control is fundamental to the prevention of gingivitis and in the maintenance of health following effective treatment. In chronic periodontitis, debridement of the root surfaces is the most effective routine approach for plaque control, although it is not possible to completely remove all of the attached microorganisms. In aggressive periodontitis, root planing may be supplemented with adjunctive systemic antimicrobial agents (see later). For caries, plaque control measures are particularly effective when combined with a reduction in the amount and frequency of sugar intake. It is difficult to alter established eating habits and to maintain a high degree of motivation for effective oral hygiene. Alternative preventive measures for caries and periodontal diseases are under development that require little cooperation from the public. Occlusal pits and fissures are the most caries-prone areas of the human dentition. Strongly adherent, self-polymerising and ultra violet (UV)-light polymerising plastic sealant materials have been applied to fissures as a barrier against microbial attack. The long-term retention of these materials in the mouth can be problematic.

Rather than regarding oral health as a state that is merely the absence of disease, approaches are being developed that are designed to actively promote oral health and well-being. The success of these approaches will depend on a greater understanding of the factors that underpin health, and promotion of oral health may require different strategies in different people.

FLUORIDE

It has been known for many decades that fluoride in the water supply can significantly reduce the incidence of caries. The caries benefit of fluoride was established from epidemiologic surveys that showed a reduced caries incidence in certain geographical locations; the factor that correlated with protection was the natural fluoride content of the water supply. The optimum concentration for maximal protection against caries is approximately 1 part per million (1 ppm), but in some water supplies it occurs naturally at higher concentrations. Fluoride is also found in tea and in the bones of fish (especially soft-boned sardines and salmon). Excessive exposure to fluoride can cause fluorosis, which in extreme cases results in discolouration of teeth. Despite its proven value in decreasing caries incidence, the addition of fluoride to drinking water remains a controversial and emotive issue. Consequently, fluoride has been used to supplement other commodities (e.g., table salt, milk, toothpastes), so consumers can have a choice as to whether or not they want to gain further caries benefit. Fluoride can also be used in mouthwashes and gels for topical use, and in tablets for supplementation of the systemic effect, and has also been incorporated into topical varnishes and slow-release capsules. High concentrations of fluoride are used to treat caries-vulnerable groups, including xerostomic and disabled patients.

The precise mechanisms behind the anticaries mechanisms of fluoride are still the subject of much debate. The original studies concluded that fluoride needed to be present preeruptively, so as to be incorporated into developing teeth. More recent evidence suggests that fluoride functions posteruptively by favourably influencing the kinetics of demineralisation and remineralisation. Thus, fluoride can exert its effect on erupted teeth both topically (e.g., following the use of fluoridated toothpastes) and systemically after ingestion (e.g., via fluoridated water or milk). Low levels of fluoride appear in oral fluids (saliva, GCF) and interact with the surface of the enamel of erupted teeth to form fluorapatite. Fluorapatite is thermodynamically more stable than apatite and resists acid dissolution to a greater extent than hydroxyapatite.

Fluoride can also inhibit the metabolism of plaque bacteria (Fig. 6.22) thereby affecting their competitiveness especially at low pH. Under acidic conditions, fluoride exists as HF, which is lipophilic and is able to easily cross bacterial membranes. The intracellular pH of bacteria is alkaline with respect to the extracellular pH; therefore, once inside the cell, HF will dissociate and H$^+$ will acidify the cytoplasm and:

(1) inhibit various enzymes with pH optima near neutrality;
(2) reduce the transmembrane pH gradient, thereby affecting some uptake and secretion processes; whereas F- will:
(3) reduce glycolysis by direct inhibition of enolase;
(4) indirectly inhibit sugar transport by blocking the production of phosphoenolpyruvate (PEP) for the phosphotransferase system (PTS; see Chapter 5); and

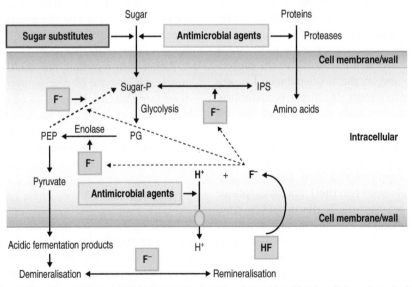

FIGURE 6.22 The site of action of some classes of inhibitors used in dentistry. *F*, Fluoride; *IPS*, intracellular polysaccharide; *PG*, phosphoglycerate; *PEP,* phosphoenolpyruvate.

(5) inhibit the synthesis of IPS compounds, especially glycogen.

Dental plaque has been found to concentrate fluoride from ingested water. In areas where the concentration of fluoride in the water supply is low, dental plaque has been found to contain 5 to 10 parts per million (ppm). In water supplies supplemented with 1 ppm fluoride, concentrations of up to 190 ppm have been found in dental plaque. Much of this fluoride is bound to organic components in plaque, but there is also evidence that it can be released when the pH falls, and be bioavailable to interfere with acid production by plaque bacteria. The sensitivity of oral bacteria to fluoride increases as the pH falls, so that concentrations of fluoride that are ineffective at resting pH values can be inhibitory at pH 5.0 or below. Mutans streptococci are particularly sensitive to low levels of fluoride at a moderately low environmental pH. Although surveys have failed to detect major changes in the qualitative and quantitative composition of plaque in humans residing in places with high or low natural levels of fluoride in the drinking water, fluoride is more likely to function prophylactically in these circumstances. Thus, mutans streptococci would be suppressed in plaque under conditions when they would otherwise be expected to flourish; the rate of change of pH in plaque following sugar metabolism would also be diminished. This influence on metabolism and pH will nullify the expected competitiveness that aciduric bacteria such as *S. mutans* and lactobacilli normally experience after sugar intake relative to organisms associated with enamel health. Studies have shown that sufficient fluoride to affect the growth and metabolism of *S. mutans* can be released by acid attack from a fluoride-containing surface. Thus, fluoride can serve to stabilise the composition of the plaque microbiota, a preventative mechanism that is consistent with the ecological plaque hypothesis. This antimicrobial effect can be enhanced by changing the counter-ion; thus, stannous fluoride is markedly more inhibitory to oral bacteria than sodium fluoride. Other antimicrobial agents will be discussed in the next section.

ANTIMICROBIAL AGENTS

For many individuals, it is difficult to maintain plaque at levels compatible with health by oral hygiene alone over prolonged periods. Consequently, the use of antimicrobial agents (not including antibiotics) to augment mechanical plaque control has been advocated for a number of years. These agents can be formulated into oral care products such as toothpastes and mouthrinses; they have been shown to reduce plaque, and some have anticaries and antigingivitis benefits. The relatively short contact time between the inhibitor delivered from the product and the mouth dictates that it is essential that the agents bind effectively to oral surfaces, especially mucosal tissues (because of their large surface area); this property is termed **substantivity**. Once adsorbed, such inhibitors are released slowly from these reservoirs back into the oral environment (especially saliva), from where they can be redistributed around the mouth. In this way, effective agents can reduce the growth or metabolism of microorganisms for prolonged periods even at sub-lethal concentrations (see Fig. 6.22). Some products are antiplaque rather than antimicrobial, for example, they detach plaque without necessarily killing the microorganisms in the biofilm. Some examples of antimicrobial agents that have been successfully formulated into oral care products are listed in Table 6.9. Some agents that are used in

TABLE 6.9 **Classes and examples of inhibitors used as antimicrobial agents in mouthwashes and toothpastes**

Class of inhibitor	Examples
Bisbiguanide	Chlorhexidine, alexidine
Enzymes	Mutanase, glucanase; amyloglucosidase-glucose oxidase-lactoperoxidase system
'Essential oils'	Thymol, eucalyptol
Metal ions	Copper, zinc, stannous
Natural molecules	Exogenous: plant and herbal extracts; propolis; polyphenols Endogenous: lactoferrin, lysozyme, immunoglobulins
Phenols	Triclosan
Quaternary ammonium compounds	Cetylpyridinium chloride
Surfactants	Sodium lauryl sulphate

mouthrinses cannot be formulated into toothpastes because of compatibility issues with other components of the dentifrice.

One of the most effective antimicrobial agents for oral use is chlorhexidine, which can be successfully formulated into a mouthrinse. This bisbiguanide has a broad spectrum of activity against yeasts, fungi, and a wide range of Gram-positive and Gram-negative bacteria. Chlorhexidine can reduce plaque, caries, and gingivitis in humans; it is not recommended for prolonged use because of side-effects such as staining of teeth and mucosal irritation. At high concentrations, chlorhexidine is bactericidal and damages the cell membrane. Chlorhexidine is substantive, and is bound to oral surfaces from where it is released gradually into saliva over many hours at bacteriostatic concentrations. At these sublethal concentrations, chlorhexidine can still:

(1) abolish the activity of the PTS sugar transport system (see Chapter 5) and thereby markedly inhibit acid production in streptococci;
(2) inhibit amino acid uptake and catabolism in some streptococci;
(3) inhibit a major protease (arg-gingipain) of *Porphyromonas gingivalis*; and
(4) affect various membrane functions, including the adenosine triphosphate (ATP)-synthase and the maintenance of ion gradients in streptococci (see Fig. 6.22).

Mutans streptococci are more sensitive to chlorhexidine than other oral streptococci, and this property has been exploited in those people at high risk of developing caries. Levels of mutans streptococci in the mouth have been reduced by the use of chlorhexidine mouthrinses whereas other oral streptococci, such as *S. sanguinis* (associated more with enamel health), were relatively unaffected. This approach has also been applied successfully to pregnant women. The suppression of mutans streptococci in mothers reduced the transmission of these potentially cariogenic organisms to the baby and delayed the onset of caries.

Chlorhexidine can be delivered either by gel (e.g., as a 1% gel in a custom-fitted vinyl applicator), as a mouthrinse, or as a varnish. Combinations of chlorhexidine with other agents such as fluoride or thymol in varnishes has resulted in additive or synergistic benefits, for example, in preventing caries in high risk patients such as those receiving radiation therapy for head and neck cancer. In these patients, the radiation therapy affects the salivary glands, and the reduced saliva flow is conducive to rampant caries.

Triclosan is a commonly used antimicrobial agent in toothpastes. Triclosan has a broad spectrum of antimicrobial activity against yeasts and a wide range of Gram-positive and Gram-negative bacteria. However, under conditions of use in the mouth (i.e., high concentrations + short contact time; low concentrations + longer contact time), Triclosan has a more selective antimicrobial profile, and preferably inhibits the obligately anaerobic, Gram-negative species that are prevalent in periodontal disease. Like chlorhexidine, Triclosan is also substantive and multi-functional in its mode of action. At sub-lethal concentrations, it can inhibit acid production by streptococci and protease (arg-gingipain) activity by *P. gingivalis*. Triclosan is also antiinflammatory, which may enhance its effectiveness in preventing gingivitis, and reduces the development of new aphthous ulcers in sufferers. The activity of Triclosan has been enhanced by combining it with either a copolymer to boost its oral retention, or with zinc citrate as a complementary antimicrobial agent. Zinc ions are also substantive and can inhibit sugar transport, acid production, and protease activity. There have been concerns raised over the widespread use of Triclosan. This compound has been found to accumulate in environmental samples, while repeated exposure to Triclosan has been linked with increased resistance of some microorganisms to important antibiotics.

Enzymes and essential oils have also been included in toothpastes. Examples include dextranases and glucanases (from fungi) to modify the plaque matrix and reduce plaque formation (see Chapter 5). One product is formulated with three enzymes [glucose oxidase + amyloglucosidase + lactoperoxidase] to boost the activity of the salivary peroxidase (sialoperoxidase) system, together with three natural host defence factors [lysozyme, lactoferrin and immunoglobulins] (see Chapter 2).

There has been an upsurge of interest in the use of natural products and traditional medicines, especially those derived from plants and herbs. Many of these compounds inhibit virulence traits of oral bacteria, such as glucan synthesis and acid production. Essential oils (menthol, thymol, eucalyptol, etc.) have been successfully formulated into a mouthwash and shown to penetrate plaque biofilms. Regular use of a mouthwash containing essential oils can reduce plaque and gingivitis over a six-month period in clinical trials, and also reduce halitosis. The oils function by disrupting bacterial cell membranes and inhibiting key enzymes. Inhibitors of mineralisation, such as polyphosphonates, zinc salts, and pyrophosphates, can reduce calculus formation (see Chapter 5).

Changes in public attitudes to the incorporation of synthetic agents in over-the-counter oral care products has led to an increased interest in exploiting the antimicrobial properties of natural compounds that are found in extracts from plants or herbs, and which have been used in traditional medicines. Many of the active ingredients are polyphenol compounds, for example, from green tea or oolong tea, coffee and so on, and not only inhibit bacterial growth but also affect metabolic traits such as glucosyltransferase activity and acid production. Propolis is produced by bees, and has some antibacterial and antifungal activity, and the active constituents include flavonoids. A challenge with the use of natural products for commercial use is their inherent seasonal and geographic variability in composition and activity.

Potentially, the regular, unsupervised use of antimicrobial agents from toothpastes and mouthrinses could lead to the disruption of the ecology of the oral microbiota by either (a) perturbing the balance among the resident organisms, which might lead to the overgrowth by potentially more pathogenic species, or (b) the development of resistance. Guidelines are now laid down to ensure that manufacturers perform long-term clinical trials to confirm that these eventualities do not occur. The reason why oral care products containing antimicrobial agents are able to deliver clinical benefit without unduly disturbing the resident microbiota of the mouth is probably because of the active agents functioning in a selective manner under the conditions of use (short contact time; increased tolerance of biofilms to inhibitors; see Chapter 5) in the oral cavity (e.g., Triclosan preferentially inhibits obligate anaerobes rather than the whole microbiota). In this way, these agents could function prophylactically to control the composition and metabolism of the biofilm without killing bacteria that might also provide benefit to the host (see Chapter 4).

In more advanced forms of periodontal disease, treatment requires professional plaque control which in some circumstances may require surgery so that clear access to the root surface is achieved. In extreme cases, not only is there a need to remove plaque and/or calculus, but also the outer surface layers of cementum (root planing), because of the possible penetration into cementum of cytotoxic or inflammatory products of subgingival bacteria, especially endotoxin (LPS). Bacteria may still persist and survive because of their invasion of epithelial cells, resulting in sites becoming repopulated rapidly leading to further loss of attachment in some pockets. Consequently, post-surgical control of microorganisms is sometimes necessary. This again can involve meticulous supragingival plaque control (to reduce the likelihood of subgingival colonisation) or the use of antimicrobial agents, such as chlorhexidine, or even systemic antibiotics, such as tetracycline, amoxicillin or metronidazole. Antibiotics should only be used in special circumstances, such as some forms of aggressive periodontitis or in refractory periodontal disease, because of the global problems of antibiotic resistance (see Chapter 10). A potential strategy to treat periodontal pockets is to locally apply antimicrobial agents such as chlorhexidine, metronidazole and tetracycline.

SUGAR SUBSTITUTES

Most humans enjoy and prefer to eat sweet substances. Unfortunately, many sweet foods are composed of monosaccharides or disaccharides, which are easily metabolised by plaque bacteria to acids and glucans, thereby predisposing teeth to dental caries. The use of inert (non-metabolisable) dietary sweeteners has been proposed to satisfy the human preference for sweet substances without causing caries. These sugar substitutes function by stimulating saliva flow in the absence of a significant acid challenge to enamel; indeed, the use of these agents can sometimes lead to the remineralisation of enamel.

Artificial sweeteners are of two types: (a) the intense type many times sweeter than sucrose, and (b) the bulk agents, which are usually not as sweet. The intense sweeteners include cyclamate, aspartame and saccharin, and are used in drinks. These sweeteners have some weak antimicrobial effects, with aspartame and saccharin being capable of inhibiting bacterial growth. The bulk agents, for example, polyols such as sorbitol and xylitol, are not as sweet as sucrose, but cannot be metabolised by the majority of plaque bacteria and are used in the confectionery industry. Other polyols include mannitol, lactitol, Lycasin® (a mixture of sorbitol, mannitol, maltotriitol, and polysaccharide alcohols), and Palatinit® (a mixture of two 12-carbon polyols). Some of these polyols have been incorporated into sugar-free chewing gums; the use of these products three or more times a day can reduce the incidence of caries, by reducing the frequency of acid attack on the enamel (see Fig. 2.3) and by stimulating saliva flow, thereby encouraging remineralisation. Xylitol has been claimed to be superior to other sugar alcohols because of its effect on bacterial metabolism. Xylitol is transported into cells of mutans streptococci by the fructose-PTS where it enters a futile cycle of phosphorylation, dephosphorylation and eventual expulsion. This futile cycle reduces the rate of growth and acid production (from exogenous sugars such as glucose) of cells, and leads to reduced levels of both mutans streptococci and caries in habitual users of xylitol-containing confectionery. The use of sugar substitutes is consistent with the ecological plaque hypothesis, because the prevention of periods of low pH in plaque between meal periods would remove opportunities for the preferential growth of acid-tolerating bacteria.

FUTURE DIRECTIONS

Replacement therapy, prebiotics and probiotics. The possibility that antagonistic microorganisms could be exploited to control pathogens and prevent disease has been proposed for over 100 years, and is termed **replacement therapy**. A major potential benefit of this approach is that it could provide lifelong protection with minimal cost or compliance on behalf of the recipient once colonisation by an effector strain has been achieved. There are two main approaches: (a) preemptive colonisation, where key ecologic niches (functions) within plaque are filled by a harmless or beneficial organism before the undesirable strain has had a chance to colonise or become established. The initial coloniser becomes integrated into the ecosystem and subsequently excludes the pathogen. Low-virulence mutants of mutans streptococci have been produced that are deficient in glucosyltransferase (GTF) activity or intracellular polysaccharide production, or which lack lactate dehydrogenase activity, and are designed to prevent subsequent colonisation by wild-type mutans streptococci. Similarly, genes encoding for alkali production are being cloned into acidogenic bacteria to reduce the acid challenge to enamel. An alternative approach is to (b) derive a more competitive strain that would displace a preexisting organism from plaque. This strategy has the advantage that it is not dependent on treatment with the effector strain at or before colonisation by the undesirable organism. Examples of strains that have been designed for this role include *S. salivarius* (strain TOVE-R), which has been shown to displace *S. mutans* from the teeth of rats and to inhibit caries. This stratagem is being evaluated in human trials using a strain of *S. mutans* that cannot make acid (lactate dehydrogenase has been replaced with alcohol dehydrogenase) and which produces a bacteriocin active against wild-type strains. Assurances over the safety of such effector strains will be required by both the authorities and by the public.

Probiotics are live microorganisms which, when administered in adequate numbers, confer a health benefit on the host. Probiotics are proving popular with consumers in improving gastric health, and are now being considered for applications in oral care. Many of the strains being evaluated are lactobacilli and bifidobacteria from the dairy industry, and they can be delivered by milk, cheese and yoghurt, or as tablets or lozenges. Studies have provided contradictory results, but a metaanalysis in relation to dental caries concluded that probiotics can decrease levels of mutans streptococci. Benefits have also been reported from the use of probiotics in patients with gingival inflammation. The mode of action of these probiotics is unclear, but they may exert their effects by the production of antimicrobial agents or by modulating innate or adaptive immunity; there is little evidence that they successfully colonise the mouth.

Prebiotics are non-digestible oligosaccharides that can stimulate the growth of beneficial resident bacteria. This approach has proved successful in improving gastric health, and similar approaches are being investigated for use in oral care.

Active and passive vaccination. The oral cavity is provided with all of the components necessary to mount an effective immune response against microorganisms (see Chapter 2). Although the microbial aetiology of dental diseases is not totally specific, evidence implicates certain organisms as major causative bacteria in both caries and advanced periodontal disease. This has led to the proposal of using active vaccination to provide life-long protection against these diseases, with most progress being made on developing a caries vaccine.

A vaccine against dental caries using mutans streptococci (whole cell vaccines), or molecules derived from these bacteria (subunit vaccines), has been proposed for many decades. Early studies used crude whole cell preparations of *S. mutans* to protect animals. Although protection against caries and a reduction in the levels of mutans streptococci was achieved, concern was expressed over possible immunologically-mediated tissue damage in humans following exposure to streptococcal antigens (as occurs in, for example, rheumatic fever). Subsequent work was directed towards characterising the antigenic composition of mutans streptococci and selecting individual purified antigens that conferred protection but lacked any potential for human tissue cross-reactivity (a subunit vaccine). Three protein antigens have received most attention; these are: (a) adhesins known as the antigen I/II family (also referred to as antigen B, P1, SpaP, Pac, SpaA, Pag), (b) glucosyltransferases (GTFs); and (c) glucan-binding proteins. Subunit vaccines have been shown to induce salivary secretory IgA and circulating IgG antibodies to antigens of mutans streptococci, and these are capable of reducing (a) colonisation by these cariogenic bacteria, and (b) the number of caries lesions. IgA antibodies can inhibit sucrose-independent and sucrose-dependent mechanisms of streptococcal attachment. Mucosal vaccination strategies have been developed that establish immune memory, and which induce high levels of salivary antibodies that can persist for long periods. A major issue for the introduction of a caries vaccine will centre around the risk-benefit analysis. There have been no major clinical trials to assess their efficacy in humans even though potential vaccines against mutans streptococci have already been manufactured to standards

that satisfy the legislative authorities. This is because the incidence of caries has fallen dramatically in most industrialised societies during the time of the development of these vaccines, probably as a result of fluoride, while the public acceptance of mass-vaccination programmes can be poor, even for serious medical infections. A major question facing health organisations is whether a vaccine is justified against a non-life threatening disease? It might be that vaccination could be considered of benefit to particular high-risk groups in the population.

Periodontal diseases represent an even more complex microbial challenge in terms of vaccination. The elevated levels of *P. gingivalis* in advanced forms of periodontitis, and its possible role as a 'keystone pathogen', have resulted in research programmes to develop a vaccine against this organism. Pilot studies in animal models, using intact killed whole cells or proteases (e.g., gingipains) as the vaccine candidate, have shown reduced bone loss, although the microbial challenge consisted only of *P. gingivalis*. It remains to be determined whether or not such vaccines would have clinical benefit in a more realistic setting, involving a polymicrobial infection.

A development arising from the studies on vaccination is the concept of using preexisting antibodies (**passive immunisation**) to control putative pathogens. When the natural levels of mutans streptococci in the mouth were suppressed by chlorhexidine, the topical application to teeth of monoclonal antibodies directed against antigen I/II was shown to prevent subsequent recolonisation by mutans streptococci in humans for up to 100 days, and protect against caries in primates. Transgenic plants have been genetically-engineered to produce a monoclonal secretory antibody with specificity for antigen I/II of mutans streptococci. The dimeric nature of this antibody enabled it to persist intact for longer periods in the mouth than the parent antibody. Application to human volunteers from whom indigenous mutans streptococci had been cleared, prevented recolonisation by *S. mutans* for up to four months. Similar benefits have been reported following the use of monoclonal antibodies targeted against *P. gingivalis*. This approach has many advantages, not least being the reduction of any of the risks (however small) that are associated with active vaccination. Antibodies could be generated against a wider number of putative pathogens, and they could be applied by dental professionals at regular intervals as part of routine visits to the dentist. In the future, this could form the basis of a novel approach to maintaining dental plaque with a microbial composition that is compatible with oral health.

Photodynamic therapy, nanotechnology, redox and antiinflammatory agents. Other novel approaches to controlling pathogens in plaque may involve photodynamic therapy or redox agents. Periodontal pathogens, including *P. gingivalis*, *A actinomycetemcomitans* and *F. nucleatum*, and cariogenic bacteria, such as mutans streptococci, are susceptible to killing by low power laser light once cells have been treated with low concentrations of a photosensitiser dye such as toluidine blue. When activated, the dye liberates free radicals, which are lethal to neighbouring cells. Photodynamic therapy can work on biofilms such as dental plaque, though penetration and distribution of the sensitiser throughout the biofilm can be a challenge. The approach is indiscriminate, and there is a potential risk for bystander damage, although selected pathogens could be targeted by coupling the dye to a molecule that binds to the pathogen.

Nanoparticles are being developed that either contain a photosensitiser or which generate reactive oxygen species when photoactivated. Nanoparticles with antimicrobial activity are also being investigated, for example, by exploiting the properties of silver or copper ions; such particles can be incorporated into materials such as denture acrylic.

Agents that can alter the redox potential (degree of anaerobiosis; see Chapter 2) of subgingival sites have been evaluated; these redox agents are designed to raise the Eh so that conditions will be less suitable for the proliferation of the obligate anaerobes that dominate in periodontal pockets. A new generation of antiinflammatory agents is being developed (e.g., lipoxins, resolvins and protectins) that could reduce bystander damage and reduce GCF flow thereby removing a key nutrient supply for periodontal pathogens, while also promoting tissue healing. These agents act as 'resolution agonists' to orchestrate the return of the tissues to health by enhancing clearance of bacteria and controlling excessive host cellular activity.

KEY POINTS

The mechanical removal of plaque by efficient oral hygiene can almost completely prevent plaque-mediated diseases. However, this commitment can be difficult to maintain for long periods by many patients, and additional strategies need to be deployed. Many toothpastes and mouthwashes are supplemented with antiplaque and antimicrobial agents (e.g., chlorhexidine, Triclosan, metal salts, essential oils, etc.), which even at sublethal concentrations can inhibit metabolic traits of plaque bacteria that are implicated in caries and periodontal diseases. The use of confectionery, drinks and chewing gums containing alternative sweeteners (e.g., polyols) that cannot be metabolised rapidly to acid can reduce the acidic challenge to teeth while stimulating saliva flow. Fluoride is the most effective strategy in reducing caries by promoting remineralisation and reducing demineralisation of teeth; fluoride can also reduce glycolysis and interfere with other key biochemical processes in cariogenic bacteria. New strategies are being developed that include photodynamic therapy, prebiotics and probiotics, replacement therapy, redox and antiinflammatory agents, and vaccination (active and passive).

CHAPTER SUMMARY

Distinct shifts in the balance of the microbiota of dental plaque occur during the development of caries and periodontal diseases. Numerous cross-sectional and longitudinal surveys have found a strong association between the levels of mutans streptococci in plaque and the initiation of enamel caries. Increased proportions of lactobacilli are found in advanced lesions. However, the relationship between mutans streptococci and caries is not absolute, and other streptococci with relevant traits will also play a role. *Actinomyces* spp., mutans streptococci and lactobacilli are also implicated with root surface caries, whereas infected dentine has a complex microbiota, with many anaerobic and proteolytic bacteria being detected.

The properties of cariogenic bacteria that correlate with their pathogenicity include the ability to rapidly metabolise sugars to acid, especially at low pH, and to survive and grow under the acidic conditions generated (i.e., cariogenic bacteria are acidogenic and aciduric). Additional properties include the ability to synthesise intracellular and extracellular polysaccharides. Strategies to control or prevent dental caries are based on: (a) reducing levels of plaque in general, or specific cariogenic bacteria in particular, for example, by antiplaque or antimicrobial agents; (b) using fluoride to encourage remineralisation and to strengthen the resistance of enamel to acid attack; and (c) reduce bacterial acid production by avoiding the frequent intake of fermentable carbohydrates in the diet, by replacing such carbohydrates with sugar substitutes, or by interfering with bacterial metabolism with fluoride or antimicrobial agents. Other strategies being developed for the future include: (i) enhancing the colonisation resistance of plaque by replacement therapy, whereby harmless strains may exclude or suppress cariogenic species, and (ii) active or passive vaccination against mutans streptococci using subunit vaccines or specific antibodies, respectively.

Periodontal diseases are a group of disorders that affect the supporting tissues of the teeth but, as with caries, there is no single or unique pathogen. There is a shift away from a sparse and mainly Gram-positive microbial community in the healthy gingival crevice to a predominantly Gram-negative, proteolytic and obligately anaerobic microbiota in disease. Gingivitis is associated with a build-up of plaque mass beyond levels that are compatible with health, resulting in the host mounting an inflammatory response. This may be sufficient to control the biofilm, but if gingivitis is not resolved then irreversible damage to the periodontium may ensue. This tissue damage is a consequence of a dysregulated and subverted inflammatory response to the accumulation of biofilm. The microbiota in disease is diverse, and includes *Porphyromonas gingivalis, Prevotella intermedia, Aggregatibacter actinomycetemcomitans, Tannerella forsythia, Dialister pneumosintes, Fusobacterium nucleatum, Eubacterium* spp. and spirochaetes. Culture-independent approaches have identified microbial communities with an even greater diversity, and many of the organisms are unculturable and represent novel taxa, whose role in disease is still to be determined. Bacterial invasion of tissues can occur, especially in some aggressive and necrotising conditions such as NUG. Risk factors for periodontal diseases include abnormalities in the functioning of the host defences, smoking, and systemic disease such as diabetes mellitus.

Periodontal diseases may also act as risk factors for more serious systemic conditions, including preterm, low birth weight babies, pneumonia, diabetes, rheumatoid arthritis, some forms of cancer and cardiovascular disease (see Chapter 11). Treatment and prevention of periodontal disease involves good oral hygiene and effective plaque control, which may be augmented by the use of antimicrobial agents.

FURTHER READING: DENTAL CARIES

Aas JA, Griffen AL, Dardis SR, et al. Bacteria of dental caries in primary and permanent teeth in children and young adults. *J Clin Microbiol.* 2008;46:1407-1417.

Chalmers NI, Oh K, Hughes CV, et al. Pulp and plaque microbiotas of children with severe early childhood caries. *J Oral Microbiol.* 2015;7:25951.

Chen L, Qin B, Du M, et al. Extensive description and comparison of human supra-gingival microbiome in root caries and health. *PLoS ONE.* 2015;10:e0117064.

Dige I, Grønkjær L, Nyvad B. Molecular studies of the structural ecology of natural occlusal caries. *Caries Res.* 2014;48:451-460.

Kassebaum NJ, Bernabé E, Dahiya M, et al. Global burden of untreated caries: A systematic review and metaregression. *J Dent Res.* 2015;94:650-658.

Kianoush N, Adler CJ, Nguyen K-AT, et al. Bacterial profile of dentine caries and the impact of pH on bacterial population diversity. *PLoS ONE.* 2014;9:e92940.

Marsh PD, Takahashi N, Nyvad B. Biofilms in caries development. In: Fejerskov O, Nyvad B, Kidd E, eds. *Dental caries. The disease and its clinical management.* 3rd ed. Oxford: Wiley Blackwell; 2015:108-131.

Mantzourami M, Gilbert SC, Sulong HN, et al. The isolation of bifidobacteria from occlusal carious lesions in children and adults. *Caries Res.* 2009;43:308-313.

Moye ZD, Zeng L, Burne RA. Fueling the caries process: carbohydrate metabolism and gene regulation by *Streptococcus mutans. J Oral Microbiol.* 2014;6:24878.

Munson MA, Banerjee A, Watson TF, et al. Molecular analysis of the microflora associated with dental caries. *J Clin Microbiol.* 2004;42:3023-3029.

Nyvad B, Crielaard W, Mira A, et al. Dental caries from a molecular microbiological perspective. *Caries Res.* 2013;47:89-102.

Sheiham A, James WPT. Diet and dental caries: The pivotal role of free sugars reemphasized. *J Dent Res.* 2015;94:1341-1347.

Schulze-Schweifing K, Banerjee A, Wade WG. Comparison of bacterial culture and 16S rRNA community profiling by clonal analysis and pyrosequencing for the characterization of the dentine caries-associated microbiome. *Front Cell Infect Microbiol.* 2014;4:164.

Tanner ACR, Kent RL, Holgerson PL, et al. Microbiota of severe early childhood caries before and after therapy. *J Dent Res.* 2011;90:1298-1305.

Tanner ACR, Sonis AL, Holgerson PL, et al. White-spot lesions and gingivitis microbiotas in orthodontic patients. *J Dent Res.* 2012;91:853-858.

Torlakovic L, Klepac-Ceraj V, Øgaard B, et al. Microbial community succession on developing lesions on human enamel. *J Oral Microbiol.* 2012;4:16125.

FURTHER READING: PERIODONTAL DISEASE

Aas JA, Barbuto SM, Alpagot T, et al. Subgingival plaque microbiota in HIV positive patients. *J Clin Periodontol.* 2007;34:189-195.

Darveau RP. Oral microbial interactions. The oral microbial consortium's interaction with the periodontal innate defense system. *DNA Cell Biol.* 2009;28:389-395.

Dashper SG, Seers CA, Tan KH, et al. Virulence factors of the oral spirochete *Treponema denticola. J Dent Res.* 2011;90:691-703.

Hans M, Hans VM. Toll-like receptors and their dual role in periodontitis: a review. *J Oral Sci.* 2011;53:263-271.

Hajishengallis G. Periodontitis: from microbial immune subversion to systemic inflammation. *Nat Rev Immunol.* 2015;15:30-44.

Hajishengallis G, Darveau RP, Curtis MA. The Keystone Pathogen Hypothesis. *Nat Rev Microbiol.* 2012;10:717-725.

Hajishengallis G, Lamont RJ. Beyond the red complex and into more complexity: the polymicrobial synergy and dysbiosis (PSD) model of periodontal disease etiology. *Mol Oral Microbiol.* 2012; 27:409-419.

Hajishengallis G, Lamont RJ. Breaking bad: Manipulation of the host response by *Porphyromonas gingivalis. Eur J Immunol.* 2014; 44:328-338.

Haubek D, Johansson A. Pathogenicity of the highly leukotoxic JP2 clone of *Aggregatibacter actinomycetemcomitans* and its geographical dissemination and role in aggressive periodontitis. *J Oral Microbiol.* 2014;6. doi:10.3402/jom.v6.23980.

Könönen E, Müller HP. Microbiology of aggressive periodontitis. *Periodontol 2000.* 2014;65:46-78.

Lourenço TGB, Heller D, Silva-Boghossian CM, et al. Microbial signature profiles of periodontally healthy and diseased patients. *J Clin Periodontol.* 2014;41:1027-1036.

Park OJ, Yi H, Jeon JH, et al. Pyrosequencing analysis of subgingival microbiota in distinct periodontal conditions. *J Dent Res.* 2015; 94:921-927.

Paster BJ, Falkler WA Jr, Enwonwu CO. Prevalent bacterial species and novel phylotypes in advanced noma lesions. *J Clin Microbiol.* 2002;40:2187-2191.

Pérez-Chaparro PJ, Gonçalves C, Figueiredo LC, et al. Newly identified pathogens associated with periodontitis: A systematic review. *J Dent Res.* 2014;93:846-858.

Socransky SS, Haffajee AD. Periodontal microbial ecology. *Periodontol 2000.* 2005;38:135-187.

Visser MB, Ellen RP. New insights into the emerging role of oral spirochaetes in periodontal disease. *Clin Microbiol Infect.* 2011;17:502-512.

Wade WG. The oral microbiome in health and disease. *Pharmacol Res.* 2013;69:137-143.

Zenobia C, Hajishengallis G. *Porphyromonas gingivalis* virulence factors involved in subversion of leukocytes and microbial dysbiosis. *Virulence.* 2015;6:236-243.

FURTHER READING: TREATMENT OF PLAQUE

Allaker RP, Douglas CWI. Non-conventional therapeutics for oral infections. *Virulence.* 2015;6:196-207.

Cheng L, Li J, He L, et al. Natural products and caries prevention. *Caries Res.* 2015;49(suppl 1):38-45.

Choi JI, Seymour GJ. Vaccines against periodontitis: a forward-looking review. *J Periodontal Implant Sci.* 2010;40:153-163.

Hasturk H, Kantarci A, van Dyke TE. Paradigm shift in the pharmacological management of periodontal diseases. *Front Oral Biol.* 2012;15:160-176.

Jeon JG, Rosalen PL, Falsetta ML, et al. Natural products in caries research: current (limited) knowledge, challenges and future perspective. *Caries Res.* 2011;45:243-263.

Konopka K, Goslinski T. Photodynamic therapy in dentistry. *J Dent Res.* 2007;86:694-707.

Laleman I, Detailleur V, Slot DE, et al. Probiotics reduce mutans streptococci counts in humans: a systematic review and meta-analysis. *Clin Oral Investig.* 2014;18:1539-1552.

Marquis RE, Clock SA, Mota-Meira M. Fluoride and organic weak acids as modulators of microbial physiology. *FEMS Microbiol Rev.* 2003;26:493-510.

Ribeiro LGM, Hashizume LN, Malz M. The effect of different formulations of chlorhexidine in reducing levels of mutans streptococci in the oral cavity: A systematic review of the literature. *J Dent.* 2007;35:359-370.

Russell MW, Childers NK, Michalek SM, et al. A caries vaccine? The state of the science of immunization against dental caries. *Caries Res.* 2004;38:230-235.

MULTIPLE CHOICE QUESTIONS

Answers on p. 249

1 *Which of the following is* not *one of the hypotheses relating the composition of dental plaque to caries or periodontal diseases?*

a. Specific plaque hypothesis

b. Non-specific plaque hypothesis

c. Homeostatic hypothesis

d. Ecological plaque hypothesis

2 *Which type of epidemiological survey will determine most accurately the role of plaque bacteria in dental disease, and establish a cause-and-effect relationship?*

a. Longitudinal

b. Observational

c. Cross-sectional

d. Prospective

3 *Which of the following has* not *provided evidence for the role of microorganisms in the aetiology of dental caries?*

a. Intervention studies using antibiotics in animal models

b. Vaccination studies in human clinical trials

c. Transmission studies in rodents colonised by mutans streptococci

d. Use of mutants of mutans streptococci in animal models

4 *Which of the following species of streptococci have been implicated in the aetiology of dental caries?*
a. *Streptococcus sanguinis*
b. *Streptococcus sobrinus*
c. *Streptococcus salivarius*
d. *Streptococcus oralis*

5 *Which of the following groups of microorganism are most linked to enamel dental caries?*
a. Mutans streptococci and *Candida* and *Propionibacterium*
b. Mutans streptococci and lactobacilli and bifidobacteria
c. Lactobacilli and *Actinomyces* and *Propionibacterium*
d. Mutans streptococci and *Actinomyces* and *Propionibacterium*

6 *The microbiota associated with root surface caries is diverse; which of the following group of bacteria are most commonly reported to be present in root surface lesions?*
a. *Actinomyces* and *Treponema* species
b. Lactobacilli and *Veillonella* and staphylococci
c. Mutans streptococci, lactobacilli and *Actinomyces*
d. Lactobacilli, *Treponema* and *Prevotella*

7 *Which of the following characteristics do not contribute to the cariogenicity of mutans streptococci?*
a. Rapid sugar transport
b. Low tolerance of external acidic pH
c. Extracellular polysaccharide (EPS) production from sucrose
d. Intracellular polysaccharide (IPS) production

8 *Implicit in the ecological plaque hypothesis is that dental caries can be controlled or prevented, by all of the following strategies, except one. Which one of the following is not a strategy that is consistent with the ecological plaque hypothesis?*
a. Directly targeting the putative pathogens
b. Stimulating saliva flow
c. Vaccination against *Streptococcus mutans*
d. Promoting the use of snacks containing sugar substitutes

9 *Which one of the following changes in local subgingival environment is associated with an inflammatory host response?*
a. A rise in the redox potential
b. A decrease in temperature
c. A decrease in flow of gingival crevice fluid (GCF)
d. An increase in pH

10 *Which of the following is not a model or hypothesis that is currently applied to the aetiology of periodontal disease?*
a. Anaerobic pathogen model
b. Keystone pathogen hypothesis
c. Polymicrobial synergy and dysbiosis model
d. Ecological plaque hypothesis

11 *Which of the following are isolated most commonly in advanced periodontal lesions?*
a. *Eikenella corrodens, Porphyromonas catoniae, Prevotella nigrescens*
b. *Porphyromonas gingivalis, Tannerella forsythia, Treponema denticola*
c. *Streptococcus intermedius, Selenomonas sputigena, Veillonella parvula*
d. *Capnocytophaga gingivalis, Prevotella intermedia, Aggregatibacter actinomycetemcomitans*

12 *The organisms associated with lesions in necrotising ulcerative gingivitis include which of the following?*
a. *Fuso-spirochaetal complex*
b. *Prevotella nigrescens* and *Porphyromonas gingivalis*
c. Mixed community of spirochaetes only
d. Mixed community of motile bacteria only

13 *The bacterial pathogen most commonly associated with localised aggressive periodontitis is:*
a. *Porphyromonas gingivalis*
b. *Tannerella forsythia*
c. *Filifactor alocis*
d. *Aggregatibacter actinomycetemcomitans*

14 *Which of the following is a virulence factor of* P. *gingivalis?*
a. Lipoteichoic acid (LTA)
b. Ammonia production
c. Gingipain production
d. Leukotoxin production

15 *What does the early response by the host against periodontal pathogens mainly involve?*
a. Antibodies
b. Matrix metalloproteinases
c. Macrophages
d. Neutrophils

16 *Which is a major virulence factor produced by* Aggregatibacter actinomycetemcomitans?
a. Gingipain production
b. Leukotoxin production
c. Lipoteichoic acid production
d. Hydrogen peroxide production

17 *The optimum concentration of fluoride supplementation in drinking water for maximal protection against caries is approximately which of the following?*
a. 1 part per million (1 ppm)
b. 10 ppm
c. 100 ppm
d. 1000 ppm

18 *The mode of action of fluoride includes inhibition of which of the following?*
a. Gingipain, lipopolysaccharide (LPS), and leukotoxin
b. Glycolysis, IPS synthesis, sugar transport
c. Glycolysis, LPS, sugar transport
d. Cell wall synthesis, IPS synthesis, sugar transport

19 *Which of the following is an example of an antimicrobial that is in the phenols class?*
a. Chlorhexidine
b. Thymol
c. Triclosan
d. Phenol

20 *Which of the following is not an artificial sweetener?*
a. Aspartame
b. Casein
c. Xylitol
d. Saccharin

Orofacial bacterial infections

As described in previous chapters, the mouth contains a rich and diverse microbiota, of which only 50–70% can be cultivated. Normally, the oral microbiota has a commensal relationship with the host. However, the composition of dental plaque can change in response to alterations in lifestyle or environmental conditions, and this can lead to the two most prevalent human diseases, namely dental caries and periodontal disease (see Chapter 6). Untreated, both of these conditions can progress into other forms of acute and chronic infection within the mouth and orofacial tissues (Fig. 7.1), and may on occasions lead to severe life-threatening situations.

Contemporary microbiological studies have revealed that the types of bacteria recovered from orofacial dental infections reflect the wide spectrum of facultatively and obligately anaerobic bacteria that comprise the host's oral microbiota. Obligate anaerobes comprise a major proportion of the microbiota within acute suppurative infections. In addition, pathogenicity experiments in animals have implicated strictly anaerobic bacterial species, in particular Gram-negative bacilli, as not only the predominant species, but also the most likely pathogens, although the reasons for this are uncertain. One possibility is the synergy of specific combinations of bacterial species, and animal models have shown that *Prevotella* species and *Fusobacterium* species are more pathogenic when in combination with members of the *Streptococcus anginosus* group than when separately inoculated (pathogenic synergism; see Fig. 6.18). It has also been proposed that microaerophilic species produce an environment that favours the proliferation of obligately anaerobic species. The detection of microaerophilic species, such as members of the *Streptococcus anginosus* group, early in the course of purulent infection, often in pure culture, lends support to this proposal. The presence of an extracellular capsule on certain bacterial strains recovered from dentoalveolar abscesses has also been implicated as a potential pathogenic determinant since

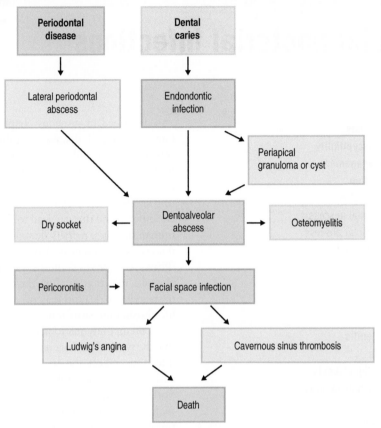

FIGURE 7.1 Interrelationship of dental bacterial infections.

this may protect bacteria from phagocytosis or intracellular killing (Fig. 7.2). Although found on fresh clinical isolates, the capsule is often lost after repeated subculture in vitro.

In an infection involving a diverse microbial community, it is likely that environmental factors such as availability of nutrients, local pH and the status of the immune defences also play major contributing roles in determining the clinical outcome and whether or not an acute suppurative process develops. The primary source of nutrients is serum-derived proteins along with some host tissue components. Bacterial species associated with the infection may produce a range of complementary enzymes, in particular glycosidases and proteases, which permit progression of the infection (see Chapters 4 and 5). *Prevotella oralis, Prevotella intermedia* and *Porphyromonas endodontalis* have been identified as being particularly effective in

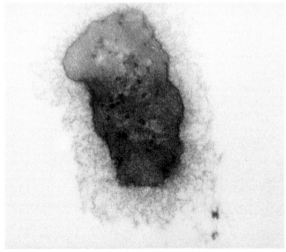

FIGURE 7.2 Transmission electron microscopy (TEM) of capsulate *Prevotella intermedia* isolated from an acute dentoalveolar abscess.

the degradation of serum proteins and immunoglobulins. These species also obtain essential growth elements such as iron and haemin from the catabolism of albumin, haptoglobin, haemopexin and transferrin. An example of the interrelationship among the bacteria within the polymicrobial community is the degradation of proteins and peptides by *Prevotella* species for bacteria such as *F. nucleatum*, *Eubacterium* species and anaerobic streptococci. These consortia also produce metabolic substances, in particular hydrogen sulphide, indoles and amines that inactivate host polymorphonuclear leukocytes and prevent complement action, in addition to acidic end products of metabolism that are cytotoxic.

Orofacial bacterial infections may present as either a localised abscess or diffuse cellulitis depending on the virulence of the bacteria, local anatomical structures and host defence mechanisms. On rare occasions, bacteria may enter the bloodstream to produce a potentially life-threatening septicaemia. An abscess is a localised collection of bacteria, inflammatory cells, tissue-breakdown products, serum-derived proteins and other organic material. Tissue destruction is predominantly caused by bacterial enzymes although some damage is host-mediated. An abscess is hypertonic in relation to the immediate environment and pressure effects result in osteoclastic activity in surrounding bone. In dentoalveolar abscesses, perforation of bone permits spread of infection into the surrounding soft tissues. Subsequent inflammation in the soft tissue is termed cellulitis, which is often accompanied by limited localised muscular movement (trismus). Bacterial metabolites, exotoxins and endotoxins along with host inflammatory substances then act on the temperature regulatory centre in the hypothalamus to raise the patient's temperature (pyrexia).

LABORATORY DIAGNOSIS

A major problem associated with the recovery of the causative microorganisms from specific orofacial infections is the high potential for sample contamination from microorganisms present in saliva. Contamination of a specimen with relatively rapidly growing bacteria, such as streptococci or staphylococci, can potentially prevent the isolation of more slowly growing and relevant species. As a basic principle, the diagnostic

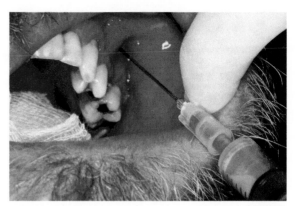

FIGURE 7.3 Aspiration of pus from an acute dentoalveolar abscess.

microbiological report can only be as good as the quality of the specimen. In view of the likely presence of oxygen-sensitive bacteria in orofacial infections, all efforts must be made to ensure successful recovery of such obligate anaerobes. Samples of pus should be obtained by aspiration to minimise the risk of contamination and protect oxygen-sensitive anaerobes from atmospheric oxygen (Fig. 7.3). If a swab is the only option for sampling, then this should be placed immediately in an appropriate transport medium. A microbiological specimen is a living sample and as such must be transferred to the laboratory for processing as rapidly as possible to minimise the loss of viable bacteria and to ensure the resulting report accurately reflects the original microbial composition of the purulent material in vivo.

On arrival at the laboratory, a Gram stain of a smear of the sample can be used to confirm that the specimen is truly pus and not another substance, such as cyst fluid. The Gram stain of pus will reveal a large number of polymorphonuclear leukocytes and frequently numerous Gram-positive and/or Gram-negative bacteria (Fig. 7.4). The sample will routinely be plated onto non-selective blood-based media, which will be incubated in an atmosphere of air plus 5% CO_2 and also anaerobically. Fastidious anaerobe agar is also used to ensure isolation of obligate anaerobes. Agars are incubated at 37°C and examined after 18 to 24 hours for primary growth, before being returned to the incubator for prolonged incubation and reexamination on a daily basis for up to 10 days. Many obligate anaerobic species, including some *Eubacterium* species, form minute, slowly growing colonies which may

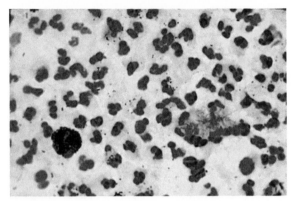

FIGURE 7.4 Gram-stained smear of pus obtained from acute dentoalveolar abscess.

take up to 10 days to become apparent. Representative colonies of any detected growth are subcultured for pure growth and determination of atmospheric requirements. Identification of obligate anaerobes within orofacial infections can take a number of days because of their slow-growing nature. This factor limits the clinical benefit of sampling such infections for the individual affected. However, the results may be of value in the management of the patient who does not respond well to the initial intervention and collectively, the results of specimen analysis are useful in surveillance of patterns of infection. Molecular-based techniques have been developed to provide rapid identification and detection of specific bacterial species in dental infections (see Chapters 3 and 4). These methods have been applied to both the rapid identification of cultured isolates and the direct analysis of clinical material without culture, often using polymerase chain reaction (PCR) targeted to previously selected known pathogens. Culture is an important element of both these approaches, but it is also known that such culture methods often fail to recover the full diversity of microorganisms within orofacial infections (see Chapter 3). Community molecular profiling, in which deoxyribonucleic acid (DNA) has been extracted from pus obtained from acute dentoalveolar abscesses and 16S ribosomal DNA (rDNA) has been amplified using universal bacterial primers, has revealed that unculturable species account for a high percentage of the microbiota in the sample when compared with results of traditional culture. Similar trends

have been reported for endodontic infections, as well as for pericoronitis and periimplantitis. Associations between the presence of some species, including as yet uncultured taxa, and distinct clinical parameters such as the presence of symptoms in endodontically treated teeth are emerging. Further work in this area, and particularly the large amount of data generated by high throughput whole genome sequencing in the context of community profiling, will add considerably to our understanding of the microbial aetiology of the individual infections described later. It is likely that as yet, uncultured and other novel bacterial species will be shown to play a critical role in dental infections. Although the exact role of the individual microorganisms and consortia is not fully understood at present, the information that is now being gathered is likely to improve the clinical usefulness of microbiology in the management of dental infections in the future, with the ultimate aim being accurate and prognostic point of care testing.

ANTIMICROBIAL SUSCEPTIBILITY

The global emergence of antibiotic resistance is of great concern, and bacteria recovered from orofacial infections are now being found to have reduced susceptibility to penicillins and other antibiotics. Historically, isolates from acute suppurative dental infections rarely demonstrated resistance to penicillin, but this is no longer the case. The incidence of resistance to penicillin has increased dramatically in Gram-negative obligately anaerobic bacilli, in particular *Prevotella* species, because of the production of β-lactamases. Studies in the United Kingdom have revealed that the incidence of penicillin resistance in acute dentoalveolar infections rose from 3% of isolates in 1986 to 23% of isolates in 1995. Similar incidences of penicillin resistance have now also been reported in the USA (33%), Sweden (38%) and Japan (39%).

Susceptibility testing is traditionally performed using a disc diffusion method on solid agar media. This technique allows a basic assessment of sensitivity to a particular drug. Calculation of the minimum inhibitory concentration (MIC) requires more labour intensive broth or agar dilution methods. In recent years, the development of a simple agar diffusion method called the E-test has permitted direct reading

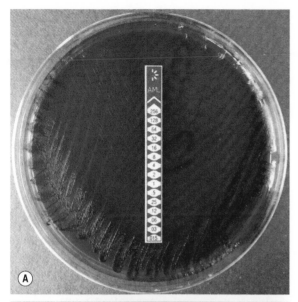

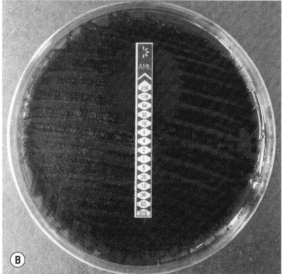

FIGURE 7.5 Incubated plate of a *Prevotella* species demonstrating susceptibility (**A**) and resistance (**B**) to penicillin using the E-test.

of antimicrobial MIC from an agar plate (Fig. 7.5), and this approach is often routinely used in diagnostic laboratories.

Molecular techniques have been developed that permit rapid detection of antimicrobial resistance genes to penicillin, erythromycin and tetracycline, and these can be applied directly to samples of pus.

These techniques may prove to be helpful in clinical management if they become more widely available in the future. The presence of penicillin-resistant bacteria has been reported to be responsible for treatment failures in head and neck infections of dental origin. The production of β-lactamases not only has a direct pathogenic role by destroying the penicillin antibiotic, but also indirectly shields non-β-lactamase producing, penicillin-sensitive bacteria within the infection. The widespread use of penicillin has contributed to this problem, because it has been shown that the administration of penicillin leads to the emergence of β-lactamase-producing bacteria, especially Gram-negative bacilli, at sites such as the oropharynx. Increased resistance to other antibiotics prescribed for dental infections is being reported in some countries, although there would appear to be no consistent pattern. Of specific interest, is the extremely low incidence of resistance to clindamycin, even in countries such as Germany and Japan, where this agent is frequently used to treat acute dental infections.

PRINCIPLES OF MANAGEMENT

The actual treatment for an individual patient will be dependent on the specific circumstances. The basic principles are the drainage of pus, if present, and removal of the source of infection, usually by pulp extirpation or extraction of the affected tooth. Consideration should be given for the need for antimicrobial therapy only when there is evidence of rapid local spread, such as cellulitis or marked lymphadenopathy, or signs of systemic infection such as pyrexia. Undoubtedly, in the past, antibiotics have frequently been prescribed either inappropriately or unnecessarily, and in some countries, dentists are responsible for prescribing up to a tenth of all antibiotics, a figure which seems disproportionately high. Such habits have contributed to the emergence of penicillin resistance in bacterial species encountered in the mouth. Despite this, if required, members of the penicillin group (amoxicillin, phenoxymethylpenicillin) given orally, remain the antibiotic therapy of first choice. Erythromycin and metronidazole are suitable alternative agents for patients with hypersensitivity to penicillins. Standard dosages are used for dental outpatients, although increased dosages and combination therapy have been recommended for severe infections. Many countries have developed prescribing guidelines as part of improved antimicrobial stewardship schemes to help limit the development of antimicrobial resistance and other adverse effects. Antimicrobial susceptibility data from a given patient specimen can be used to inform changes of drug in the case of the non-improving patient and, when collated as part of a surveillance scheme, will record local patterns and inform empirical prescribing. For this reason, it is considered good practice to always send purulent material to a microbiology laboratory for analysis.

The concept of a complete course of antibiotics is obsolete and patients should take the drug for as short a time as possible, in practical terms until symptoms have resolved. A short course of two 3g administrations of amoxicillin 12 hours apart has been found to be effective for acute dentoalveolar abscesses. The range of other antimicrobial agents that have been suggested for the treatment of orofacial infections include cephalosporin, azithromycin, spiramycin, amoxicillin-clavulanate and clindamycin, although many of these broad spectrum drugs are not recommended as first-line agents, as they increase risk of infection with *Clostridium difficile*, meticillin-resistant *Staphylococcus aureus* (MRSA) and resistant microorganisms (see Chapter 10).

ENDODONTIC INFECTION

The presence of microorganisms in root canals immediately before and during endodontic treatment has been studied extensively in recent years. Different sampling techniques and identification methods have been used and this, in part, probably explains the wide spectrum of bacteria recovered. Overall, the microbiota encountered is similar to that found in acute dentoalveolar abscesses. In recent years, culture and sequencing techniques have revealed over 400 unique bacterial taxa in endodontic infection and root canals typically contain between 7 to 20 different species, in particular *Olsenella profusa*, *P. gingivalis*, *Dialister* species and anaerobic streptococci. *Enterococcus faecalis* has received special attention since it had been proposed that this species was specifically associated

with endodontic failures. Molecular studies have revealed that *E. faecalis* is frequently present in necrotic pulps before treatment as well as following failed endodontic therapy. Molecular community profiling of periapical lesions and adjacent root apices has revealed distinct microbial profiles in these locations, highlighting the complexity of the infected root canal environment. Phylogenetic analysis of bacterial and archaeal 16S ribosomal ribonucleic acid (rRNA) has detected a *Methanobrevibacter oralis*-like species along with *Treponema denticola*. Furthermore, animal studies have implicated *Treponema denticola* as being the cause of disseminating infection from the root canal to distant organs. In addition to the identification of bacteria, studies have quantified the presence of endotoxins within root canals; higher levels of lipopolysaccharide have been found in teeth with clinical symptoms compared with asymptomatic teeth. These contemporary studies indicate a complex polymicrobial community within endodontic infections and substantiate the link between oral disease and systemic conditions (see Chapter 11).

DENTOALVEOLAR INFECTION

The term dentoalveolar infection can be used to describe pyogenic (pus-forming) conditions that affect the teeth and supporting structures, and includes lateral periodontal abscess and acute dentoalveolar (periapical) abscess.

LATERAL PERIODONTAL ABSCESS

The lateral periodontal abscess can be differentiated from the dentoalveolar abscess by the fact that the tooth that it is associated with has a vital pulp. The periodontal abscess develops as a result of blockage, occasionally because of the presence of foreign material such as a fish bone or toothbrush bristle, in an established periodontal pocket. Clinically, the abscess develops rapidly producing localised swelling and erythema. Pus is likely to discharge from the gingival margin. Obtaining a true sample without contamination of the specimen is almost impossible. Not surprisingly, studies have reported the presence of those bacterial species that are also associated with subgingival biofilms, in particular, *Porphyromonas* species,

Prevotella species, *Fusobacterium* species, haemolytic streptococci, *Actinomyces* species, *Capnocytophaga* species and spirochaetes. The abscess should be treated by drainage and irrigation with an antiseptic mouthwash, such as 0.2% chlorhexidine. An assessment should be made in relation to the long-term prognosis of the tooth, since on many occasions there is advanced periodontal disease and loss of supporting bone, which are indications for extraction. Antibiotic therapy is rarely required.

ACUTE DENTOALVEOLAR ABSCESS

Acute dentoalveolar abscess is the most frequently occurring orofacial bacterial infection. This condition represents the onset of a suppurative process at the apex of the root of a tooth with necrotic pulp. Pulp death usually occurs because of invasion of bacteria from advanced dental caries. However, occasionally the pulp may have become necrotic because of loss of its blood supply as a result of trauma (e.g., from a blow to the tooth) to the apical vessels. The majority of acute dentoalveolar abscesses are preceded by a period of chronic infection and development of periapical granulation tissue that may persist for many months or years. Evidence of a long-standing inflammatory process at the apices of the roots is seen radiographically as an area of radiolucency at that site on radiographs (Fig. 7.6). Interestingly, microscopic examination of periapical granuloma, obtained in the absence of acute symptoms, has revealed the presence of low numbers of bacteria in the tissues, often within macrophages.

Bacteria probably gain access to the apical tissue by one of three routes: direct spread from the pulp chamber, through the periodontal membrane on the root surface or by seeding from local blood vessels (anachoresis). The mechanisms that cause a chronic asymptomatic lesion to change into an acute suppurative process are unknown, but the occurrence of specific combinations of bacteria or the sudden provision of nutrients via local tissue damage is involved. The onset of acute inflammation produces the characteristic symptom of severe pain. Other signs and symptoms will depend on the individual case. However, clinical examination often reveals a carious or discoloured tooth that is tender to touch with localised

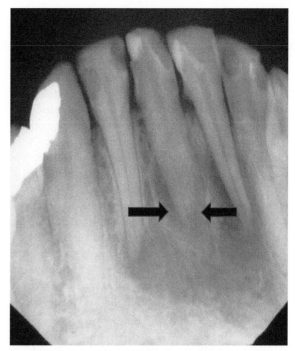

FIGURE 7.6 Intraoral radiograph showing periapical radiolucency because of bone loss associated with dentoalveolar infection (*arrows*).

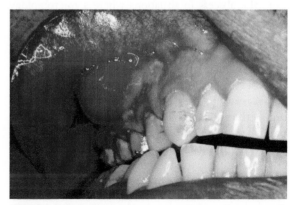

FIGURE 7.7 Dentoalveolar abscess presenting as a fluctuant swelling in the buccal sulcus.

swelling, erythema and trismus (Fig. 7.7). The onset of raised body temperature and malaise are a response to circulating inflammatory cytokines, interleukins and tumour necrosis factor, in response to bacterial endotoxins.

Investigations using culture and molecular methods have confirmed the polymicrobial nature of this infection, which usually involves five or six bacterial species. The most frequently recovered facultatively anaerobic isolates are streptococci, in particular members of *S. anginosus* group and *Actinomyces* species, whilst the predominant obligately anaerobic isolates are anaerobic streptococci, *Veillonella, Prevotella, Porphyromonas* and *Fusobacterium* species. Quantitative studies have revealed the viable microbiota of acute dentoalveolar abscess to be between 10^6 to 10^8 colony forming units (CFU)/ml of pus. The number and proportions of obligately anaerobic species encountered in dentoalveolar abscesses are greater than the number of facultatively anaerobic species. Obligate anaerobes are not only the predominant species, often accounting for four or more of the six or seven species encountered within the microbial consortia, but they also comprise 80% to 90% of the overall cultivable microbiota. Molecular approaches often detect species that are difficult to grow by traditional culture techniques, and some novel species have been found.

The majority of cases of dentoalveolar abscess can be managed successfully by establishing surgical drainage alone. This should involve aspiration of pus from the abscess in situations where a microbiology service is available for culture before incision of the soft tissues, extirpation of the pulp or removal of the tooth. However, occasions do arise when adequate drainage cannot be achieved, or the patient has clinical signs of systemic upset. In these circumstances, it may be necessary to provide antimicrobial therapy. Selection of the antimicrobial agents to be used is based on published susceptibilities rather than identification of the causative organisms and determination of antimicrobial sensitivity in a specific patient. A pus specimen from an individual patient cannot be processed fast enough by traditional methods to be of value in making treatment decisions, since information is rarely available to the clinician within the first 48 hours. Agents in the penicillin group, principally amoxicillin and phenoxymethylpenicillin, are still the antimicrobials of choice in the treatment of acute dental infections whereas metronidazole or a macrolide such as erythromycin or clarithromycin should be used as an alternative agent for patients with hypersensitivity to penicillins. Clindamycin is used as the antibiotic of first choice in some parts of the world (see Chapter 10).

SEVERE ODONTOGENIC INFECTION

Immediate referral to a specialist is required when a patient presents with symptoms of cellulitis, difficulty in swallowing, tachycardia, hypotension, raised temperature, lethargy or dehydration. Specialist care may also become necessary when standard outpatient treatment fails to result in symptomatic improvement. Infection may spread into a number of tissue spaces, and this is influenced by the local anatomy, in particular, muscle attachment and their relationship to the position of the apices of the tooth involved (Fig. 7.8, A and B). Spread into the facial spaces of the neck may lead to difficulty in swallowing. Hospitalisation permits the provision of intravenous antibiotics and fluids. There is also the ability to secure the airway with a tracheostomy, if required. Rarely, infection from dentoalveolar infection in the maxilla may spread into the facial air sinuses via the facial vein and cause cavernous sinus thrombosis, a condition that is associated with high mortality.

An inadequately treated dentoalveolar infection can progress to cause widespread swelling of the tissue spaces (submental, sublingual and submandibular) in the head and neck with the spread of infection through fascial spaces to the mediastinum, a situation referred to as Ludwig's angina.

The tissues of the neck become markedly swollen and tense leading to difficulty in breathing. Hence, the use of the term angina, which literally means choking. Death from Ludwig's angina still occurs, especially in developing countries, because of late intervention or treatment failure. Airway management, involving intubation or tracheostomy, is usually required. The bacterial species most frequently encountered in Ludwig's angina include *Prevotella* species, *Porphyromonas* species, *Fusobacterium* species and anaerobic streptococci, and occasionally, staphylococci, enterobacteria and coliforms have been recovered. Awareness of the potential presence of these bacterial species is important to ensure appropriate antibiotic therapy. Initial treatment must include intravenous delivery of broad spectrum antibiotic therapy, such as a combination of ceftriaxone and metronidazole.

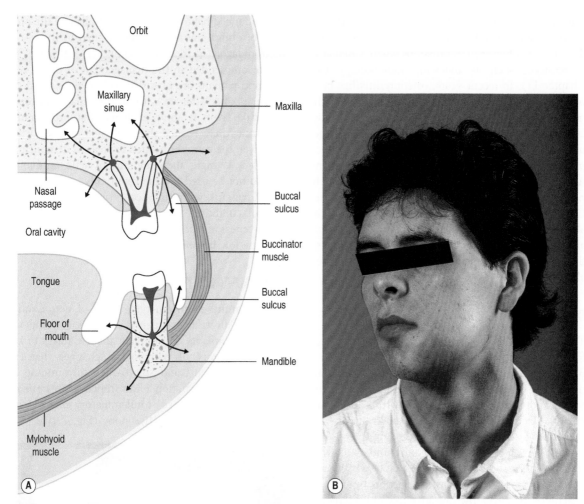

FIGURE 7.8 Pathways by which infection may spread from the periapical region. Muscle attachments and local anatomy (**A**) influence whether the swelling presents intraorally or extraorally. (**B**) Extraoral fluctuant swelling caused by an abscess on a lower second molar.

KEY POINTS

The aetiological agents of purulent orofacial infection are most frequently a polymicrobial mix of endogenous bacteria including microaerophilic organisms and obligate anaerobes. Molecular approaches confirm the prevalence of these pathogens in infection and highlight possible roles for others including as yet uncultivated species. The fundamental principle of management is the establishment of drainage and removal of the source of infection, that is, the pulp or the tooth. It is good clinical practice to send infected material to the microbiology laboratory for analysis, including antimicrobial susceptibility testing of microbial isolates. Antibiotics should only be prescribed if there are signs of local or systemic spread of infection.

OSTEOMYELITIS

Osteomyelitis is defined as inflammation of the medullary bone within the maxilla or mandible with possible extension into the adjacent cortical bone and overlying periosteum. This condition may be acute or chronic and can be extremely difficult to treat effectively. It is perhaps surprising that there are not more cases of osteomyelitis in the jaws following tooth extraction when the potential for members of the oral microbiota to gain access to the underlying bone is considered. The good blood supply to the jaws is probably responsible for the low incidence of osteomyelitis at this site. This concept is supported by the observation that the rare cases of osteomyelitis that do occur are often seen in situations where vascularity is reduced, such as following radiotherapy (see Chapter 11). In recent years, osteomyelitis has been observed in patients taking bisphosphonates for the treatment of osteoporosis or a range of malignant diseases (see Chapter 11). Although it is unclear whether infection is a primary or secondary condition, when present, typical isolates include obligate anaerobes and *Actinomyces* species. Treatment is based on local debridement and topical antiseptic on exposed areas. Clindamycin is often recommended because of its ability to achieve therapeutic levels within bone, although the risks of *Clostridium difficile* associated diarrhoea must be considered in this group of vulnerable patients.

DRY SOCKET

This extremely painful condition, which is a localised form of alveolar osteitis, occurs after approximately 3% of routine extractions and 20% of surgical extractions. Risk factors include a previous history of a dry socket and extraction from an area with reduced vascularity. Examination will reveal an empty socket at the site of extraction in the preceding 2 to 3 days (Fig. 7.9). The aetiology is not fully understood but involves fibrinolysis of the blood clot, which may occur because of opportunistic infection by obligate anaerobes. However, the causative role of bacteria has not been conclusively established. Clinically, there is

a pronounced halitosis which has implicated the presence of obligate anaerobes and has led to the use of metronidazole in treatment. However, antibiotics are not recommended in the management of this condition and patients are provided with analgesia and the socket is often dressed with an obtundant antiseptic material. There is some evidence that preoperative antibiotics may reduce the incidence of dry socket. However, the number needed to treat to demonstrate an effect is high, therefore prophylactic antibiotics should not be used routinely and only considered for those patients with significant risk factors for this painful condition. There is some evidence for the effectiveness of placing chlorhexidine gel in the extraction site for the prevention of dry socket.

PERIIMPLANTITIS

Periimplantitis is an emerging form of periodontitis that is a direct consequence of the increasing use of dental implants. Periimplant disease refers to the general category of pathological changes that can occur in the hard and soft tissues surrounding an implant. The integration of an implant can be jeopardised by the presence of inflammatory changes that cause loss of the supportive bone (Fig. 7.10). Most

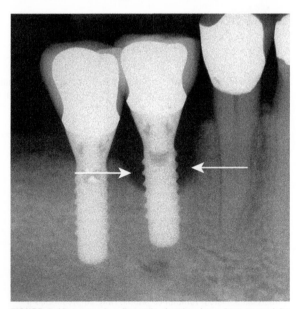

FIGURE 7.10 Intraoral radiograph showing bone loss caused by periimplantitis around a single tooth implant (*arrows*).

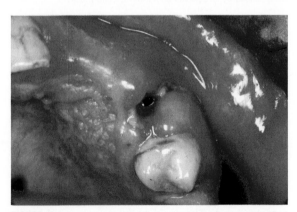

FIGURE 7.9 Dry socket following extraction of an upper first premolar.

periimplant disease is plaque-induced, and cultural analysis reveals that the spectrum of bacterial species recovered in dentate patients is comparable to that encountered in adult periodontitis, namely *A. actinomycetemcomitans, P. gingivalis, P. intermedia* and *F. nucleatum* (see Chapter 6). However, molecular community profiling studies are suggesting that the communities associated with periimplantitis may be distinct to those of periodontitis. Interestingly, but perhaps not surprisingly, the microbiota encountered with healthy stable implants in edentulous individuals is similar to that found on the mucosa and includes Gram-positive facultatively anaerobic streptococci. For dentate individuals the microbiota associated with periimplantitis has been shown to have considerably lower bacterial diversity and appears less complex structurally in comparison to that found in periodontal disease. *Staphylococcus aureus*, enteric bacteria, *Candida* species and asaccharolytic anaerobes such as *Eubacterium* species have been isolated more frequently from cases of periimplantitis than periodontitis.

Periimplantitis has been shown to respond to local mechanical and chemical means of reducing the microbiota in the immediate vicinity of the implant. However, consideration has to be given to the possibility of causing physical damage to the surface of the implant. Irrigation with an antiseptic, such as 0.2% chlorhexidine, has been found to be beneficial. Alternatively, the provision of systemic antimicrobial therapy, such as amoxicillin, metronidazole, ornidazole or tetracycline, has also been recommended.

PERICORONITIS

Inflammation of the soft tissues covering or immediately adjacent to the crown of a partially erupted tooth can cause extreme pain, particularly when the opposing teeth cause additional trauma (Fig. 7.11). This condition occurs fairly frequently in relation to erupting lower third molar teeth in young adults, and is due to infection in the space between the tooth and overlying soft tissue. Obligate anaerobes, in particular *P. intermedia*, anaerobic streptococci and *Fusobacterium* species, are often present, and more contemporary studies have also isolated *Aggregatibacter actinomycetemcomitans* and *Tannerella forsythia*. Molecular studies have suggested that certain species, for example, *Dialister*

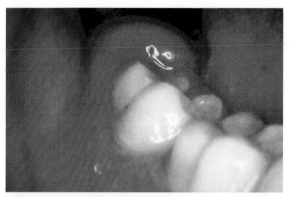

FIGURE 7.11 Localised inflammation leading to pericoronitis over a lower right third molar tooth.

invisus and *Fusobacterium nucleatum,* are present at greater abundance at sites with clinical symptoms. Treatment is local irrigation, but if the opposing tooth is non-functional then it should be extracted. In cases with evidence of local spread or systemic involvement, it may be necessary to prescribe metronidazole or amoxicillin.

BACTERIAL SIALADENITIS

Inflammation of the salivary glands is termed sialadenitis, and this may arise because of either bacterial or viral infection. Historically, suppurative sialadenitis was regarded as an infection principally caused by *S. aureus*, and the condition was a recognised postoperative complication in hospitalised patients undergoing general surgery. However, this postoperative parotitis is now rare because of a better understanding of maintaining fluid balance and the reduced likelihood of *S. aureus* colonisation of the mouth because of improved oral hygiene measures. Sialadenitis within the parotid gland is usually caused by the presence of underlying xerostomia, because of Sjögren syndrome or previous radiotherapy, whereas sialadenitis in the submandibular gland is most frequently secondary to blockage of the duct by a salivary stone. The clinical presentation involves painful swelling of the infected gland and discharge of pus from the duct orifice (Fig. 7.12).

Knowledge of the microbiology of suppurative sialadenitis has become clearer because of the use of improved sampling techniques. Ideally, pus should be collected by aspiration of the duct orifice to minimise

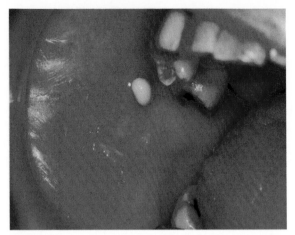

FIGURE 7.12 Discharge of pus from the right parotid salivary gland duct.

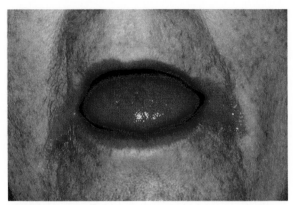

FIGURE 7.13 Angular cheilitis presenting as erythema at both angles of the mouth.

the risk of sample contamination from the oral microbiota. If a swab technique is used, then great care should be taken to avoid sample contamination from the adjacent oral mucosa. On rare occasions, pus may also spread extraorally, and a sample can be obtained by external aspiration. Quantitative microbiological studies of suppurative parotitis have revealed a viable microbiota of 10^6 to 10^8 CFU/ml comprising a wide spectrum of bacterial species, such as alpha-haemolytic streptococci, *Haemophilus* species, *Eikenella corrodens, Prevotella* species and obligate anaerobic Gram-positive cocci. Very occasionally, *Mycobacterium tuberculosis* and atypical mycobacteria are encountered in parotitis.

Antimicrobial therapy should be prescribed, with amoxicillin the agent of choice and erythromycin used in patients with a hypersensitivity to the penicillins. If microbiological investigation reveals the presence of obligate anaerobes then the use of metronidazole could be considered.

Recurrent parotitis of childhood is a relatively rare condition in which sufferers develop a purulent discharge from one of the parotid glands about two or three times a year. The microbiology of the infection is similar to that encountered in other forms of suppurative sialadenitis. It has been suggested that patients would benefit from long-term antibiotic therapy, although most patients are managed adequately with the provision of amoxicillin or erythromycin as and when acute symptoms develop.

ANGULAR CHEILITIS

This condition represents an area of inflammation that is localised to the angles of the mouth (Fig. 7.13). Angular cheilitis is usually bilateral, although only one side of the mouth may be affected on occasions. The inflammatory changes are associated with the presence of *S. aureus*, including MRSA, or *Candida* species, either alone or in combination. Streptococci are also recovered from approximately a third of cases. As a generalisation, staphylococci are usually encountered in dentate individuals whereas *Candida* are found in patients with dentures or an orthodontic appliance. The reservoir of staphylococcal infection is often the anterior part of the nose, whilst the mouth is the source of the *Candida*. Treatment should involve not only the angles, but also the appropriate reservoir of infection. In the case of staphylococci, fusidic acid cream can be prescribed, with one tube for the angles and a separate tube for the nose. Miconazole cream is also useful in cases where there is uncertainty about the microorganism that may be present since this agent has activity against *Candida* and Gram-positive cocci. An antifungal agent should be given in cases involving *Candida* (see Chapter 8).

CERVICOFACIAL ACTINOMYCOSIS

Actinomycosis is an example of an opportunistic infection caused by members of the *Actinomyces* genus. A range of *Actinomyces* species are encountered in plaque biofilms, dentinal caries and dentoalveolar

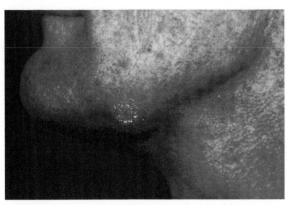

FIGURE 7.14 The clinical appearance of cervicofacial actinomycosis.

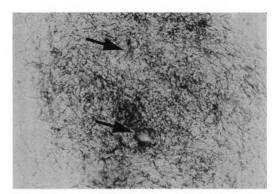

FIGURE 7.15 A Gram-stained film of *Actinomyces israelii* (original magnification × 100). Note the branching filaments and the tendency to form granular masses (*arrows*).

abscess (see Chapters 5 and 6). However, in cervico-facial actinomycosis, which characteristically presents as a submandibular swelling, *A. israelii* is encountered in 90% of cases. Occasionally, *A. bovis* or *A. naeslundii* may be isolated either alone or in combination with *A. actinomycetemcomitans, Haemophilus* species, *Propionibacterium* species or *Prevotella* species, any of which may account for up to 25% of the microbiota. It has been proposed that the aetiology involves the introduction of these bacterial species into the deeper tissues following trauma or extraction of a tooth. The characteristic swelling at the angle of the mandible, which may be either localised or diffuse, progresses slowly until multiple sinuses develop within an indurated overlying skin (Fig. 7.14). Pus expressed from the sinuses is thick and yellow with granular particles consisting of calcified aggregates of *Actinomyces* filaments that are referred to as sulphur granules. Diagnosis is based on Gram-staining of these granules combined with an eosin counterstain that produces a clubbing effect on the peripheral filaments (Fig. 7.15). Cultures should be incubated anaerobi-cally for up to 14 days; colonies of *A. israelii* on blood agar are sometimes described as being shaped like molar teeth. Although the submandibular region is by far the most frequently affected area, cases of actino-mycosis have also been reported in the maxillary antrum, tongue and major salivary glands. This infec-tion induces a granulomatous reaction in the sur-rounding tissues, which results in multiple pus-filled pockets within the tissues. This particular aspect of actinomycosis has implications for treatment since it

is essential to break these pockets down surgically to allow drainage. Amoxicillin is the antibiotic of choice although erythromycin or clindamycin should be used if the patient is hypersensitive to penicillins. Therapy may have to be prolonged (4 to 6 weeks) because of failure to achieve adequate drug levels in the granula-tion tissue.

STAPHYLOCOCCAL LYMPHADENITIS

Infections in the head and neck region can cause enlargement and pain in the regional lymph nodes. Although this is a general observation in a number of infections, there is a specific condition in which a patient (usually a child) develops a localised painful swelling of the facial lymph node. This is because of infection involving a *Staphylococcus* spp. which has spread from colonisation within the nose. Flucloxacil-lin should be used systemically to treat the lymphad-enitis and topical fusidic acid should be applied to the anterior part of the nose to eliminate the source of infection.

FACIAL LACERATIONS

Superficial lacerations involving the face, neck and scalp have the potential to become infected with members of the commensal skin microbiota, such as *Staphylococcus epidermidis* and *Propionibacterium acnes*. Soft tissue wounds should be treated within 24 hours by thorough cleaning before suturing. Infection in lac-erations is rare, and there is seldom a need to prescribe antibiotics. If infection develops in a wound, a swab should be taken and sent for culture. In these circumstances an antibiotic with known activity against staphylococci, such as flucloxacillin, can be provided empirically. Wounds that cannot be closed by sutures or adhesive strips, and/or which may become infected, benefit from applications of a topical agent such as 2% mupirocin ointment or 2% fusidic acid cream, which may be applied two or three times daily. There is interest in the use of semiocclusive wound dressings, many of which incorporate antimicrobial agents, to improve wound healing and reduce scarring, which is of particular aesthetic importance in the management of facial wounds.

CHAPTER SUMMARY

Orofacial bacterial infections are usually opportunistic polymicrobial conditions involving microbial species that are also regarded as members of the host commensal microbiota, particularly obligate anaerobes. Wherever possible, samples should be obtained by aspiration to minimise the risk of contamination from saliva and other oral surfaces. Specimens need to be transported to the laboratory promptly for processing. The use of molecular microbiological techniques has revealed that many unculturable bacterial species are often present and these approaches will considerably increase our understanding of the composition of clinical material and potentially highlight significant

disease associations. The reason why these microorganisms become pathogenic is uncertain, but synergistic relationships between some species are likely to be involved. The formation of such consortia is likely to protect infecting microorganisms from the host defences. Antibiotic resistance is relatively rare in dental infections although reduced susceptibility to penicillins because of β-lactamase production, particularly by Gram-negative obligate anaerobic bacilli, is increasingly being encountered. Treatment of such infections should be based on local measures to drain and clear infection. Antibiotic therapy is rarely required and should only be given if symptoms of systemic involvement are present.

FURTHER READING

Kuriyama T, Absi EG, Williams DW, et al. An outcome audit of the treatment of acute dentoalveolar infection: impact of penicillin resistance. *Br Dent J.* 2005;199:759-763.

Kuriyama T, Karasawa T, Nakagawa K, et al. Incidence of β-lactamase production and antimicrobial susceptibility of anaerobic gram-negative rods isolated from pus specimens in orofacial odontogenic infections. *Oral Microbiol Immunol.* 2001;16:10-15.

Mitchell DA. *An introduction to oral and maxillofacial surgery.* Oxford: Oxford University Press; 2006.

Robitaille N, Reed DN, Walters JD, et al. Periodontal and periimplant diseases: Identical or fraternal infections? *Mol Oral Microbiol.* 2015; doi: 10.1111/omi.12124.

Siqueira JF Jr, Rôças IN. Diversity of endodontic microflora revisited. *J Dent Res.* 2009;88:969-981.

Siqueira JF Jr, Rôças IN. Microbiology and treatment of acute apical abscesses. *Clin Microbiol Rev.* 2013;26:255-273.

Stefanopoulos PK, Kolotronis AE. The clinical significance of anaerobic bacteria in acute orofacial infection. *Oral Surg Oral Med Oral Pathol Oral Radiol Endod.* 2004;98:398-408.

MULTIPLE CHOICE QUESTIONS

Answers on p. 250

1 *Studies have revealed that the types of bacteria isolated from orofacial infections reflect which of the following?*

a. Polymicrobial infections, with a wide spectrum of facultatively anaerobic and obligately anaerobic bacteria

b. Obligately anaerobic bacteria only

c. Gram-positive anaerobic bacteria only

d. Gram-negative anaerobic bacteria only

2 *What is the most appropriate sampling technique for the investigation of a purulent orofacial infection?*

a. Moist swabs placed immediately into phosphate-buffered saline (PBS)

b. Moist swab directly into reduced transport fluid

c. Aspiration of pus by syringe

d. Whole saliva

3 *What is the bacterium most commonly isolated from cases of cervicofacial actinomycosis?*
a. *Actinomyces naeslundii*
b. *Actinomyces actinomycetemcomitans*
c. *Actinomyces bovis*
d. *Actinomyces israelii*

4 *Which of the following is the reason that identification of bacteria within orofacial infections can take a number of days?*
a. Time taken in plating the bacteria onto selective and non-selective agar plates
b. Slow-growing nature of obligate anaerobes
c. Lack of knowledge of optimal culture conditions
d. Sample contamination with saliva

5 *The reduced* in vitro *antimicrobial susceptibility to penicillins and other antibiotics of bacteria recovered from orofacial infections is caused by which of the following?*
a. Contamination of cultures
b. Emergence of antibiotic resistance
c. Availability of nutrients and complementary enzymes
d. Reduced activity of penicillins and other antibiotics

6 *A lateral periodontal abscess can be differentiated from a dentoalveolar abscess by which of the following?*
a. Necrotic pulp is evident at the apex of the root
b. The tooth has a vital pulp
c. The tooth requires urgent antibiotic therapy
d. The tooth does not have a vital pulp

7 *What is the drug of choice to treat staphylococcal lymphadenitis?*
a. Metronidazole
b. Flucloxacillin
c. Amoxicillin
d. Tetracycline

8 *The majority of cases of dentoalveolar abscesses can be managed successfully by which of the following?*
a. Intravenous antibiotics
b. Prescribing oral antibiotic therapy
c. Establishing drainage of pus and removal of the source of infection
d. Using antimicrobial rinses

9 *Osteomyelitis in the jaw is rare, but is sometimes a consequence of which of the following?*
a. Radiotherapy
b. Trauma
c. Periimplantitis
d. Xerostomia

10 *Which of the following is an emerging form of periodontitis associated with tooth replacement?*
a. Bacterial sialadenitis
b. Denture stomatitis
c. Periimplantitis
d. Sjögren syndrome

11 *Which of the following statements is correct?*
"In comparison to periodontitis, periimplantitis .."-
a. Is more complex structurally
b. Is less diverse microbiologically
c. Is less likely to be associated with asaccharolytic anaerobes such as *Eubacterium* species
d. Is less likely to be associated with *Candida* spp

12 *Pericoronitis occurs because of which of the following?*
a. Herpetic lesions
b. Trauma
c. Erupting lower third molar teeth in young adults
d. Inflammation found in periodontal pockets

13 *Sialadenitis within the parotid gland is usually caused by the presence of underlying xerostomia often associated with which of the following?*
a. Pericoronitis
b. Sjögren syndrome
c. Gingival inflammation
d. Alveolar osteitis

14 *Which of the following describes the condition presenting as an area of inflammation localised to the angles of the mouth?*
a. Angular cheilitis
b. Stomatitis
c. Herpetic lesion
d. Alveolar osteitis

15 *Which of the following is a specific condition in which a patient, usually a child, develops a localised painful swelling of the facial lymph node?*
a. Pericoronitis
b. Lymphadenitis
c. Cervicofacial actinomycosis.
d. Angular cheilitis

Oral fungal infections

*C*andida are fungi that are frequently encountered in the mouths of healthy individuals and as such are considered members of the normal oral microbiota. The incidence of oral candidal carriage is between 35% and 55% in healthy individuals, depending on the population group studied. Traditionally, other fungi, including species of *Saccharomyces*, *Geotrichum* and *Cryptococcus* have also been isolated from the mouth (Table 8.1), but their numbers are generally limited and they are not normally implicated in oral infection. However, with the advent of new high-throughput sequencing technology, it has become apparent that the oral microbiota is much more complex than culture-based methods would imply. Indeed, studies using pyrosequencing approaches have now detected in excess of 85 fungal genera from the mouths of individuals, a diversity that is much higher than encountered at other body sites. Nevertheless, even using contemporary molecular methods of detection, *Candida* species are still the predominant fungi encountered in the mouth.

Although *Candida* species are normally harmless commensals, when conditions in the mouth alter to one that favours proliferation of *Candida*, a shift to a pathogenic relationship with the host may occur. As such, *Candida* infection is invariably an opportunistic occurrence and dependent upon some form of underlying host predisposition. Infection with *Candida* is described in the literature as a candidosis (candidoses, pl) or candidiasis (candidiases, pl). Both terms are widely used, although candidosis is often preferred because of its consistent use of the osis stem with the terminology for other fungal infections. The term *Candida* originates from the Latin word *candidus*, meaning white. Since *Candida* are eukaryotic cells, they do have a high level of similarity with the mammalian cells of the human host. Nevertheless, there are some key differences, and the presence of a thick cell wall outside the cell membrane of *Candida* is perhaps the most notable difference. The cell wall of *Candida*

TABLE 8.1   Fungal species recovered from the human mouth

Candida species	Other fungal species (rare)
Candida albicans	Paracoccidioides brasiliensis
Candida glabrata	Aspergillus spp.
Candida tropicalis	Cryptococcus neoformans
Candida krusei	Histoplasma capsulatum
Candida lusitaniae	Mucor spp.
Candida dubliniensis	Saccharomyces spp.
Candida kefyr	Geotrichum spp.
Candida guilliermondii	Rhizopus spp.
Candida parapsilosis	

is a two-layered structure comprised mainly of carbohydrates such as mannans, β-glucans and chitin, and proteins are also present. The inner cell wall is afforded strength through the abundance of chitin and β-glucans, whilst the mannans of the outer wall give an open and more porous structure. Since the cell wall is the *Candida* structure that first comes in contact with the host, it is important in terms of antigenicity and adherence to host surfaces (see later sections). In addition, the components within the cell wall, both from a synthesis and structural perspective offer potential targets in the development of antifungal therapies.

PATHOGENIC *CANDIDA* SPECIES

In 2011, the *Candida* genus contained 314 different and ubiquitously distributed species. However, to highlight the dynamic nature of *Candida* taxonomy, by 2014, the classification of a total of 434 yeast species in the *Candida* genus was under discussion. However, it is important to recognise that only a few of these *Candida* species are associated with human infection.

The most prevalent *Candida* species recovered from both healthy and infected human mouths is *Candida albicans*, and it is estimated that this species is responsible for over 80% of oral yeast isolates. In terms of oral prevalence, *C. albicans* is followed by *C. glabrata*, *C. krusei*, *C. tropicalis*, *C. guilliermondii*, *C. kefyr* and

C. parapsilosis, with *C. inconspicua*, *C. lusitaniae*, *C. norvegensis* and *C. rugosa* being less frequently detected. In recent years, the importance of non-*Candida albicans* *Candida* species in human disease has increasingly been recognised. Although these species typically lack the range of virulence factors encountered with *C. albicans*, they have come to prominence because of their enhanced resistance to commonly used antifungal agents. *Candida dubliniensis* was first described in 1995, following its co-isolation with *C. albicans* from cases of oral candidosis in HIV-infected individuals. As *C. dubliniensis* shares a number of unique phenotypic characteristics with *C. albicans*, its misidentification as *C. albicans* has been commonplace.

CANDIDA VIRULENCE FACTORS

The transition of *Candida* from a harmless commensal to a pathogen is complex and most likely relates to local environmental changes in the host that promote either increased growth of *Candida* or altered expression of its virulence factors (Table 8.2). It is likely that the combined effect of both host and candidal factors contribute overall to the development of oral infection. In addition, it is increasingly recognised that as well as interaction between host factors and *Candida*, the bacterial component of the oral microbiota is also important with regards to development of oral candidosis. In categorising *Candida* virulence factors, it is important to note that a number of these do not directly induce damage to host tissues, but will influence lifestyle of *Candida*, which indirectly promote pathogenicity.

ADHERENCE

To cause oral candidosis, *Candida* has to be retained within the mouth. Consequently, a key virulence attribute of *Candida* is its ability to adhere to host surfaces. In the oral cavity, this allows *Candida* to resist removal from the effects of salivary flow and swallowing. Adherence can be to the oral epithelium or surfaces of prosthetic devices including dentures and orthodontic appliances. In the case of oral epithelium, as cells are sloughed off, *Candida* can be removed. Therefore, its ability to grow on the surface at a rate that at least is in equilibrium to loss of cells is vital to its persistence. Furthermore, mucosal surfaces can

TABLE 8.2 Putative virulence factors associated with *Candida albicans*

Virulence factor	Effect
Adherence	**Promotes retention in the mouth**
• Relative cell surface hydrophobicity	• Non-specific adherence process
• Expression of cell surface adhesin molecules	• Facilitates specific adherence mechanisms
Evasion of host defences	**Promotes retention in the mouth**
• High frequency phenotypic switching	• Antigenic modification through frequent cell surface changes
• Hyphal development	• Reduces likelihood of phagocytosis; allows phagocytosed yeast to escape phagocyte
• Secreted aspartyl proteinase production	• Secretory IgA destruction
• Binding of complement molecules	• Antigenic masking
Invasion and destruction of host tissue	**Enhances pathogenicity**
• Hyphal development	• Promotes invasion of oral epithelium
• Secreted aspartyl proteinase production	• Host cell and extracellular matrix damage
• Phospholipase production	• Damage to host cells

IgA, Immunoglobulin A.

readily be recolonised from reservoirs of *Candida* on prosthetic devices, which of course lack the ability to remove *Candida* by surface renewal.

Adherence mechanisms can be specific or non-specific, the latter involving electrostatic or hydrophobic interactions, together with the simple physical entrapment of the microorganism at locations in the mouth. The process of *Candida* adherence is a complex and multifactorial one that is dependent on host and candidal characteristics.

The cell surface molecules on *Candida* involved in specific adherence are described as adhesins (see Chapter 5). The host cell components that these adhesins interact with are referred to as receptors. Perhaps the most frequently cited adhesins of *C. albicans* are the agglutinin-like sequence (ALS) proteins, Hyphal wall protein 1 (Hwp1) and more recently, the EAP1 (enhanced adherence to polystyrene) protein. There are currently eight ALS proteins that are designated ALS1 to ALS7, and ALS9. All have a related three-domain structure and are associated with β-1,6-glucan in the cell wall of *C. albicans*. In the case of Hwp1, glutamine residues in the N-terminal domain are cross-linked to host proteins through the action of host trans-glutaminases leading to covalent attachment between the yeast and host surface. The *EAP1* gene encodes a glycosylphosphatidylinositol-anchored, glucan-cross-linked cell-wall protein that facilitates *C. albicans* adhesion to epithelial cells. Receptors on host surfaces for *Candida* adhesins are thought to include components of serum, extracellular matrix (ECM), and immobilised ligands such as cadherins or integrins. In addition, candidal adhesins may also indirectly bind to the host via interaction with other adherent microorganisms.

MORPHOLOGY

A number of *Candida* species are dimorphic or polymorphic. For example, *C. albicans* and *C. dubliniensis* can both grow as yeast cells, pseudohyphae (elongated chains of yeast cells), and true hyphae (Fig. 8.1). Pseudohyphae and hyphae are distinguishable as the former contains constrictions between filaments as opposed to septa-defined filament divisions. Other *Candida* species grow only in the yeast form or may also produce pseudohyphae. Once attached to host surfaces, *Candida* and in particular *C. albicans* can switch from its yeast morphology to a filamentous form, which may facilitate epithelial penetration, and this, coupled with an increased resistance to

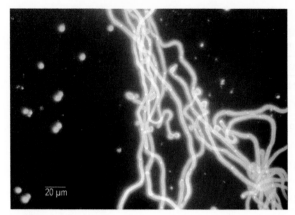

FIGURE 8.1 Fluorescent microscopy image of *Candida albicans* illustrating a mixture of yeast and filamentous growth forms.

phagocytosis, will promote persistence of *Candida* in the mouth. A number of environmental triggers are thought to contribute to the production of hyphal elements including elevated temperature (37°C), CO_2 concentration, alkaline pH, the presence of serum, and limited availability of certain nutrients. Several genes generate positive regulators for hyphal production in *C. albicans* including *HGC1* (hyphae-specific G1 cyclin), *Efg1* (elongation factor G), and *Cph1*. Importantly, mutant strains lacking such functional regulator proteins exhibit an inability to generate hyphae and often, such strains are avirulent.

PHENOTYPIC SWITCHING

High-frequency switching describes the ability of *C. albicans* to rapidly change its cell morphology, and *in vitro* this is seen as reversible changes in colony morphotypes which are induced by exposure to various environmental stimuli. Switching has multiple effects on *Candida* and is associated with altered gene expression affecting surface antigenicity, adhesiveness, drug susceptibility and phagocytosis resistance. The extent of switching mode is a strain-dependent trait and therefore may also subsequently influence strain virulence.

HYDROLYTIC ENZYMES

Destruction of host tissues by *Candida* might be induced by the physical effect of hyphal ingrowth into tissues. However, it is also thought that release of extracellular hydrolytic enzymes into the local environment can also facilitate tissue damage. The enzymes

most frequently implicated in the virulence of *C. albicans* are secreted aspartyl proteinases (SAPs) and phospholipases.

SECRETED ASPARTYL PROTEINASES

Currently, 10 different genes have been identified that encode for SAPs in *C. albicans*. Expression of these *SAP* genes occurs under different conditions and three (*SAP4*, *SAP5* and *SAP6*) appear to be expressed specifically during hyphal development. All SAPs exhibit a number of common characteristics including an activity largely restricted to an acidic environment and one that is inhibited by pepstatin A (a hexapeptide originally isolated from *Actinomyces* species). The *Candida* SAPs provide essential physiologic roles in acquiring nutrition, adapting cell morphology and facilitating growth. The role of these enzymes in virulence is perhaps less clear. However, the ability of SAPs to break down tissue barriers, cleave immune proteins (*e.g.*, immunoglobulins, antimicrobial peptides, complement and cytokines) and facilitate adherence would be obvious features that would enhance pathogenicity. Other species of *Candida* apart from *C. albicans* can produce SAPs, but these enzymes are generally in lower quantities and may differ in activity and antigenicity.

PHOSPHOLIPASES

In addition to SAPs, enzymes categorised as phospholipases (PLs) may also serve as virulence factors of *Candida*. Phospholipases hydrolyse phospholipids into fatty acids, and four classes of phospholipases (A, B, C, and D) have been defined depending upon the type of ester bond cleaved. The production of all classes of phospholipase has been described for *Candida* and these could contribute to host cell membrane damage, promoting cell lysis or exposure of receptors to facilitate adherence.

KEY POINTS

Several *Candida* species are recognised as important opportunistic pathogens of humans and the ability to cause disease is dependent upon the delicate balance that exists between host defences, the composition of the oral microbiota and expression of virulence factors by the infecting *Candida*. No single predominant virulence factor for *Candida* is recognised, although there are a number of putative factors implicated in *Candida* infection. These include attributes involved in the adhesion of *Candida* to oral surfaces (*e.g.*, relative cell surface hydrophobicity and the presence of specific adhesin molecules), *Candida* morphology, the ability to resist host immune defence mechanisms (*e.g.*, high frequency phenotypic switching and morphologic transition) and the release of hydrolytic enzymes (*e.g.*, secreted aspartyl proteinases and phospholipases) that can induce damage to host cells.

ORAL CANDIDOSIS

Candidosis has been referred to as a disease of the diseased, highlighting the importance of host debilitation in the development of infection. This is perhaps most evident from the high incidence of oral candidosis in human immunodeficiency virus (HIV)-positive individuals and those suffering from acquired immunodeficiency syndrome (AIDS). However, less obvious is when infection is triggered by subtle changes within the oral environment and there are many such predisposing factors that are currently recognised (Table 8.3).

It is important to recognise that oral candidosis is not a single infection entity, and traditionally, four distinct forms of primary oral candidoses are described based on clinical presentation (Fig. 8.2). The reasons why individuals suffer from one form of infection as opposed to another are unclear especially as all these infections are seemingly caused by the same fungus.

TABLE 8.3 Host-related factors associated with oral candidosis

Suggested host factor
Local host factors
• Denture wearing
• Steroid inhaler use
• Reduced salivary flow
• Carbohydrate-rich diet
Systemic host factors
• Extremes of age
• Endocrine disorders, *e.g.*, diabetes
• Immunosuppression
• Receipt of broad spectrum antibiotics
• Nutritional deficiencies

Host factors are, however, likely to be instrumental in determining the occurrence of a particular form of oral candidosis. What is also evident is that *C. albicans* is an extremely heterogeneous species, whose strains differ markedly, both phenotypically and genotypically. Thus, candidal strain variation could be a factor in determining which type of infection develops, whether the host actually manages to clear the colonising strain or whether the strain is retained as a commensal. It is conceivable that strain variation could promote pathogenesis through elevated expression of virulence determinants and by affecting the nature of host immune responses.

The four primary forms of oral candidosis will now be described in more detail.

PSEUDOMEMBRANOUS CANDIDOSIS

Pseudomembranous candidosis (Fig. 8.2, A) is characterised by white plaque-like lesions on the oral mucosa and occurs most frequently in neonates and elderly individuals. The relatively high incidence in these groups likely stems from an age-related weakened immune system, or age-related factors that promote *Candida* colonisation. The infection is synonymous with the term oral thrush and the pseudomembranes associated with the condition can be seen on the surface of the labial and buccal mucosa, hard and soft palate, and tongue. These lesions can be removed by gentle scraping (which is a diagnostic feature of the infection) to reveal an underlying erythematous mucosa. When viewed by light microscopy, pseudomembranes contain desquamated epithelial cells and fungal elements.

Pseudomembranous candidosis is generally considered an acute infection resulting from underlying host predisposition. Management and correction of host-related factors frequently leads to resolution of the condition. However, with the advent of HIV infection and AIDS, chronic occurrence of pseudomembranous candidosis occurs that can persist for several months, if not years. Furthermore, in such immunocompromised individuals, progression of oral infection leading to oesophageal involvement is often evident, and this may result in added complications such as difficulties in swallowing and chest pain. The increased prevalence of steroid inhaler use, particularly in young adults as part of asthma management, has also been

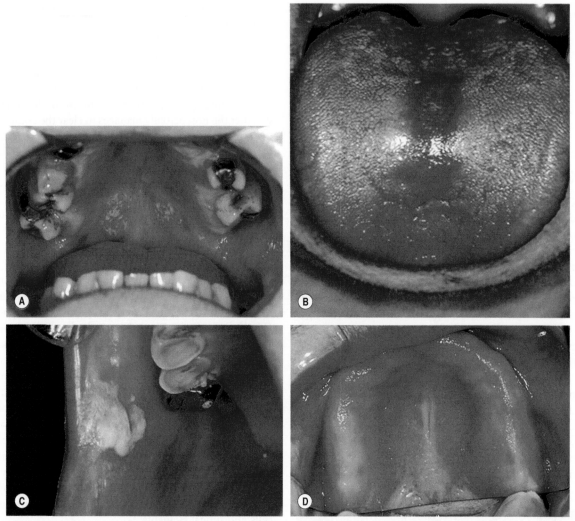

FIGURE 8.2 Clinically distinct forms of oral candidosis (**A**) pseudomembranous candidosis (thrush), (**B**) acute erythematous candidosis, (**C**) chronic hyperplastic candidosis, (**D**) chronic erythematous candidosis.

associated with cases of pseudomembranous candidosis in the soft palate.

ACUTE ERYTHEMATOUS CANDIDOSIS

Acute erythematous candidosis (Fig. 8.2, B) manifests as painful, reddened patches on the oral mucosa, typically on the dorsum of the tongue. The infection is primarily associated with prior receipt of a broad-spectrum antibiotic and particularly when the patient also uses a steroid inhaler. It is believed that antibiotic use decreases the bacterial community within the oral microbiota, allowing *Candida* numbers to increase. Cessation of antibiotic treatment generally results in resolution of the lesion. The relationship between antibiotic therapy and this form of oral candidosis explains its alternative name of antibiotic sore mouth.

CHRONIC HYPERPLASTIC CANDIDOSIS

Chronic hyperplastic candidosis (CHC; Fig. 8.2, C) is a comparatively rare form of oral candidosis and mainly occurs in middle-aged men who are also smokers or have a high rate of alcohol consumption.

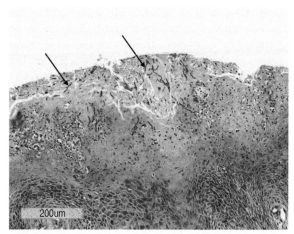

FIGURE 8.3 Periodic acid–Schiff (PAS) staining method detecting hyphal invasion (*arrowed*) of *C. albicans* in chronic hyperplastic candidosis lesions. Image provided by Dr Adam V Jones, School of Dentistry, University of Cardiff.

CHC is often asymptomatic and if left untreated, some cases (5% to 10%) proceed to exhibit dysplasia, with subsequent development of oral cancer at the lesional site. Unlike other forms of oral candidosis, CHC is characterised by *Candida* hyphal invasion of the oral epithelium (Fig. 8.3). Lesions may occur at any oral mucosal site, but are most frequently evident as bilateral white patches in the buccal commissure regions of the mouth. Importantly, the lesions cannot be removed by gentle scraping without bleeding, which distinguishes CHC from pseudomembranous candidosis. Two CHC lesional types are described based on clinical appearance. Homogeneous lesions are smooth and white, and these are distinct from heterogeneous lesions where there are areas of erythema giving a nodular or speckled appearance. Some studies suggest that heterogeneous lesions are more prone to malignant transformation. The potential role of *Candida* in promoting malignancy in CHC is unclear and debate exists on whether occurrence of *Candida* in premalignant lesions reflects a secondary infection or whether *Candida* can instigate malignant change. It has been reported that a higher incidence of cancer occurs in white patch lesions (leukoplakias) that contain *Candida*, and animal models have demonstrated *Candida*-induced epithelial hyperplasia. *Candida* can generate carcinogenic nitrosamines from salivary precursors and importantly, strains exhibiting high nitrosation potential have been recovered from lesions exhibiting advanced precancerous changes.

CHRONIC ERYTHEMATOUS CANDIDOSIS

Chronic erythematous or *Candida*-associated denture stomatitis is the most frequently encountered oral candidosis (Fig. 8.2, D). This infection is seen as reddening (erythema) of the mucosa beneath the fitting surface of a denture. Up to 65% of denture wearers show signs of this infection, although the sufferer is often unaware. The condition develops under any acrylic denture or intra-oral appliance, but is almost invariably seen on the palate rather than on the mandibular mucosa. Inadequate oral hygiene (including poor compliance to denture cleansing and/or not removing the denture at night while sleeping) or the presence of a poor-fitting denture, are both strongly associated with chronic erythematous candidosis. Unlike chronic hyperplastic candidosis, invasion of the epithelium by *Candida* hyphae is not a feature of this infection.

OTHER SECONDARY FORMS OF ORAL CANDIDOSIS

In addition to the primary oral candidoses, other *Candida*-associated lesions are recognised including angular cheilitis, median rhomboid glossitis and chronic mucocutaneous candidosis.

ANGULAR CHEILITIS

Angular cheilitis presents as erythematous lesions at the corners of the mouth (Fig. 8.4). The infection is often seen with other forms of oral candidosis and particularly chronic erythematous candidosis. Although *Candida* are detected from lesional sites, the exact role of the organism in the infection is difficult to ascertain because bacteria such as *Staphylococcus aureus* or streptococci are also frequently present.

MEDIAN RHOMBOID GLOSSITIS

Median rhomboid glossitis manifests as a symmetrical-shaped area in the midline of the dorsum of the tongue. The infection is a chronic one and presents as atrophy of the filiform papillae. Recovery of *Candida* from this area is high and the infection is strongly associated with smoking and use of inhaled steroids.

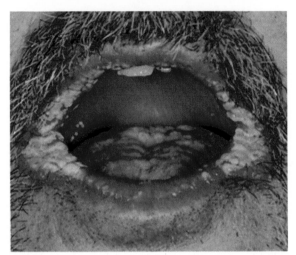

FIGURE 8.4 *Candida*-associated lesions as illustrated by angular cheilitis.

CHRONIC MUCOCUTANEOUS CANDIDOSIS

Chronic mucocutaneous candidosis (CMC) manifests as a collection of *Candida* infections confined to the skin, mucous membranes and nails of an individual. A number of relatively rare congenital conditions are associated with CMC, and the key predisposing factor would appear to be an impaired cellular immunity against *Candida*.

KEY POINTS

Oral candidosis is not a single disease entity and four clinically distinct primary infections are described. These include pseudomembranous candidosis and acute erythematous candidosis, which are typically acute infections. Chronic forms of candidoses are chronic erythematous candidosis and chronic hyperplastic candidosis. With the advent of the AIDS epidemic and long-term use of steroid inhalers, chronic forms of pseudomembranous candidosis are more frequently encountered. Each infection has a distinct clinical presentation and associated host predisposing factors.

HOST RESPONSE TO ORAL CANDIDOSIS

Efficient host immunity is essential in prevention of oral candidosis. Innate immunity is first encountered in the oral cavity in the form of antimicrobial peptides (AMPs), also referred to as host defence peptides (HDPs; see Chapter 2) that are found in saliva or released by oral epithelial cells. The latter occurs when *Candida* binds to a particular group of receptors on epithelial cell surfaces. These receptors are termed pattern-recognition receptors, of which Toll-like receptors (TLRs) are a major class. In humans, TLR2 and TLR4 are responsible for recognising fungal pathogens resulting in activation of intracellular pathways leading to cytokine production, activation of the innate immune response and release of AMPs. Furthermore, the β-glucan component of the *Candida* cell wall can be recognised by a lectin receptor expressed on certain epithelial and host defence cells; this receptor is called dectin-1.

Examples of AMPs include lactoferrin, α- and β-defensins, histatins, lysozyme, secretory immunoglobulin A, mucins, sialoperoxidase and transferrin (see Chapter 2). The primary function of AMPs is to kill *Candida* or limit its adherence to oral surfaces. Histatins are largely specific to the mouth and have anticandidal activity. Reduced histatin levels have been linked with elevated *Candida* colonisation of the oral mucosa.

Also of importance in early host defence is the phagocytotic clearing of *C. albicans* by polymorphonuclear cells (PMNs) and monocytes. Stimulation of macrophages may occur through direct contact with candidal cell-wall molecules. After phagocytosis, killing of *C. albicans* involves reactive oxygen and nitrogen intermediates. Phagocyte-dependent protection is promoted or impaired by cytokines released by T-helper (Th) cells. The importance of an appropriate Th response in protecting against oral candidosis is highlighted by the high incidence of oral candidosis in HIV-positive individuals, where decline in T-cell activity occurs. The type of Th response generated is influenced by interaction of *Candida* with antigen-presenting cells (APCs), such as dendritic cells (DCs), that perform a sentinel role within the oral mucosa. After contact with *Candida*, or its products, DCs migrate into the draining lymph node where they mature and direct CD4+ T cells to develop subsets of T helper (Th) cells (*e.g.*, Th1, Th2, Th17, Treg cells) by *Candida* antigen presentation and cytokine production. Polarised T cell maturation towards Th1 and Th17 types is considered protective against *Candida* through promoting cell-mediated immunity and phagocytosis, whereas Th2 responses are linked with B cell development and *Candida* mucosal infection.

Evidence suggests that the environment of initial DC stimulation may be important in determining the Th response. Studies in mice indicate that early release of proinflammatory cytokines such as interferon-γ (IFN-γ) and tumour necrosis factor-α (TNF-α) by macrophages, and interleukin-12 (IL-12) by DCs are important in directing Th cell maturation towards the Th1 type. In contrast, release of IL-4 and IL-10 would appear important for Th2 cell development. Different strains of *C. albicans* could theoretically influence this process by stimulating tissues to produce particular cytokine profiles, or affecting the DC phenotype and thus the influence of DCs on naïve T cell maturation. There is evidence suggesting that the latter occurs with the different morphologic forms of *C. albicans*, as DCs have been shown to discriminate between yeast and hyphal forms of *C. albicans*, which respectively promote Th1 and Th2 responses. Development of regulatory T cells (CD4⁺CD25⁺ T lymphocytes; Treg cells) is promoted by IL-10 and transforming growth factor β (TGFβ), and it has been suggested that Treg cells suppress the normally protective Th1 responses.

Recently, it has been reported that epithelial cells can also differentiate between the hyphal and yeast forms of *C. albicans* after the adherence process. Oral epithelial cells respond to *C. albicans* through NF-κB (nuclear factor kappa-light-chain-enhancer of activated B cells) and MAPK (mitogen-activated protein kinase) signalling. Regardless of morphology, *C. albicans* activates NF-κB with a subsequent transient MAPK response. This then activates a transcription factor termed c-Jun. However, in the case of hyphae a much stronger MAPK response occurs, with subsequent activation of a transcription factor called c-Fos and production of the MAPK phosphatase MKP1. This hyphal-induced response triggers production of proinflammatory cytokines. Furthermore, the response is also dependent on hyphal bioburden and therefore it constitutes a protective mechanism that is only initiated when a significant pathogenic threat is present.

Antibody-driven (humoral immunity) protection against oral candidosis is first seen in the form of secretory IgA, which is an important inhibitor of *Candida* (and indeed other oral microbial) adhesion to oral surfaces. Serum antibodies probably constitute a secondary defence line and become important once either tissue penetration or systemic infection occurs.

KEY POINTS

Host defence against oral candidosis initially involves a complex combination of non-specific antimicrobial molecules found in saliva and gingival crevicular fluid, the phagocytic clearing activity of polymorphonuclear and monocytic cells, and classical cell-mediated defence mechanisms. Host epithelial cells and immune cells are thought to have the ability to differentiate between candidal yeast and hyphae and elicit different responses accordingly. In the event of tissue penetration, antibody-based protection will become more prominent. A deficiency in the functioning of any of these defence mechanisms has the effect of predisposing an individual to *Candida* infection.

DIAGNOSIS OF ORAL CANDIDOSIS

Diagnosis of oral candidosis is frequently done based on clinical features, although microbiologic specimens should be taken to identify and quantify any *Candida* that may be present and provide isolates for antifungal sensitivity testing. Identification of infecting agents is important as the emergence of species with reduced sensitivity to frequently administered antifungals is increasingly evident.

ISOLATION OF *CANDIDA* FROM THE ORAL CAVITY

Oral samples can be obtained by a variety of methods (Table 8.4) with the most common approaches being the taking of swabs, imprint cultures, oral rinses and the collection of whole saliva. Each method has merits and drawbacks, and the most appropriate technique is dependent on the lesion type. When there is an accessible and defined lesion, a direct sampling approach, such as a swab or imprint is often preferred, as these provide information on the organisms at the lesion itself. Where no obvious lesions are present, or when the lesion is difficult to access, indirect analysis based on culture of saliva or an oral rinse is more acceptable.

In chronic hyperplastic candidosis, a biopsy of the lesion is necessary for subsequent detection of invading *Candida* by histologic staining using the periodic acid-Schiff (PAS) technique or Gomori methenamine silver stains (Fig. 8.3).

Quantitative estimation of fungal load at the lesion has been justified as a means of differentiating between commensal carriage and pathogenic involvement of oral *Candida*, with higher numbers considered likely

TABLE 8.4 Methods of recovering *Candida* from the oral cavity

Isolation method	Advantages	Disadvantages
Culture of whole saliva	Sensitive; viable organisms isolated	Problems may occur with collection of sample; not site specific
Concentrated oral rinse	Quantitative; viable cells isolated	Some patients have difficulty in using rinse; not site specific
Swab	Simple to use; viable cells isolated; site specific	Difficult to standardise
Smear	Simple to use; not reliant on culture	Viable cells not determined; species identity not readily confirmed
Imprint culture	Quantitative; viable cells isolated; site specific	Some sites difficult to sample
Biopsy	Essential for chronic hyperplastic candidosis	Invasive; not appropriate for other forms of candidosis

in the latter. On this basis, the imprint culture and the oral rinse offer advantages over the other approaches.

Samples for *Candida* detection are traditionally cultured on Sabouraud dextrose agar (SDA), which supports growth of oral *Candida* species, with the added benefit of suppressing bacterial growth because of a relatively low pH. Occasionally, microbiologists will incorporate antibiotics into SDA to further increase selectivity. Other differential media, *e.g.*, CHROMagar® *Candida* (Fig. 8.5), have been developed and provide presumptive identification of certain *Candida* species based on colony appearance and colour following primary culture. The advantage of such media is that multiple *Candida* species in a single infection can be determined, which may be important in selecting subsequent treatment options.

Definitive identification of *Candida* can be made through a variety of supplemental tests such as those based on morphologic and physiologic characteristics of isolates. As previously mentioned, *C. albicans* and *C. dubliniensis* are the only species that produce true hyphal growth, and this trait is exploited for identification through the germ-tube test. In the germ-tube test, the organism is subcultured in horse serum at 37°C for 2 to 4 hours, and then examined by light microscopy for germ-tubes (rudimentary hyphae; Fig. 8.6).

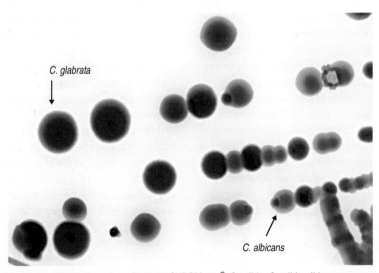

C. glabrata

C. albicans

FIGURE 8.5 Mixed *Candida* species differentiated by culture on CHROMagar® *Candida*. *Candida albicans* appear as green colonies, non-C. *albicans* species frequently present with purple or alternative colouration.

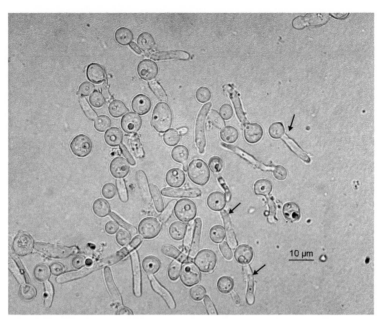

FIGURE 8.6 Germ-tube production (*arrowed*) by *C. albicans* cultured in horse serum at 37°C for 2–4 hours.

Candida albicans and *C. dubliniensis* can also be identified from other species based on chlamydospore production. Chlamydospores are refractile, spherical structures generated at the ends of hyphae following culture on nutritionally poor media such as cornmeal agar. Isolates are inoculated in a crosshatch pattern on the agar, overlaid with a sterile coverslip and incubated for 24 to 48 hours at 37°C; chlamydospores are then detected microscopically (Fig. 8.7).

Biochemical identification of *Candida* is primarily based on carbohydrate assimilation, with a range of commercial systems now available to facilitate such tests. Isolate identification is determined by the profile of carbohydrates able to support growth of the test organism. Traditional testing would have involved culture of test isolates on a basal agar lacking a carbon source. Carbohydrate solutions would then be placed within wells of the seeded agar or upon filter paper discs located on the agar surface. Growth in the vicinity of the carbon source would indicate utilisation. Commercial systems such as the API 32C system are based on the same principle, but test carbohydrates are housed in plastic wells located on a test strip. Growth in each well is read by changes in turbidity or colour changes in certain kit systems. Numerical codes obtained from the test results are used to identify the test organism based on database comparison.

Increasingly, molecular-based methods are used, with a number of species-specific polymerase chain reaction (PCR) approaches for *Candida* available. Several target genes have been reported for *Candida* species discrimination, although the most frequently used are regions of the ribosomal ribonucleic acid (rRNA) operon. Identification is obtained based on PCR product size as determined by electrophoretic mobility, or PCR product sequence determined by direct sequencing or through use of restriction fragment analysis following cleavage of PCR sequences with restriction endonucleases. Molecular-based technologies such as pulsed field gel electrophoresis (PFGE), random amplified polymorphic deoxyribonucleic acid (RAPD) analysis and REP (repeat sequence amplification) PCR have been used to genotype *Candida* species in epidemiologic studies of oral candidosis.

MANAGEMENT OF ORAL CANDIDOSIS

Since oral candidosis is an opportunistic infection, identification and elimination of underlying predisposing host factors (Table 8.3) is key to patient management.

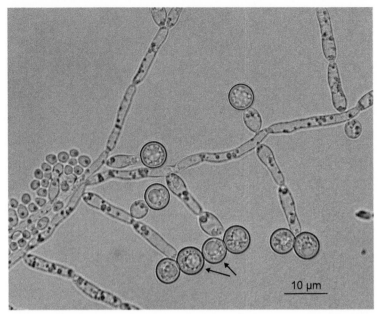

FIGURE 8.7 Chlamydospores (arrowed) produced by *Candida albicans* on cornmeal tween 20 agar.

KEY POINTS

In recent years, greater emphasis has been placed on the reliable identification of *Candida* from human clinical samples. A key driver to this has been the recognition that different *Candida* species are associated with human infection and importantly, these may vary in both pathogenic potential and susceptibility to administered antifungal agents. Since *Candida* are frequent components of the microbiota in health, appropriate sampling methods are required to assist in ascertaining the exact location of the organisms in the mouth together with their number. There are a wide variety of phenotypic methods available for identifying isolated *Candida* including differential agar media, morphologic culture tests and biochemical screening panels. These methods have recently been supplemented with more sophisticated molecular tests involving analysis of the DNA of isolated organisms.

Consideration of the patient's medical history is highly important in developing a management regime for a patient with oral candidosis, and predisposing factors need to be identified and resolved wherever possible. In many cases these goals are achievable as exemplified by improving the oral hygiene of denture wearers who have chronic erythematous candidosis, which is paramount to management of this condition. Stopping smoking of sufferers with CHC or median rhomboid glossitis should also be targeted, together with educating asthmatics using steroid inhalers about the importance of rinsing their mouths after administration of the inhaler. Haematological tests may reveal deficiencies in vitamins and minerals, and such situations may be addressed through management of diet and/or the use of supplements. Undiagnosed or poorly controlled diabetes is a recognised predisposing factor to oral candidosis and therefore assessment of blood glucose may be required.

In some instances, predisposing factors cannot be resolved, as seen for individuals who are immunosuppressed through the receipt of an immunosuppressant drug required for the treatment of a cancer, or to avoid organ rejection following transplant surgery. In these cases, the role of antifungal therapy in management of candidosis has added importance.

The range and use of antifungal drugs in the management of oral candidosis is covered in detail in Chapter 10. The development of such agents has been limited compared with antibiotics, and this has been attributed to the inherent problems of developing effective agents active against a eukaryotic fungal cell without having toxicity to eukaryotic host cells. In addition, it is only relatively recently that diagnostic procedures have highlighted the significant role that fungi have in human disease and indeed their increasing occurrence, largely because of medical interventions increasing host susceptibility. Antifungal resistance is also increasing and may either be intrinsic (present without previous exposure to the antifungal) or inherent, where resistance develops in a previously susceptible organism following exposure. The two major groups of antifungal drugs are the polyenes (*e.g.*, nystatin and amphotericin) and the azoles (*e.g.*, fluconazole and itraconazole). Polyene antifungals exhibit their activity through interaction with the ergosterol component of the fungal cell membrane that generates pores, and induces cell leakage with loss of cytoplasmic content. Azole antifungals inhibit ergosterol biosynthesis by interfering with the fungal enzyme, lanosterol demethylase, leading to a depletion of ergosterol in the fungal cell membrane. Azole antifungals are fungistatic rather than fungicidal and consequently, it is important to simultaneously address underlying host conditions to provide the best chance of infection resolution.

In recent years, several new classes of antifungals have been developed that target the fungal cell wall. For example, the echinocandins (caspofungin, micafungin, and anidulafungin) inhibit synthesis of β1,3 D-glucan, whereas nikkomycins inhibit biosynthesis of chitin.

KEY POINTS

> Management of oral candidosis involves the identification and control of host factors that predispose to the infection. In addition, a range of antifungal agents is available to directly combat infecting *Candida*. The variety and number of these agents is low compared with traditional antibiotics that target bacteria, which is in part because of the difficulties in developing an antifungal agent that is effective against its targeted organism and has no toxic effects against host cells. Suitable antifungal strategies include either directly targeting the ergosterol component in the fungal cell membrane (polyene antifungals) or the enzymes involved in its biosynthesis (azole antifungals). More recently, constituents of the fungal cell wall such as chitin (target site of nikkomycins) and glucan (echinocandin antifungals) have received attention, although the use of these agents is currently limited with regard to oral candidosis.

CHAPTER SUMMARY

Several species of *Candida* are frequently encountered as harmless members of the normal oral microbiota of humans. In instances where host debilitation occurs, these fungi can cause infection, which may manifest as several forms of oral candidosis, each with distinct clinical presentations.

Candida albicans is the most frequently isolated species from the oral cavity and although it also represents the principal species associated with oral candidosis, several other species can also cause oral infection.

Candida albicans expresses a number of putative virulence factors that contribute to its pathogenicity. The ability to switch from yeast to hyphal morphology is linked with protection against host immune defences and invasion of the oral epithelium. In addition, a number of hydrolytic enzymes including the secreted aspartyl proteinases and phospholipases are implicated in causing host cell damage and degradation of defence molecules. Expression of these virulence factors alone is not sufficient to cause infection and needs to be coupled with a lowering of host defence mechanisms.

Significant advances have been made in developing methods aimed at identifying *Candida*. These advances also correlate with the increasing incidence of all forms of candidosis as the proportions of debilitated and immunosuppressed people have elevated. The reasons for such increases in human candidosis have largely been attributed to the wider use of invasive surgical procedures, immunosuppressive therapies and the spread of HIV and AIDS infection.

An important aspect of patient management of oral candidosis is to address any underlying host predisposing factor. This may take the form of advising patients on aspects of oral hygiene or denture cleansing, administration of appropriate therapeutics or correcting any nutritional deficiencies. In many cases however, antifungal therapy will be required, particularly when any underlying host factors cannot be identified or modulated.

In recent years there has also been much emphasis on the development of antifungal agents used in the management of candidosis. Such development has again been in response to the increasing incidence of candidosis and is also a reflection of the more prevalent detection of non-*Candida albicans Candida* species in human infection. Although these species are often considered to be inherently less pathogenic than *C. albicans*, they frequently exhibit greater resistance to certain antifungal agents.

FURTHER READING

Additional resources on the clinical aspects of oral candidosis include the historical works of Samaranayake & MacFarlane (1990), Oral candidosis, Wright, London, United Kingdom; and the reference book of Odds (1988), *Candida* and candidosis: a review and bibliography, Bailliere Tindale, London, United Kingdom. More contemporary and specific references on aspects covered in this chapter are listed below.

Butts A, Krysan DJ. Antifungal drug discovery: something old and something new. *PLoS Pathog.* 2012;8:e1002870.

Li L, Redding S, Dongari-Bagtzoglou A. *Candida glabrata:* an emerging oral opportunistic pathogen. *J Dent Res.* 2007;86: 204-215.

Mayer FL, Wilson D, Hube B. *Candida albicans* pathogenicity mechanisms. *Virulence.* 2013;4:119-128.

Naglik JR, Moyes DL, Wächtler B, et al. *Candida albicans* interactions with epithelial cells and mucosal immunity. *Microbes Infect.* 2011;13:963-976.

Soysa NS, Samaranayake LP, Ellepola ANB. Antimicrobials as a contributory factor in oral candidosis - a brief overview. *Oral Dis.* 2008;14:138-143.

Wei XQ, Rogers H, Lewis MA, et al. The role of the IL-12 cytokine family in directing T-cell responses in oral candidosis. *Clin Dev Immunol.* 2011;697340.

Williams DW, Kuriyama T, Silva S, et al. *Candida* biofilms and oral candidosis: treatment and prevention. *Periodontol 2000.* 2011;55:250-265.

Williams DW, Lewis MA. Isolation and identification of *Candida* from the oral cavity. *Oral Dis.* 2000;6:3-11.

MULTIPLE CHOICE QUESTIONS

Answers on p. 250

1 Which of the following fungal genera is most often considered as part of normal oral microflora?
a. *Saccharomyces*
b. *Aspergillus*
c. *Candida*
d. *Cryptococcus*

2 Which Candida *species is most frequently isolated from the human mouth?*
a. *Candida dubliniensis*
b. *Candida parapsilosis*
c. *Candida albicans*
d. *Candida guilliermondii*

3 Which of the following host factors does not promote oral candidosis?
a. A reduced flow of saliva
b. A weakened immune system
c. The use of broad-spectrum antibiotics
d. Infection with herpes simplex virus 1 (HSV-1)

4 Which one of the following is a Candida albicans virulence factor?
a. Expression of antibiotic resistance
b. Secretion of aspartyl proteinases
c. Replication in the yeast morphology
d. Production of acid from fermentation of sucrose

5 Acute erythematous candidosis is characterised by which of the following?
a. White patch lesions
b. Pseudomembranes
c. Difficulty in swallowing
d. Painful reddened patches on the palate

6 Which one of the following is considered a secondary Candida infection?
a. Periodontal infection
b. Hairy leukoplakia
c. Dentoalveolar abscess
d. Angular cheilitis

7 Which one of the following forms of oral candidosis has an association with oral cancer?
a. Acute erythematous candidosis
b. Median rhomboid glossitis
c. Chronic hyperplastic candidosis
d. Chronic erythematous candidosis

8 *Host protection from oral candidosis first involves which of the following?*
  a. Preventing adherence by antimicrobial molecules in saliva
  b. Phagocytic responses by macrophages
  c. T-cell derived inflammatory cytokines
  d. The removal of adhered *Candida* by high epithelial cell turnover.

9 *Which of the following approaches provides a sample for quantifying* Candida *in the mouth?*
  a. Oral rinse
  b. Swab
  c. Biopsy
  d. Mucosal smear

10 *Which of the following antifungal agents inhibits ergosterol synthesis?*
  a. Nystatin
  b. Itraconazole
  c. Nikkomycins
  d. Echinocandins

CHAPTER 9

Orofacial viral infections

It has been estimated that 90% of adults harbour viruses that have been acquired as a result of infection during earlier life. Many viruses have the property of latency and may reside in the tissues asymptomatically for the remainder of the patient's life. The orofacial tissues are a frequent site for symptomatic primary infection and also reactivation of latent viruses. The presence of these viruses often becomes apparent at times when the host's immune defence is compromised. The clinical signs and symptoms may range from recurrent episodes lasting a few days in otherwise healthy individuals to prolonged lesions in patients with human immunodeficiency virus (HIV).

Viruses are some of the smallest microorganisms (100 to 300 nm) consisting of a core (genome) containing either deoxyribonucleic acid (DNA) or ribonucleic acid (RNA) surrounded by a protein shell (capsid) (Fig. 9.1), and can cause a range of important human diseases. Certain viruses also possess an outer lipoprotein coat derived from infected host cells. Viruses are obligate intracellular parasites in that they require the protein synthesising apparatus (ribosomes) of the host cell. Viral replication is a complex process but comprises a number of recognised steps including adsorption/penetration into the host cell, uncoating, transcription, synthesis of viral components, assembly and finally, release of new virions (Fig. 9.2).

DIAGNOSIS OF VIRAL DISEASE

A variety of laboratory methods have been developed for the detection, isolation and identification of viruses within clinical samples (Table 9.1). These techniques involve microscopy, culture, serology and nucleic acid amplification. However, the most appropriate method of sampling depends on the nature of the suspected infection.

Electron microscopy can be used to provide a provisional identification based on the morphological appearance of viral particles, but this approach has

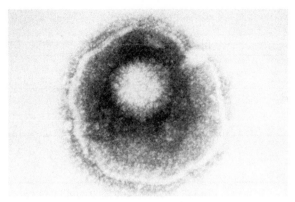

FIGURE 9.1 Photomicrograph of HSV-1 showing central capsid and surrounding envelope (original magnification × 100 000).

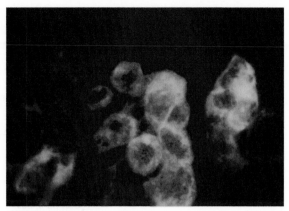

FIGURE 9.3 Immunofluorescence of a smear showing presence of herpes simplex virus-1.

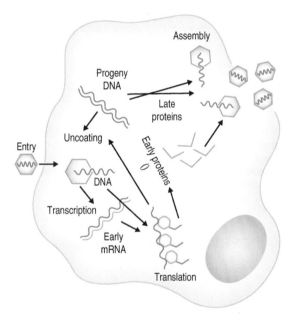

FIGURE 9.2 Stages of herpes simplex virus replication within a host cell.

low specificity and requires additional tests. Routine light microscopy can be used in conjunction with immunofluorescence and monoclonal antibodies to detect the presence of specific viruses (Fig. 9.3). This is a relatively rapid method, giving a result within 30 minutes, but the technique is not widely available.

Historically, the confirmation of the clinical presence of a particular virus has been based on growth in tissue culture, usually involving baby hamster or monkey kidney fibroblasts. A swab of the lesion should be placed in viral transport medium, which contains at least two antibiotics, usually penicillin and streptomycin, to prevent bacterial growth, combined with an antifungal, such as amphotericin, to eliminate any fungal contamination. The transport medium should also contain serum and a buffer to maintain virus viability. The specimen should be sent to the laboratory promptly although it will not be processed for 24 hours to allow the antimicrobials mentioned earlier time to have an effect. The first stage of processing is inoculation into a monolayer of tissue culture. The presence of virus is determined in the laboratory by detection of a cytopathic effect, which is seen as the development of multinucleate giant cells. This may take up to 10 days, although the cytopathic effect occurs more rapidly in the presence of high numbers of virus particles.

Alternatively, diagnosis may be confirmed retrospectively by the detection of a 4-fold rise in antibody titre between acute and convalescent sera taken from the patient. However, this technique has limited clinical benefit in diagnosis because of the prolonged time involved in obtaining a result.

Molecular methods, based on real-time polymerase chain reaction (PCR), to detect viral DNA or messenger RNA (mRNA), have been developed for the detection of specific viruses in clinical samples and are now being used for the diagnosis of infection due

TABLE 9.1 Special investigations used in the diagnosis of orofacial viral infection		
Investigation	**Advantages**	**Disadvantages**
Electron microscopy of vesicular fluid	Easy to sample Rapid result	Insensitive Not specific
Light microscopy of lesional smear	Easy to sample smear Widely available Rapid result	Not specific
Light microscopy of lesional smear with immunofluorescence	Easy to sample Rapid result Specific	Not routinely available
Culture of swab of lesion	Easy to sample Can be specific Widely available	Result may not be available for up to 10 days
Antibody titre in venous blood	Requires paired venous samples	Two haematological samples required. Result not available for at least two weeks
Polymerase chain reaction amplification of vesicular fluid or swab of lesion	Easy to sample Rapid result Cost effective	Previously not widely available

to herpes simplex viruses (HSVs) and varicella zoster virus (VZV). These methods can be used on a variety of clinical specimens, including the sample of choice for orofacial tissues, namely, a swab from the lesion placed in viral transport fluid. Saliva samples, collected on cotton wool rolls, can also be used. Several multiplex systems have been employed for the detection of HSV-1, HSV-2 and VZV, and a range of kits are available commercially. Not only are these more sensitive than the traditional methods of detection but the total test-to-result time can be less than 1 hour. The rapid availability of a result provides a huge clinical advantage over any other method of detection. Commercially available molecular PCR assays are now being approved by regulatory bodies and are being employed routinely in diagnostic virology laboratories.

KEY POINTS

The majority of adult individuals in the Western world have suffered from primary viral infections and harbour latent viruses in the orofacial tissues.

Detection of the presence of viruses can be achieved by a variety of methods although most of these are associated with long delays before results are available, which limits their clinical usefulness. Molecular-based methods, that provide relatively rapid confirmation of the presence and identification of viruses, are becoming more widely used and this will assist patient management.

MANAGEMENT OF VIRAL INFECTIONS

Viral infection that leads to clinical signs and symptoms within the orofacial tissues can either be a primary infection caused by initial infection or secondary infection caused by reactivation of latent virus within the tissues. In the vast majority of cases of a primary infection, the patient will recover relatively quickly because of the production of specific antibodies by their immune system. Treatment in these circumstances is palliative and can be limited to provision of antiinflammatory therapy that is aimed at reducing symptoms of pain and raised temperature. Assessment of the patient's general health and immune status is an important principle of management because the presence of underlying systemic disease or reduced host defence mechanisms will influence the choice of additional therapy. Immunodeficiency and immunosuppression, either inherent or drug induced, are important considerations influencing the use of antiviral agents. Only a small number of drugs with direct antiviral action have been developed (see Chapter 10). The use of antiviral therapy should be considered carefully because the principle action of these drugs is prevention of viral replication and therefore maximum benefit is gained early in infection. Little additional benefit is gained by the drugs once the infection is established and the host immune system is producing antibodies. However, the use of an antiviral agent should be considered in situations where the patient is immunocompromised, either because of underlying disease or immunosuppressive therapy, such as systemic steroids.

KEY POINTS

A number of viruses can cause orofacial signs and symptoms. If the patient is otherwise healthy, the management of viral infections is essentially palliative. The use of specific antiviral drugs should be reserved for patients who have underlying medical conditions that are associated with impaired immunity.

HERPES VIRUSES

The name herpes comes from the Greek word *herpein,* which means to creep (chronic, recurrent). Although more than 100 herpes viruses have been isolated in nature, only eight herpes viruses have been described in humans and these are classified according to their biological properties into three subfamilies: Alphaherpesvirinae, Betaherpesvirinae and Gammaherpesvirinae (Table 9.2), all of which may be encountered in orofacial tissues.

HERPES SIMPLEX TYPE 1

Primary infection

Primary infection with herpes simplex type 1 (HSV-1) usually occurs during the first few years of life, and antibody markers to the virus are found almost universally in the population in the Western world by 15 years of age. Orofacial signs and symptoms are characterised by the rapid development of generalised oral discomfort and widespread gingivostomatitis. These features are relatively mild and often

TABLE 9.2 Nomenclature of human herpes viruses (*herpesviridae*)

Name	Trivial name	Acronym
Alphaherpesvirinae		
Human herpesvirus 1	Herpes simplex virus 1	HSV-1
Human herpesvirus 2	Herpes simplex virus 2	HSV-2
Human herpesvirus 3	Varicella zoster virus	VZV
Betaherpesvirinae		
Human herpesvirus 5	Cytomegalovirus	HCMV
Human herpesvirus 6		HHV-6
Gammaherpesvirinae		
Human herpesvirus 4	Epstein-Barr virus	EBV
Human herpesvirus 7		HHV-7
Human herpesvirus 8	Kaposi sarcoma herpesvirus	HHV-8

mistakenly diagnosed as an episode of teething in young children. However, it has been estimated that clinical changes are severe in up to 10% of cases and manifest as blood-crusted lips (Fig. 9.4), gingival swelling, multiple oral ulcers, lymphadenopathy and pyrexia. Regardless of the severity of the primary infection, all signs and symptoms resolve within 10 days. The signs and symptoms of primary herpetic gingivitis are often sufficiently characteristic that a diagnosis can be made on the findings of clinical presentation alone. However, if definitive diagnosis of HSV-1 infection is required, this can be made by detection of the virus from a swab of a lesion using either culture or preferably a molecular assay. Large numbers of virus are present not only on the ulcerated mucosa but also within saliva.

Treatment is supportive although a decision must be made on the need to provide the patient with antiviral therapy. The agent of choice is aciclovir, preferably as a suspension, because the tablet form is difficult to swallow in the presence of widespread oral

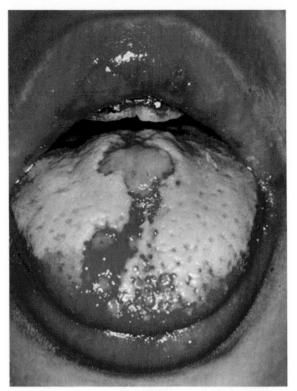

FIGURE 9.4 Blood-encrusted lips and oral ulceration of primary herpes simplex virus-1 infection.

ulceration. Aciclovir (200 mg) should be given five times daily for 5 days. Children under the age of 2 years should receive a half-dose, whereas those over 2 years of age should receive the adult dose. Regardless of the use of an antiviral agent, HSV-1 is not eliminated from the body following resolution of the acute symptoms, and the virus remains within the tissues in a latent form and can reactivate.

Secondary infection

Up to 40% of HSV-1 positive individuals suffer from recurrent episodes of secondary infection. Reactivation of latent HSV-1 is related to either a breakdown in local immunosurveillance or an alteration in local inflammatory mediators. Traditionally, it has been thought that reactivated HSV-1 migrates from the trigeminal ganglion to the peripheral tissues of the lips or face. Although this is true, it is becoming increasingly apparent that HSV also resides more locally in neural and other tissues.

Reactivation of HSV-1 characteristically produces herpes labialis, known more commonly as a cold sore or fever blister (Fig. 9.5). The symptoms of herpes labialis characteristically begin with a tingle or burning sensation (prodrome) in a localised region of the lips at the vermillion border. However, approximately 25%

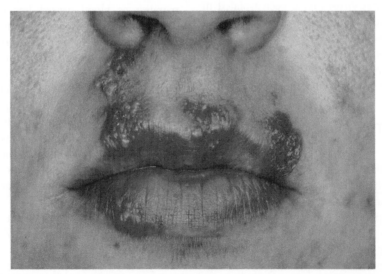

FIGURE 9.5 Recurrent herpes labialis (cold sore) caused by reactivation of herpes simplex virus-1.

of episodes have no prodromal stage and the lesion initiates as vesicles. Within 48 hours the vesicles rupture to leave an erosion, which subsequently crusts over and eventually heals within 7 to 10 days. The clinical appearance is so characteristic that diagnosis is based on this alone. However, if necessary, the presence of HSV can be confirmed by sending a lesional swab for either tissue culture or molecular assay. Alternatively, HSV can be detected by immunofluorescence on a smear of the lesion. Factors that predispose to the development of herpes labialis in susceptible individuals include sunlight, trauma, stress, fever, menstruation and immunosuppression. A sunscreen applied to the lips can also be effective in reducing the frequency of sunlight-induced recurrences. The topical application of aciclovir or penciclovir can reduce the duration of the outbreak. Individuals with severe or frequent recurrences can benefit from the prophylactic use of systemic aciclovir (200 mg two or three times daily).

Reactivation of HSV-1 can also produce recurrent intra-oral ulceration. In a similar way to herpes labialis, the patient with an intraoral lesion is usually aware of prodromal tingling. The mucosa of the hard palate (Fig. 9.6) is the site most frequently involved. It is also recognised that HSV-1 is asymptomatic and shed periodically in the saliva of up to 70% of the population at least once a month. Such shedding represents a risk of spread of the virus and, in part, explains the widespread nature of HSV-1 in the community. Reactivation of HSV-1 has also been implicated as an aetiological factor in periodontal disease and erythema multiforme.

HERPES SIMPLEX TYPE 2

It has traditionally been taught that herpes simplex type 2 (HSV-2) is only encountered in the genital region. However, it is becoming increasingly apparent that on rare occasions HSV-2 can cause oral lesions clinically identical to those of secondary HSV-1 infection. This observation is probably because of the more frequent transmission of virus as a result of direct contact during orogenital sexual practices but may, in part, also reflect the more widespread use of typing methods for suspected orofacial herpetic infections. The presence of HSV-2 can be confirmed by molecular methods or, if available, direct immunofluorescence on a smear. Aciclovir is the agent of first choice for treatment of HSV-2 infection. At present HSV-2 is associated with an increased risk of cervical cancer, but a similar association has not been shown for mouth cancer.

VARICELLA ZOSTER VIRUS
Primary infection

VZV, the third member of the herpes group of viruses, spreads by droplet infection and the primary infection occurs most frequently in childhood causing

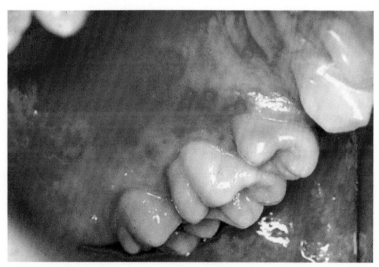

FIGURE 9.6 Localised cluster of ulcers in the palate caused by reactivation of herpes simplex virus-1.

chickenpox. The skin rash of chickenpox appears 2 to 3 weeks after infection and may occasionally be accompanied by the development of vesicles in the palate and facial region, which rapidly rupture to produce small ulcers (2 to 4 mm). The diagnosis is made from the history and characteristic appearance of the cutaneous lesions. Culture of the virus is difficult and, therefore, if a microbiological diagnosis is required, this needs to employ molecular methods. Treatment is supportive, although aciclovir, valaciclovir or famciclovir may be used if the patient is immunocompromised.

Secondary infection

Reactivation of latent VZV in sensory nerve ganglia produces the clinical condition of herpes zoster, which is more commonly described as shingles. Herpes zoster is characterised by the onset of a unilateral area of severe pain which is accompanied within a few days by the development of vesiculobullous lesions (Fig. 9.7). The trigeminal nerve is affected in about 15% of cases of herpes zoster, and involvement is limited to one division of the nerve. Although the diagnosis can be made on the basis of clinical presentation alone, confirmation of herpes zoster can be made by demonstration of the presence of VZV by immunofluorescence on a smear, if this method is available, or more routinely now by molecular techniques.

Antiviral treatment should be instituted as early as possible, preferably within the first 48 hours of symptoms, and should constitute either famciclovir 250 mg every 8 hours (or 750 mg once daily) for 10 days, or valaciclovir 1 g every 8 hours for 10 days. Postherpetic neuralgia may be a subsequent problem in these patients, and this is why it is recommended that antiviral therapy should be provided for at least 10 days to reduce the likelihood of this extremely painful condition.

EPSTEIN–BARR VIRUS

The fourth member of the herpes group is Epstein–Barr virus (EBV), named after the two virologists who first observed it. EBV has been subsequently associated with a number of infections that affect the orofacial region, including infectious mononucleosis, Burkitt's lymphoma, oral hairy leukoplakia, nasopharyngeal carcinoma and post-transplant lymphoproliferative disease. The virus is prevalent in the population with approximately 70% of adults carrying the virus by the age of 30 years. Similar to HSV, this virus is also periodically and asymptomatically shed in the saliva.

Infectious mononucleosis

Infectious mononucleosis, also known as glandular fever, is an acute infectious disease that is spread most frequently during kissing. The onset of a painful throat

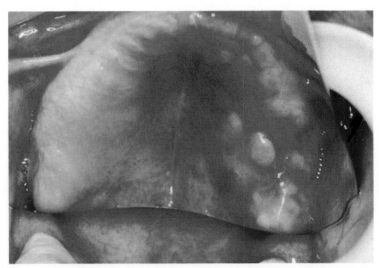

FIGURE 9.7 Unilateral ulceration in the palate caused by reactivation of herpes zoster virus (shingles).

and submandibular lymphadenopathy is accompanied by fine petechial haemorrhages in the hard and soft palate. A white pseudomembrane may develop on the tonsils. Diagnosis is supported by demonstration of a lymphocytosis and atypical mononuclear cells (Downey cells) in a blood film or, alternatively, by detection of heterophile antibodies (monospot test), EBV specific antibody using immunofluorescence methods, or EBV DNA by PCR.

Hairy leukoplakia

Hairy leukoplakia was first described in the 1980s in the mouths of men who have sex with men and was a novel oral manifestation of HIV infection. Subsequently, hairy leukoplakia has been reported in non-HIV-positive individuals who are immunosuppressed because of other causes, usually drug therapy. Characteristically, hairy leukoplakia presents as a corrugated white lesion on the lateral border of the tongue, although it has also been described on the dorsum of the tongue and the buccal mucosa. EBV has been demonstrated in lesional tissue by in situ hybridisation with appropriate DNA probes. Although the exact role of EBV in hairy leukoplakia is still uncertain, temporary clinical resolution of the condition can occur following provision of high doses of aciclovir. Imprint cultures of hairy leukoplakia often yield candidal species, but it is likely that this represents opportunistic secondary infection.

Burkitt lymphoma and nasopharyngeal carcinoma

EBV is regarded as an oncogenic virus and is associated with Burkitt's lymphoma, an aggressive tumour of the jaws seen in areas where malaria is also prevalent, and nasopharyngeal carcinoma, especially in China and Southeast Asia.

HUMAN CYTOMEGALOVIRUS

Although human cytomegalovirus (HCMV), the fifth herpes group virus, is widespread in the community, it has only rarely been associated with the presence of oral symptoms similar to those seen in infectious mononucleosis. It can be detected by direct immunofluorescence. HCMV is a potential pathogen in the developing foetus and immunodeficient individuals. Ganciclovir and foscarnet are two antiviral agents used in management of serious HCMV infection.

HUMAN HERPES VIRUS 6

Human herpes virus 6 (HHV-6) is found in latent form in lymphoid tissue but is also asymptomatically shed in the saliva of most adults. The virus is implicated in infectious mononucleosis-like symptoms and skin rashes (roseola infantum). It has also been suggested that HHV-6 is the cause of erythematous papules in the soft palate and uvula (Nagayama spots) seen in these children.

HUMAN HERPES VIRUS 7

Human herpes virus 7 (HHV-7) has been found in saliva, but its role in human disease is unknown at present.

HUMAN HERPES VIRUS 8

Human herpes virus 8 (HHV-8) has been encountered in all forms of Kaposi's sarcoma and is believed to be the aetiological agent of this condition. Kaposi's sarcoma is a proliferation of endothelial cells producing a tissue swelling, particularly in association with HIV infection but, occasionally, also in other immunosuppressed patients. Small lesions can be excised, treated with low-dose radiotherapy or by the injection of chemotherapeutic drugs, such as vinblastine. Larger lesions may require the use of systemic chemotherapy. HHV-8 has also been associated with sarcoidosis.

KEY POINTS

The herpes group of viruses contains eight viruses that have been implicated in a range of human diseases, many of which affect the orofacial tissues. The nature of the signs and symptoms of these infections is extremely variable and differs depending on whether it is primary or secondary infection. Herpes simplex type 1 is by far the most frequent member of the herpes group virus that is encountered in the mouth and perioral tissues. A history of primary infection with HSV type 1 is almost ubiquitous in the adult population of the Western world. A high percentage of individuals suffer from reactivation of latent herpes simplex virus and varicella zoster virus. The use of specific antiviral drugs can limit the clinical impact of infections caused by these viruses.

Other members of the herpes group are associated with a range of relatively rare primary and opportunistic secondary infections.

COXSACKIE VIRUSES

The Coxsackie viruses are enteroviruses that affect the gut and are named after the village in New York where they were first detected. Several subspecies of type A and type B are now recognised, and some may cause orofacial infection. These viruses are highly infectious and are widespread in the community because of transmission by the faecal–oral route or by nasopharyngeal secretions.

HAND, FOOT AND MOUTH DISEASE

Hand, foot and mouth disease is usually caused by Coxsackie virus subspecies A16, but may also be because of infection with types A4, A5, A9 and A10. As the name of the condition implies, the distribution of lesions involves macular and vesicular eruptions on the hands, feet and mucosa of the pharynx, soft palate, buccal sulcus or tongue. The cutaneous lesions of hand, foot and mouth disease are transient, lasting only 1 to 3 days, and are unlikely to cause any significant symptoms. The diagnosis of hand, foot and mouth disease is usually made on the basis of the characteristic clinical signs. Viral culture for Coxsackie infections is not widely available, and therefore if confirmatory diagnosis is required, this has to be based on demonstration of an increase in convalescent antibody levels. Antimicrobial treatment is rarely required.

HERPANGINA

Herpangina is caused by infection by either Coxsackie virus subspecies A2, A4, A5, A6 or A8. This condition occurs predominantly in children and presents as sudden onset of fever and sore throat with subsequent development of papular, vesicular lesions on the oral mucosa and pharyngeal mucosa. Severity of symptoms is variable, but clinical resolution usually occurs within 7 to 10 days, even in the absence of treatment. The diagnosis of herpangina is usually made on the basis of the characteristic clinical signs and symptoms. Viral culture for Coxsackie infections is not widely available and, therefore, if required, confirmatory diagnosis is based on demonstration of an increase in convalescent antibody levels. Treatment consists of bed rest and the use of an antiseptic mouthwash, such as 0.2% chlorhexidine gluconate two or three times daily. Patients should be encouraged to maintain adequate fluid intake.

KEY POINTS

Members of the Coxsackie group of viruses have been identified as the cause of two types of viral infection that involve the orofacial tissues. Although highly infectious, both conditions are self-limiting and associated with mild symptoms.

HUMAN PAPILLOMA VIRUSES

More than 170 serological types of human papilloma virus (HPV) have been described, some of which have been encountered in benign conditions although others have been implicated in the aetiology of cancer at various body sites, in particular the cervix in women.

VERRUCA VULGARIS

HPV types 2 and 4 are frequently encountered in mucosal warts (Fig. 9.8). Development of orofacial lesions may be associated with transmission from warts on the hands. Alternatively, the oral lesions may arise from orogenital contact, where HPV types 6, 11 and 16 are more prevalent. The labial and lingual mucosa are the most frequent sites for oral warts which present as small localised growths. The clinical appearance is characteristic but most lesions are removed and, therefore, histopathological findings can confirm the diagnosis. Histologically, the structure of the lesion is similar to papilloma but there are large clear cells (koilocytes) in the prickle cell layer. Immunostaining may be used to detect presence of papilloma virus. Excision is usually curative and recurrence is uncommon except in immunocompromised individuals.

FOCAL EPITHELIAL HYPERPLASIA (HECK'S DISEASE)

Heck's disease is a benign condition first described in Native Americans and the Inuit but also now seen in other populations. An infectious aetiology because of human papilloma viruses (HPV types 13 and 32) has been shown by both epidemiological and molecular studies. The lesions appear as discrete or clustered, smooth-topped pink papules most frequently on the buccal mucosa, labial mucosa, tongue and gingivae. The diagnosis is made on ultrastructural studies that show 50 nm viral particles of the HPV within biopsy material.

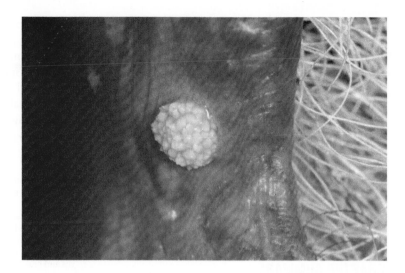

FIGURE 9.8 Human papillomavirus positive verruca vulgaris on the buccal mucosa.

OROPHARYNGEAL CARCINOMA

In recent years it has become accepted that HPV types 16 and 18 have a role in the aetiology of oropharyngeal carcinoma, as a result of oral sexual practices. The recognised association of HPV in cervical cancer resulted in 2007 in the vaccination against HPV in girls at the age of 12 years. It is likely that this will result in not only a reduction in cancer of the cervix but also oropharyngeal cancer in vaccinated women. In the UK in 2014, it was recommended that vaccination be extended to include men who have sex with men. There is now a campaign to provide a gender neutral vaccination programme, to include all adolescent boys in addition to girls, because this will provide a uniform protection against a range of HPV associated cancers. Such an approach has been adopted in Australia and some other countries.

KEY POINTS

Human papilloma viruses, of which there are many types, are frequently encountered in localised epithelial proliferations at a variety of body sites, including the orofacial tissues. The vast majority of these wart-like lesions are benign and of little importance. However, it is generally accepted that HPV type 16 and type 18 are involved in the malignant condition, oropharyngeal carcinoma. There is now sufficient evidence to support population-based vaccination against these two types of HPV.

PARAMYXOVIRUSES

The paramyxoviruses are enveloped RNA viruses that comprise four groups: parainfluenza virus, mumps virus, measles virus and respiratory syncytial virus.

MUMPS

Mumps (endemic parotitis) is traditionally associated with painful swelling of the major salivary glands. Diagnosis can usually be made on the basis of clinical symptoms; mumps can be differentiated from suppurative sialadenitis by the absence of a purulent discharge from the salivary duct orifice. However, if there is doubt, then serological investigation to demonstrate the presence of specific immunoglobulin M (IgM) antibody can be used. In addition, a sample of saliva, collected by cannulation of the parotid duct, can be examined by electron microscopy or tissue culture to demonstrate the presence of virus. Treatment is supportive, and it should be remembered that antibiotic therapy is not required.

MEASLES

Measles, a common disease of childhood, is spread by droplet infection and is highly infectious. The MMR (mumps, measles and rubella) vaccine provides immunity but in areas of low uptake or non-availability of the vaccine, measles still presents a serious illness because of potentially life-threatening bronchopneumonia or encephalomyelitis. In Saharan Africa, the virus has also been implicated in gross destruction of the orofacial tissues (noma) in malnourished individuals (see Chapter 6). In more typical milder cases, the characteristic skin rash and fever may be accompanied by transient small discrete macules in the buccal mucosa (Koplik spots).

KEY POINTS

> Paramyxoviruses are associated with two well-recognised human infections, namely measles and mumps. On rare occasions, these conditions may involve clinical signs and symptoms within the orofacial tissues although these are of little consequence and do not require specific management.

CHAPTER SUMMARY

Viruses within the herpes group, which contains eight distinct viruses, are encountered frequently in the orofacial tissues. Evidence of infection with HSV-1, which causes primary herpetic gingivostomatitis, is found in the majority (80% to 90%) of the adult population and subsequent reactivation of latent HSV-1 produces herpes labialis (cold sores) in approximately a third of these at some time in their life. Other members of the herpes group, Coxsackie A viruses, human papilloma viruses and paramyxoviruses can cause a range of signs and symptoms within the orofacial tissues, particularly in immunocompromised individuals. HPV types 16 and 18 have an established association with oropharyngeal carcinoma. A relatively small number of antiviral agents are available, and their use should be determined on an individual patient basis.

FURTHER READING

Balasubramaniam R, Kuperstein AS, Stoopler ET. Update on oral herpes virus infections. *Dent Clin North Am.* 2014;58:265-280.

Campsi G, Panzarella V, Giuliana M, et al. Human papilloma virus: its identity and controversial role in oral oncogenesis, premalignant lesions and malignant lesions. *Int J Oncol.* 2007;30:813-823.

Chattopadhyay A, Weatherspoon D, Pinto A. Human papillomavirus and oral cancer: a primer for dental public health professionals. *Community Dent Health.* 2015;32:117-128.

Dockrell H, Roitt IM, Zuckerman M, et al. *Mims' medical microbiology (Trauma Manual).* 4th ed. London: Mosby; 2007.

Fan F, Day S, Xuedong L, et al. Laboratory diagnosis of HSV and Varicella Zoster Virus infections. *Future Virology.* 2014;9:721-731.

Nair RG, Salajegheh A, Itthagarun A, et al. Orofacial viral infections-an update for clinicians. *Dent Update.* 2014;41:518-520, 522-4.

Woo SB, Challacombe SJ. Management of recurrent oral herpes simplex infections. *Oral Surg Oral Med Oral Pathol Oral Radiol Endod.* 2007;103:S12.e1-S12.18.

MULTIPLE CHOICE QUESTIONS

Answers on p. 250

1 What is the percentage of adults who are estimated to harbour viruses that have been acquired as a result of prior infection?
- a. 10%
- b. 30%
- c. 60%
- d. 90%

2 What is the approximate size of a virus?
- a. 5 to 50 nm
- b. 100 to 300 nm
- c. 400 to 600 nm
- d. 650 to 850 nm

3 Which of the following viruses (also known as the fifth Herpes virus) has been associated with defects in the developing foetus?
- a. EBV
- b. HCM
- c. CVM
- d. CMV

4 Regardless of the use of an antiviral agent, HSV-1 is not eliminated from the body following resolution of the acute symptoms and the virus remains within the tissues in which of the following states?
- a. Prodromal
- b. Resistant
- c. Latent
- d. Active

5 *Traditionally, it has been thought that reactivated HSV-1 migrated to the peripheral tissues of the lips or face in which nerve?*

a. Hypoglossal nerve

b. Trigeminal nerve

c. Facial nerve

d. Glossopharyngeal nerve

6 *Varicella zoster virus (VZV) primary infection occurs most frequently in childhood causing which of the following?*

a. Whooping cough

b. Chickenpox

c. Respiratory infection

d. Pinkeye

7 *Reactivation of latent VZV in sensory nerve ganglia produces the clinical condition of herpes zoster, which is more commonly described as which of the following?*

a. Shingles

b. Cold sores

c. Hand, foot and mouth disease

d. Glandular fever

8 *Characteristically, which of the following presents as a corrugated white lesion on the lateral border of the tongue?*

a. Aphthous ulcer

b. Hairy leukoplakia

c. Median rhomboid glossitis

d. Lichen planus

9 *An aggressive tumour of the jaw associated with the EBV oncogenic virus is which of the following?*

a. Hodgkin lymphoma

b. Burkitt lymphoma

c. Basal cell carcinoma

d. Non-Hodgkin lymphoma

10 *Human herpes virus 8 is associated with which of the following conditions?*

a. Oropharyngeal carcinoma

b. Kaposi sarcoma

c. Hairy leukoplakia

d. Acquired immune deficiency syndrome (AIDS)

11 *Herpangina is caused by which of the following?*

a. Human herpes virus 8 (HHV-8)

b. Human herpes virus 7 (HHV-7)

c. Epstein–Barr virus

d. Coxsackie virus subspecies

12 *Approximately, how many serological types of human papilloma virus have been described?*

a. 10

b. 70

c. 100

d. 170

CHAPTER 10

Antimicrobial agents

The terms antimicrobial and antibiotic are often, but incorrectly, used interchangeably. Antimicrobial is a general term and refers to agents that are active against a range of microorganisms including bacteria, viruses, fungi and protozoa. The term antibiotic, in its strictest sense, refers to substances produced by microbes which in low concentration inhibit the growth of other microbes. Penicillin was the first antibiotic discovered and was isolated from *Penicillium notatum* by Alexander Fleming in 1928. Since then, hundreds of antimicrobial agents have been developed and licensed for clinical use. Antimicrobials may be natural or synthetic in origin. *Streptomyces* species produce many natural antibiotics including tetracycline and streptomycin, although chloramphenicol is produced by a synthetic process. Many antimicrobials, including derivatives of penicillin and cephalosporins, are produced by a semisynthetic process whereby the molecule produced by the microorganism is modified chemically to enhance its properties.

Antimicrobials have had a major impact on our ability to prevent and manage infection and have facilitated increasingly complex medical interventions that would otherwise be compromised by infection. This chapter will provide an overview of the types of antimicrobials available including antibacterial, antiviral and antifungal agents and the principles of their use in both the prevention and management of orofacial infection. Antimicrobials are an important resource and must be used sparingly and appropriately. The empirical overuse of antibiotics in the last few decades has been accompanied by an enormous increase in the emergence of microbial resistance; this has made some antimicrobials ineffective in the treatment of some common diseases. Against this background, the importance of accurate microbiologic diagnosis and optimal antimicrobial stewardship in the management of oral infection will be highlighted.

ANTIMICROBIAL THERAPY

ANTIBACTERIAL AGENTS

Antibacterials may be classified in a number of ways including on their chemical structure, spectrum of activity, mode of action and predominant clinical use. Table 10.1 provides an overview of the main antibacterial groups based on mechanism of action. Antimicrobials are less likely to exhibit toxic side effects if they selectively target microbial processes that are not present in the human host cells. Targets include cell wall synthesis, cell membrane function and nucleic acid replication machinery. Protein synthesis, although similar to eukaryotes, is sufficiently different to provide targets for disruption, and tetracyclines and aminoglycosides target subunits of the microbial ribosome. Agents may either kill bacteria (bactericidal) or prevent their division (bacteriostatic). With a few exceptions, those that target protein synthesis are more likely to be bacteriostatic, whereas those which disrupt the cell wall are generally bacteriocidal.

Antibacterials in Orofacial Infection

Penicillins. Penicillin-based antimicrobials contain a nucleus of a β-lactam ring which is necessary for antibiotic activity. The basic ring structure has been modified to produce antimicrobials with different spectra of activity (Table 10.2). For example, antistaphylococcal penicillins such as flucloxacillin possess bulky side chains that prevent their inactivation by β-lactamases, enzymes which are produced by a range of bacteria including staphylococci and *Prevotella* species. A consequence of the modification is more limited penetration of the agent into certain bacteria and a reduced spectrum of activity. However, this group of agents remains very useful for staphylococcal wound infections. Aminopenicillins are broader spectrum penicillins and some, such as amoxicillin, exhibit excellent oral absorption. However, they are destroyed by β-lactamases including those produced by *Escherichia coli* and *Prevotella* species. Penicillins have been developed with an extended spectrum to include activity against *Pseudomonas* species. *Pseudomonas* is an uncommon primary pathogen in orofacial infections, but may present in immunocompromised or hospitalised patients.

β-Lactamase Inhibitors. Many bacteria produce enzymes that destroy the ring structure of β-lactam antibacterials, thus inactivating the agents (Fig. 10.1). β-lactamase inhibitors, such as clavulanic acid, are compounds that have no antibacterial activity themselves, but which act as suicide inhibitors of β-lactamases. They are released slowly and result in irreversible inhibition of the enzymes to protect the penicillin agents from degradation. Other examples are sulbactam and tazobactam.

Cephalosporins. Cephalosporins are another class of antibacterial agents that target the bacterial cell wall. There are several generations of cephalosporins and as a rule, the activity of each successive generation increases against Gram-negative and decreases against Gram-positive organisms. Although the spectrum of activity correlates with the pathogens present in purulent orofacial infections, and they have been used successfully for these conditions, their use as a first-line agent in the management of orofacial infections is not encouraged. This is because of their broad-spectrum nature which increases the risk of antibiotic-associated diarrhoea, the emergence of meticillin-resistant *Staphylococcus aureus* (MRSA) and other resistant infections.

Macrolides. The macrolide antibiotics which include erythromycin and clarithromycin are bacteriostatic agents. They have an antibacterial spectrum that is similar, but not identical to that of penicillin and are thus an alternative in patients allergic to penicillin. In addition, the macrolides are not affected by β-lactamases. Clarithromycin is a semisynthetic macrolide similar in structure to erythromycin but modified for better gastrointestinal tolerance, improved tissue penetration and increased half-life; consequently, it is often prescribed in preference to erythromycin. However, increasing resistance of oral pathogens to macrolides is being reported in many countries, and this may limit the usefulness of this group of agents.

Metronidazole. Metronidazole is a nitroimidazole which inhibits bacterial deoxyribonucleic acid (DNA) synthesis. It has good activity against obligate anaerobes and is widely used in the management of orofacial infections for patients who are allergic to penicillin

TABLE 10.1	Antibacterial agents classified by mechanism of action	
	Class	**Examples**
Inhibition of cell wall	**Penicillins**	
	Natural penicillins	penicillin G, penicillin V
	Aminopenicillins	ampicillin, amoxicillin
	Antistaphylococcal	flucloxacillin, oxacillin
	Extended spectrum	piperacillin
	Cephalosporins	
	First generation	cephalexin, cefradine
	Second generation	cefoxitin, cefuroxime
	Third generation	cefotaxime, ceftriaxone, ceftazidime
	Fourth generation	cefepime
	Fifth generation	ceftobiprole
	unclassified	cefaloram
	Carbapenems	imipenem, meropenem
	Glycopeptides	vancomycin, teicoplanin
Inhibition of cell membrane	Lipopeptides	daptomycin
Protein synthesis		
30S ribosome subunit	Aminoglycosides	gentamicin
	Tetracyclines	tetracycline, doxycycline
	Glycylcycline (tRNA binding)	tigecycline
50S ribosome subunit	Oxazolidinones (initiation inhibitors)	linezolid
	Peptidyl transferase	chloramphenicol
	Macrolides (MLS; transpeptidase/ ranslocation)	erythromycin clarithromycin azithromycin
	Lincosamides	clindamycin
	Streptogramins	quinupristin/dalfopristin
Elongation Factor-G	Steroid antibacterials	fusidic acid
Nucleic acid synthesis	**Quinolones**	
	First generation	ciprofloxacin
	Second generation	ciprofloxacin
	Third generation	moxifloxacin
	Fourth generation	gemifloxacin
	Polypeptides	colistin, bacitracin, polymyxin B
DNA gyrase	Imidazoles	metronidazole
RNA polymerase	Lipiamycins	fidaxomicin

DNA, Deoxyribonucleic acid; *MLS*, macrolides, lincosamides, streptogramins; *RNA*, ribonucleic acid; *tRNA*, transfer ribonucleic acid.

TABLE 10.2   Antibacterial agents used in orofacial infection

Antibacterial agent	Spectrum of activity relevant to orofacial pathogens	Notes
Penicillin V	Gram-positive cocci (staphylococci, streptococci; not β-lactamase producers) Gram-negative cocci, Gram-positive bacilli Obligate anaerobes Spirochaetes	First-line agent in management of orofacial infection
Amoxicillin	Wide range of activity similar to Penicillin V but slightly wider Gram-negative spectrum.	Similar range of activity in the context of likely oral pathogens although amoxicillin range extended to more activity against Gram-negative organisms which may be of significance in compromised hosts.
Metronidazole	Gram-positive and Gram-negative obligate anaerobes	Often used as first line in the management of orofacial purulent infections, in penicillin allergic patients or those who have recently received penicillins Disulfiram reaction with alcohol causing nausea and vomiting
Erythromycin Clarithromycin	Gram-positive cocci (staphylococci and streptococci) Variable activity against Gram-negative cocci Spirochaetes Clarithromycin more activity than Erythromycin against Gram-negative bacilli	Clarithromycin increasingly used in preference to Erythromycin (improved range, tolerance and compliance) May be used for purulent orofacial infections
Tetracycline	Gram-positive and negative facultative and obligately anaerobic organisms Spirochaetes	Broad spectrum Useful agent for bacterial sinusitis Often used for topical application in management of periodontitis treatment although clinical benefit uncertain Resistance increasing Not to be used under 12 years of age because of staining and hypoplasia of teeth
Clindamycin	Gram-positive cocci, most obligate anaerobes (both Gram-positive and negative)	Good bone and salivary gland penetration In common with other broad spectrum agents, may cause *Clostridium difficile*-associated diarrhoea
Fusidic acid	Staphylococci (including many MRSA isolates) streptococci	Frequently used topically in the management of angular cheilitis

MRSA, Meticillin-resistant *Staphylococcus aureus*.

and for infections because of β-lactamase-producing anaerobes. Metronidazole has been used successfully for many decades with very little emergence of resistance.

Tetracyclines. The tetracyclines are broad-spectrum agents and are effective against oral anaerobes. However, their role in the treatment of oral infections has been surpassed by other agents because of the development of resistance, particularly by oral streptococci. They are still regarded as useful agents in the management of bacterial sinusitis. Tetracycline preparations are often recommended for the management of refractory and destructive forms of periodontal disease but the clinical benefit and defined role have yet to be established with certainty. Their use is to be

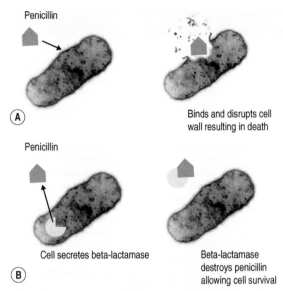

Penicillin

(A)

Binds and disrupts cell wall resulting in death

Penicillin

Cell secretes beta-lactamase

(B)

Beta-lactamase destroys penicillin allowing cell survival

FIGURE 10.1 (**A**) Penicillin, an antibiotic with a beta-lactam ring structure, binds to the cell wall and kills the microorganism. (**B**) The enzyme beta-lactamase produced by some bacteria will disrupt the beta-lactam structure and inactivate penicillin.

avoided in children under 12 years of age because they are deposited in growing bones and teeth, causing staining and occasionally dental hypoplasia.

Clindamycin. Clindamycin is a lincosamide antimicrobial which targets the 50S ribosomal subunit of bacteria to inhibit protein synthesis. It has a good spectrum of activity against oral pathogens and exhibits excellent bone and salivary gland penetration. However, the broad-spectrum nature of the agent, and its predisposition to antibiotic-associated colitis, requires that this useful antibiotic is reserved for infections that have not responded to first-line agents such as penicillin or metronidazole.

Fusidic Acid. Fusidic acid is a steroid antibacterial often used topically in the management of angular cheilitis caused by staphylococci including MRSA.

Principles of Antibacterial Therapy

The first and most fundamental principle of antimicrobial use is to establish that an antimicrobial is needed. This requires confirmation that an infection has been diagnosed and that the infection has failed to respond to appropriate local measures. For orofacial infections, this may include the drainage of pus (dentoalveolar abscess) or irrigation with antiseptic solutions (pericoronitis; see Chapter 7). The narrowest spectrum agent known to target the likely pathogens should be prescribed and in the case of purulent orofacial infections, the most frequent isolates are facultatively anaerobic organisms, microaerophilic streptococci and obligate anaerobes. It is considered good clinical practice to sample infected material and send it for microbiologic analysis and antibiotic susceptibility testing of the isolated bacteria. Currently, the time required for microbiologic analysis means that the results are unlikely to be available for the immediate management of the patient, so antibiotic choice is empirical. However, the results may be available for those patients who fail to respond to the first-line choice of antimicrobial. In addition, the pathogens isolated and the antimicrobial susceptibility profiles will provide useful surveillance data to inform local and national empirical choices. The antimicrobial must be given in the appropriate dose and dosing schedule and for the correct duration. The patient should be reviewed for resolution of infection and possible side effects of therapy. There is evidence that antimicrobials may be stopped after 3 days for dentoalveolar abscess infections with no increase in adverse events. Patient factors to consider when prescribing antimicrobials include history of allergies, renal and hepatic function, age, weight, compliance issues and status of the immune system. Immunocompromised patients and those who are debilitated by chronic disease, hospitalisation or previous antibiotic therapy may be predisposed to infections by bacteria such as Gram-negative organisms and multidrug-resistant pathogens.

Antibacterials will have a significant effect on the host microbiota both in the oral cavity and elsewhere in the body. One serious side effect of many antibacterial agents is *Clostridium difficile*-associated diarrhoea and although this can be initiated by a large number of different types of antibiotics, it is more commonly associated with broad-spectrum agents such as the cephalosporins, quinolones, clindamycin and penicillins combined with β-lactamase inhibitors such as amoxicillin and clavulanic acid. These broader spectrum agents are generally not recommended as first-line agents in the management of orofacial infections, and narrower spectrum antimicrobials such as penicillin and metronidazole are still effective in the majority of uncomplicated infections.

KEY POINTS

Many antibacterial agents are available and have been developed either from natural products or via chemical synthesis. The most widely used classification of antibacterial agents is based on the mechanism of action, and agents are developed to preferentially target microbial processes thus limiting host toxicity. Targets include cell wall synthesis (penicillins and carbapenems), protein synthesis (tetracyclines and macrolides) and nucleic acid synthesis (metronidazole). Bacteria may rapidly develop resistance to antibacterial agents and antimicrobials must therefore be used appropriately to extend their clinical effectiveness. They should only be prescribed when an infection has been diagnosed and the narrowest spectrum agent known to target the likely pathogens should be used. It is good clinical practice to send infected material for microbiological analysis; this will assist management of cases in which the first line, empirical antibiotic choice has not been effective and the resulting surveillance data will inform future prescribing.

ANTIFUNGAL AGENTS

In comparison with antibiotics, the development of antifungal agents has been relatively slow. This can be attributed to several factors including the inherent problems in developing an effective agent that acts upon a eukaryotic fungal cell type without toxicity to eukaryotic host cells. In addition, it is only relatively recently that diagnostic procedures have highlighted the significant role of fungi in disease and their increasing occurrence, largely because of medical interventions leading to host susceptibility.

The classification of antifungal drugs is currently based on their target of activity (Table 10.3) and the use of these agents often varies with the type of infection and condition of the patient (Table 10.4). Resistance to antifungal drugs is an increasingly recognised phenomenon and can be defined clinically as the persistence of signs and symptoms of the infection despite adequate delivery of a normally appropriate and tolerable level of the drug. Depending on the drug and the fungal species, the mechanism of antifungal resistance can either be intrinsic (present without previous exposure to the antifungal) or inherent, where resistance

TABLE 10.3 Antifungals used in the management of candidosis

Antifungal	Mode of action	Administration
Polyenes	Disruption of fungal cell membrane	
• Nystatin		topical
• Amphotericin		topical
Azoles	Inhibition of ergosterol synthesis	
• fluconazole	systemic	
• miconazole	topical	
• ketoconazole	topical/systemic	
• clotrimazole	topical	
• itraconazole	systemic	
• voriconazole	systemic	
• posaconazole	systemic	
5-flucytosine	Inhibition of DNA and protein synthesis	systemic, often in combined therapy with amphotericin
Echinocandins	Inhibition of β1,3 D-glucan synthesis	intravenous
• caspofungin		
• micafungin		
• anidulafungin		

DNA, Deoxyribonucleic acid.

develops in a previously susceptible organism following exposure.

Polyene Antifungals

Polyene antifungals are fungicidal because of their ability to interact with the ergosterol component within the fungal cell membrane to generate pores within the membranes causing cell leakage and loss of cytoplasmic content. The principal polyene antifungals are amphotericin B and nystatin, and these agents are generally regarded as having the broadest spectrum of antifungal activity. These agents are frequently used

TABLE 10.4 Recommended antifungal therapy for primary forms of oral candidosis

	PMC	AEC	CEC	CHC
Topical delivery				
Nystatin			Yes	
Amphotericin			Yes	
Miconazole			Yes	
Clotrimazole			Yes	
Systemic delivery				
Ketoconazole	Yes	Yes		Yes
Fluconazole	Yes	Yes		Yes
Itraconazole	Yes	Yes		Yes

Nystatin is available as both an ointment and oral
  suspension
Amphotericin is available as a lozenge
Miconazole is available as an oral gel and cream
Clotrimazole is available as a cream and pessary
Other antifungals are available and these may be more
  frequently used in hospitalised patients
AEC, Acute erythematous candidosis; *CEC*, chronic
  erythematous candidosis; *CHC*, chronic hyperplastic
  candidosis; *PMC*, pseudomembranous candidosis.

topically and can be administered in a variety of oral formulations in the treatment of oral candidosis (see Chapter 8) including suspensions, lozenges and pastilles. Polyenes are very poorly absorbed through the gut and as such their use is relatively limited. In cases of serious invasive fungal infections, intravenous administration of amphotericin B is often the preferred treatment option for hospitalised patients.

Azole Antifungals

Azole antifungals inhibit the biosynthesis of ergosterol by interference with the fungal enzyme, lanosterol demethylase. A key function of this enzyme is to convert lanosterol to ergosterol and inhibition leads to a depletion of the sterol in the fungal cell membrane. Azole antifungals have a fungistatic rather than fungicidal activity; consequently, it is important to simultaneously address any underlying host conditions during azole therapy to provide the best chance of disease resolution. The two azole agents that have been used most

frequently to treat oral candidosis are fluconazole and itraconazole. The major benefit of these drugs is that they can be given orally and are well absorbed from the gut. Fluconazole is especially effective because it is secreted in saliva and the salivary levels are almost equal to those achieved in the blood. In contrast, itraconazole is a lipid-based drug that achieves excellent tissue levels. Emergence of *Candida* resistance against the azoles has been described and can be either inherent or acquired. Several mechanisms of azole resistance are known and include (a) overproduction or an alteration in the demethylase enzyme targeted by azoles, (b) removal of the azole drug from the cytoplasm via multidrug transporters or (c) compensation by other sterol synthesis enzymes involved in membrane synthesis.

5-Flucytosine

The antifungal 5-Flucytosine (5-FC) was originally synthesised in 1957 when the drug was used as a cytosine analogue treatment in patients with leukaemia. Several years later the antifungal properties of 5-FC became evident. The drug enters the fungal cell through a cytosine permease and is then converted by the fungus into 5-fluorouracil. This nucleoside analogue becomes incorporated into ribonucleic acid (RNA) molecules and that serves to interfere with the synthesis of DNA and the manufacture of proteins within the fungal cell. Human cells are not affected because of the lack of cytosine permease in the cell membrane.

Future Strategies for Anticandidal Therapy

In recent years, several new antifungals have been developed that act upon cell wall targets. The synthesis of β1,3 D-glucan is one such target as this represents a key component in the fungal cell wall. The basis of the activity is through interference with the enzyme β1,3 D-glucan synthetase. The antifungals demonstrating this mechanism of action are referred to as the echinocandins and three such drugs (caspofungin, micafungin and anidulafungin) demonstrate activity against *Candida* species. Another cell wall component that offers an attractive antifungal target is chitin which is a polysaccharide absent from host cells but which is an essential component of fungal cell walls where it provides structural support.

Nikkomycins represent a class of drug that inhibits the enzyme chitin synthase and although good activity is evident against certain fungal species which have cell walls rich in chitin, for example, *Histoplasma capsulatum* and *Blastomyces* species, current drug forms appear to have limited or modest action against *Candida* species. A number of studies do, however, indicate synergistic activity of nikkomycin with azole drugs against *Candida*.

KEY POINTS

Management of fungal infections including oral candidosis has to involve the identification and control of any host factor that may be predisposing to the infection. In addition, a range of antifungal agents are available to directly combat the infecting fungus. The variety and number of these agents is low when compared with traditional antibiotics against bacteria due in part to the difficulty in developing an antifungal agent that is effective against its targeted organism and is devoid of toxic effects against host cells. Suitable antifungal strategies include either directly targeting the ergosterol component in the fungal cell membrane (polyene antifungals) or the enzymes involved in its biosynthesis (azole antifungals). More recently, constituents of the fungal cell wall such as chitin (target site of nikkomycin antifungals) and glucan (echinocandin group antifungals) have received attention, although the use of these agents is currently limited with regard to oral candidosis.

ANTIVIRAL AGENTS

Knowledge of the different steps in viral replication has been the principle basis for the development of the antiviral drugs. Relatively few antiviral agents have been developed when compared with the number of antibacterial drugs that are available. The intracellular nature of infection and the ability of viruses to establish latent forms have contributed to the difficulty in designing effective antiviral drugs.

The development of aciclovir was a milestone in antiviral therapy, representing the first true specific antiviral agent, recognised by the award of the Nobel Prize for Medicine in 1988. Aciclovir is a nucleoside analogue drug that has activity against members of the herpes group of viruses, in particular herpes simplex virus type 1 (HSV-1) and herpes simplex virus type 2 (HSV-2). Viral enzymes, within HSV-infected cells, phosphorylate aciclovir to monophosphate and the

agent becomes cell bound. Subsequent further phosphorylation to aciclovir triphosphate produces an analogue to deoxyguanosine triphosphate that inhibits viral DNA synthesis and prevents further viral replication (Fig. 10.2).

Because aciclovir acts by blocking viral replication, a decision to provide the drug should be made at an early stage, preferably within 48 hours of the onset of acute symptoms in herpes simplex or varicella zoster infections. Antiviral therapy started later than this time is unlikely to produce any significant clinical benefit, and therefore is not justified unless the patient is otherwise medically compromised.

Aciclovir may be applied topically or given systemically in severe infection. Other antiviral agents used for orofacial herpes simplex and varicella zoster infections include valaciclovir (which is given systemically and has a longer intracellular half-life than aciclovir), penciclovir (available only in topical form) and famciclovir (the oral prodrug of penciclovir). These agents act essentially in the same way as aciclovir. Resistance to aciclovir and related antiviral agents is rare but may develop in patients on chronic antiviral therapy such as transplant recipients or individuals with human immunodeficiency virus (HIV). Docosanol is a saturated fatty alcohol traditionally used as a thickener in cosmetics which has been shown to reduce the duration of cold sores caused by herpes simplex virus. It is thought to alter the cell membrane to inhibit fusion of the host cell with the viral envelope and because of this mode of action there would appear to be little risk of the development of drug resistance. Ganciclovir and foscarnet are two other antiviral agents that are used in specialist units for treatment of infections caused by cytomegalovirus.

KEY POINTS

A relatively small number of effective antiviral agents are available for the management of orofacial viral infections. Aciclovir and related compounds may be used either topically or systemically in the treatment of infections because of herpes simplex virus, including cold sores. Docosanol is an alternative agent which has been shown to reduce the duration of cold sores and works to prevent fusion of the virus with the host cells. Fortunately, at the present time, resistance to antiviral agents is rare, but this may develop in individuals undergoing prolonged therapy.

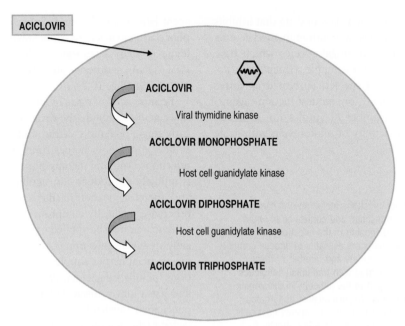

FIGURE 10.2 Viral activation of the antiviral agent aciclovir.

ANTIMICROBIAL RESISTANCE

The development of resistance by microbes to antimicrobials is a natural evolutionary response and resistance to penicillin was documented very shortly after the introduction of this agent into clinical use. The emergence of resistance to virtually every antimicrobial group developed is being detected and antimicrobial resistance is now regarded as one of the most significant global challenges to healthcare. Although there are problems with fungal and viral resistance, the more urgent problem is with bacterial resistance. In parallel with the threat of increasing antibacterial resistance has been the significant reduction in the number of new antimicrobial agents becoming available. The World Health Organisation (WHO) has highlighted the challenges of the global threat of antimicrobial resistance and governments in many countries are acting to facilitate the fast-tracking of novel antimicrobials to clinical use.

There is evidence that bacterial isolates from orofacial infection are displaying reduced susceptibility to the commonly used antimicrobials. In particular, an increase in the isolation of β-lactamase producers and bacteria resistant to macrolides and tetracyclines has been reported. This has implications in the context of both orofacial and systemic infection. The oral cavity has been shown to act as a reservoir for potential pathogens, including respiratory pathogens, and as a source of antimicrobial resistance genes which are exchanged with significant pathogens such as pneumococci (see Chapter 11). Correspondingly, there is a pressing need for comprehensive well-coordinated surveillance schemes to monitor the resistance of oral isolates from both hospital and community sources at national and international levels.

ANTIMICROBIAL STEWARDSHIP

In response to the problem of antimicrobial resistance, there has been a concerted effort in many countries to ensure antimicrobials are used appropriately. Antimicrobial stewardship is the term used to describe efforts to educate and persuade prescribers of antimicrobials to follow evidence-based prescribing, to reduce inappropriate use of antimicrobials. Measures include education of the public and healthcare professionals, the use of local policies for the restriction and/or rotation of antimicrobial agents, and the timely auditing of prescribing practices.

It is hoped that such measures will reduce the emergence and spread of resistant pathogens and extend the useful life of existing antimicrobials until novel drugs and strategies are available. New approaches which show promise include modulation of the host microbiota via probiotics and biofilm manipulation technologies, the use of bacteriophages, antimicrobial peptides and microbial drug transporter inhibitors. Technological advances in chairside diagnostics to ensure rapid and accurate diagnosis of infection will reduce the use of antimicrobials and promote appropriately targeted narrow spectrum therapy.

KEY POINTS

> Antimicrobial resistance is currently one of the most challenging global health issues. Microorganisms, and bacteria in particular, rapidly develop or acquire resistance to antimicrobials. The pipeline of new antimicrobial agents has slowed significantly in the last decade or so and patients are succumbing to infections that were previously amenable to treatment. Healthcare professionals and the public have an obligation to ensure that antimicrobials are used only when required. Research communities within many countries are prioritising the development of novel antimicrobial agents and antiinfective strategies.

ANTIMICROBIAL PROPHYLAXIS

The use of antimicrobials in the prevention of disease is called prophylaxis and is controversial. In many cases, the use of prophylactic antimicrobials in oral surgery is a matter of clinical habit rather than sound evidence-based clinical science. There are four occasions when prophylactic antimicrobials are indicated and these are:

- When the risk of postoperative infection is high;
- When wounds are contaminated with soil or dirt (e.g., after road traffic accidents) and there is a risk of infection (e.g., *Clostridium tetani*);
- Where the consequences of infection are serious or life threatening; and
- When a person's defences against infection are compromised (see Chapter 11).

This chapter will concentrate on the first and third indications for prophylactic antimicrobials where oral operations are concerned.

POSTOPERATIVE INFECTION

The majority of postoperative infections occur at the time of surgery. Secondary infection can occur following surgery (e.g., if a wound is disturbed or sutures are lost), but this is not usual. In a series of animal experiments in the 1960s, it was demonstrated that postoperative infections were usually infected at the time of surgery. The source of the postoperative infection can either be endogenous or exogenous. Endogenous infections are derived from the patient's own microbiota and are introduced at the time of the operation; they then proliferate and an infection results. The commonest time when endogenous postoperative infection occurs is when the surgery is undertaken on a site already infected with the person's own microbiota. Ideally, surgery should not be performed on areas that are infected, but this is not always possible. Exogenous wound infections arise from microorganisms being introduced into the mouth from a source outside the oral cavity, and are usually caused by poor aseptic technique or by non-sterile instruments. Exogenous wound infections can often be prevented by careful preparation of the operation site with judicious use of antiseptics.

There are two types of postoperative infection: immediate or late. Immediate postoperative infections occur in the first 2 to 3 days following the operation. Late infections can occur weeks or months after the operation and are because of microorganisms remaining quiescent within the site and then being reactivated. Late infections of this kind are particularly associated with implants or surgically-placed prostheses and are often called latent infections.

HOW DOES PRESURGICAL ANTIMICROBIAL PROPHYLAXIS WORK?

The mechanism of antimicrobial prophylaxis is still controversial. Most antimicrobial agents work best on actively dividing microorganisms which does not usually apply to most immediate wound infections. Successful antimicrobial prophylaxis does appear to suppress microbial growth. A number of other mechanisms could explain how prophylactic antimicrobials work and include:

- Antimicrobials attaching to the surface of the microorganism and forming complexes that increase phagocytosis;
- Antimicrobial/microorganism complexes increasing opsonisation;

- Antimicrobial/microorganism complexes increasing complement activation by either the classical or alternative pathways; and
- Antimicrobials preventing microorganisms from directly attaching to prostheses by blocking binding sites.

The above explanations all have some experimental evidence to support them, but it is all derived from in vitro experiments. The lack of any direct experimental evidence of the mechanism has led many people to question whether antimicrobial prophylaxis is necessary at all, especially with oral surgical operations where the incidence of postoperative infection is very low.

TIMING OF ANTIMICROBIAL PROPYLAXIS

Despite the evidence that infection occurs at the time of operation, many clinicians still give courses of antimicrobial prophylaxis at times that are inappropriate and will miss the critical time when antimicrobial protection is required. For example, antimicrobials are frequently prescribed following surgical extraction of a tooth (required when previous extraction with forceps has failed). Often it is many hours after the operation when the antimicrobials are dispensed. All the available clinical evidence has shown that giving antimicrobials sometime after the operation has little effect on the outcome. There are now a large number of double-blind clinical trials that have shown that only an antimicrobial given before the operation (in sufficient time for serum and tissue concentrations to be maximal) will have a prophylactic effect on post-surgical infection.

One important factor to consider when selecting the antimicrobial agent is that it should be able to penetrate the tissues concerned, especially bone. Clindamycin, the cephalosporins and metronidazole all penetrate bone well, but amoxicillin does not and is not licensed for use in this tissue. The macrolides also do not have good bone penetration. Amoxicillin is by far the most commonly prescribed prophylactic antimicrobial and because of its poor tissue penetration, must be given in high doses to reach appropriate concentrations in bone. This is not the case with clindamycin, the cephalosporins and metronidazole where standard adult doses give high and prophylactic concentrations in bone. Most antimicrobial agents that penetrate bone do so rapidly in the oral skeletal structures, usually attaining maximal concentrations within one hour.

ANTIMICROBIAL PROPHYLAXIS FOR ORAL SURGERY

One branch of surgery where the chances of postoperative infection could be high is oral surgery, as this is inevitably done at sites where many millions of potential infectious agents could be present. In practice, the rates of postoperative infection in oral surgery are extremely low. Most simple soft-tissue surgery within the oral cavity does not require any antimicrobial prophylaxis. The current consensus of opinion is that the rate of postoperative infectious complications is so low that antimicrobial prophylaxis cannot be justified and would not affect the outcome. For example, in simple periodontal surgery, where numerous potential pathogens are present (see Chapter 6), the elimination of pocket stagnation does not require antimicrobial prophylaxis, although it is often given. Antimicrobials given before deep root planing or extensive scaling possibly have some effect on healing, but the difference between those given prophylaxis and those without is not statistically significant.

Third Molar Surgery

The use of prophylactic antimicrobials for the removal of third molars has always been controversial. Until quite recently, third molars were removed whether or they gave symptoms. The extraction of unerupted third molars often involves the removal of bone and, as a consequence, pain, swelling and trismus (restriction of mouth opening) can occur. Postoperative infection is rare following third molar surgery, but the swelling associated with this procedure is often mistaken for infection. It is a common practice to give antimicrobial agents before and after third molar surgery and there is a strong cadre of surgeons who still perpetuate this practice. There have been nine double-blind randomised trials of a variety of prophylactic antimicrobial agents given before and after third molar surgery. All of these trials have come to the same conclusion that antimicrobial agents have no statistically significant effect on swelling, pain, trismus or postoperative infection. One trial also measured the effect of prophylactic antimicrobials on C-reactive protein and alpha-1 trypsin serum levels, which could be indicators of inflammation or infection. The antimicrobials were found to have no effect on the serum concentrations of these markers. This evidence would strongly support the contention that antimicrobials should not be given prophylactically for third molar removal.

Joint Replacements

The replacement of joints such as hips and knees with artificial prostheses is now common orthopaedic practice. Some orthopaedic surgeons believe that the bacteria that enter the bloodstream following dental procedures can pose a threat of early or late infections in the prosthesis. The consequences of infection in an orthopaedic prosthesis can be extremely serious. An infected hip prosthesis would require another surgical replacement operation and has an approximate 25% chance of being successful. This means that a person with an infected hip has only a 25% chance of being able to satisfactorily walk again. Some orthopaedic surgeons insist that persons with implanted prostheses have prophylactic antimicrobials before all dental treatment. The prophylactic antimicrobial recommended is usually amoxicillin, which is ironic, because this probably does not penetrate joints, has no proven prophylactic action in this site and is not licensed for this purpose. A risk assessment and review of the literature reveals a paucity of proven cases where infected joint replacement prostheses have been linked with dental treatment. The use of prophylactic antimicrobials for dental patients with implanted orthopaedic prostheses, therefore, is not recommended or justified scientifically.

Dental Implants

The pioneering work of Bränemark devised techniques for the placement of dental implants that integrated with bone. The use of such implants has revolutionised prosthetic dentistry and many thousands of dental implants are placed successfully each year. The surgical placement of dental implants is an elective operation done under aseptic conditions and, therefore, should not require antimicrobial use, but many surgeons around the world insist that they are given before and after implant placement. There have now been a number of double-blind placebo controlled randomised trials on the use of prophylactic antimicrobials and implant placement. Most studies were unable to show an effect. However, one trial provided

some evidence of the effectiveness of preoperative antimicrobial prophylaxis. Some national guidelines now include a recommendation for the use of preoperative prophylaxis before implant placement. However, the relative risks and benefits of the provision of an antimicrobial must be carefully considered in all cases.

ANTIMICROBIAL PROPHYLAXIS AGAINST INFECTIVE ENDOCARDITIS

One potential postoperative infection following dental procedures that could be serious and life-threatening is infective endocarditis. Infective endocarditis is often associated with oral microorganisms (see Chapter 11) and in view of the high morbidity and mortality of this infection, much research has been undertaken to determine whether it can be prevented. One possible preventative method is to give antimicrobials before certain types of dental treatment with the intention of preventing the infection. Animal studies, particularly in the rabbit, have been used to simulate the disease. If large doses of antimicrobials are given before the susceptible rabbit is inoculated, then 90% of the animals can be protected against infective endocarditis. The protection is not 100% effective in animals and this is also true for humans where infective endocarditis is not completely prevented by administration of prophylactic antimicrobials. For humans, there is no agreement as to the exact dose of antimicrobial agent required, and 2 or 3 g of amoxicillin (given orally) are being used is different countries.

There are over 44 interrelated conditions that can be associated with a susceptibility to infective endocarditis but some of these are rare. Thus there is confusion as to which patients should receive antimicrobial prophylaxis. Also there is doubt as to whether or not antimicrobial prophylaxis works at all, because the animal studies do not completely simulate human infective endocarditis. For this reason, expert groups have met around the world and issued guidelines as to which patients should receive antimicrobial prophylaxis and for which types of dental treatment.

There have also been large numbers of authorities that are questioning whether antimicrobial prophylaxis should be given at all before dental treatment for patients susceptible to infective endocarditis.

The largest review summating all the evidence was done by the National Institute for Clinical Excellence

(NICE) in the UK in 2008. Using all the available data from studies around the world they concluded there were four groups of patients that were particularly susceptible to infective endocarditis: those with acquired valvular damage, structural congenital heart disease, valve replacements and cardiomyopathy. These four groups alone could justify antimicrobial prophylaxis. NICE also looked at the effects of antimicrobial prophylaxis on bacteraemias and concluded that the effect was impossible to measure. NICE therefore recommended from March 2008 that no further antimicrobial prophylaxis should be given before any dental treatment in any group of patients susceptible to infective endocarditis in the UK. However, more recently, an increase in the incidence of infective endocarditis has been documented. Although it is not clear that the cessation of provision of antimicrobial prophylaxis has resulted in this increase, the underlying reasons will need to be determined and guidelines possibly reviewed if an association is confirmed.

CHAPTER SUMMARY

Antimicrobial agents are available to target a wide range of pathogens. They are a valuable resource and their appropriate use is paramount to ensure effective safe treatment and to reduce the impact of antimicrobial resistance. The penicillins, macrolides and metronidazole are still relatively effective against the range of pathogens encountered in orofacial infection and are considered suitable first line agents. Antimicrobials are also available for the treatment of fungal and viral infections, although the number of such agents tends to be less than that available for bacterial infections.

Antimicrobial prophylaxis is not justified for patients who have received hip replacements, minor oral surgery or third molar removal. There is some evidence for the effectiveness of antimicrobial prophylaxis during the placement of implants. The UK has also recommended that antimicrobial prophylaxis is not given before dental treatment for patients susceptible to infective endocarditis, although in some other countries prophylaxis is still given to patients at highest risk of disease.

FURTHER READING

Keenan JR, Veitz-Keenan A. Antibiotic prophylaxis for dental implant placement? *Evid Based Dent.* 2015;16:52-53.

Infective endocarditis. The NICE recommendations. National Institute for Clinical Research, 2008.

Martin MV, Kanatas AN, Hardy P. Antibiotic prophylaxis and third molar surgery. *Br Dent J.* 2005;198:327-330.

Rodrigues WC, Okamoto R, Pellizzer EP, et al. Antibiotic prophylaxis for third molar extraction in healthy patients: Current scientific evidence. *Quintessence Int.* 2015;46:149-161.

Seymour RA. Antibiotics in dentistry-an update. *Dent Update.* 2013;40(4):319-322.

WHO 2014. Antimicrobial resistance: Global report on surveillance. <www.who.int/drugresistance/documents/surveillancereport/en/>.

MULTIPLE CHOICE QUESTIONS

Answers on p. 250

1 *Select the correct statement regarding antimicrobial agents.*
   a. All antibacterial agents are antibiotics
   b. Penicillin was derived from a natural product, however, currently, all antibacterial agents are manufactured from a purely synthetic process
   c. The most effective antibacterial agents target processes that are shared between the host and the microbial cell
   d. Antimicrobial is a term that includes agents active against a range of microorganisms including bacteria viruses and fungi

2 *Select the false statement. The β-lactam ring of penicillin:*
   a. Is responsible for antibiotic activity
   b. Is inactivated by enzymes produced by Gram-negative and -positive bacteria
   c. Is absent in the aminopenicillins, such as amoxicillin
   d. May be protected from enzyme inactivation by modification of side chains

3 Select the false answer from the following statements regarding cephalosporins.
a. They target the bacterial cell wall
b. They have been used successfully in the management of orofacial infections
c. They are associated with a severe disulfiram reaction when taken with alcohol
d. They predispose to antibiotic associated diarrhoea because of their broad spectrum activity

4 Which of the following statements about the macrolide antibacterials is true?
a. They target nucleic acid synthesis
b. Clarithromycin has better tissue penetration in comparison to erythromycin
c. Macrolides are bacteriocidal agents
d. Macrolides are destroyed by β-lactamases

5 Select the false statement regarding metronidazole.
a. It is often used for the management of pericoronitis
b. It has good antianaerobic activity
c. It is an imidazole antibiotic
d. It possesses a β-lactam ring

6 Which of the following antifungal agents is an azole which is often used systemically in the management of chronic hyperplastic candidosis?
a. Fluconazole
b. Caspofungin
c. Nystatin
d. Amphotericin

7 Which of the following antiviral agents is thought to act by preventing fusion of the virus with the human host cell?
a. Aciclovir
b. Penciclovir
c. Famciclovir
d. Docosanol

8 Which of the following is not one of the four occasions when prophylactic antimicrobials are indicated?
a. When the risk of postoperative infection is high
b. When wounds are contaminated with soil or dirt (e.g., after road traffic accidents) and there is a risk of infection (e.g., Clostridium tetani)
c. To meet patient demand
d. When a person's defences against infection are compromised

9 A risk assessment and review of the literature reveals which of the following with regard to the link between dental treatment and the proven cases of infected joint replacements?
a. There is a significant relationship between dental treatment and proven cases of infected joint replacements
b. A paucity of proven evidence shows there is no relationship between dental treatment and infected joint replacements
c. There is an inconclusive link between dental treatment and proven cases of infected joint replacements
d. Ongoing research is needed to determine the role that dental treatment plays in postoperative infected joint replacements

10 When do the majority of postoperative infections occur?
a. Within the first 12 hours
b. Within the first 48 hours
c. Time of surgery
d. Within the first 24 hours

11 *A number of mechanisms could explain how prophylactic antimicrobials work and include which of the following?*

a. They form complexes that increase phagocytosis

b. They make conditions unfavourable for microbial growth

c. They eliminate opportunistic microorganisms

d. They are partially effective against environmental microorganisms

12 *The necessity of prophylactic antimicrobial use for oral surgical operations has been questioned because of which of the following?*

a. Endogenous infections are not affected by antimicrobials

b. Low incidence of postoperative infections

c. High antimicrobial effect of saliva

d. Increased vasculature in the oral cavity enhances surgical wound healing

13 *The empirical overuse of antibiotics has been accompanied by an enormous increase in the emergence of microbial resistance; which of the following describes what impact this has had on the use of antimicrobials?*

a. Antiseptics are used as an alternative to antibiotics

b. Antibiotics are used for shorter treatment courses

c. Antibiotics are ineffective for many common diseases

d. Antibiotics should never be used as they exacerbate bacterial resistance

14 *In the context of antimicrobial stewardship which of the following statements is false?*

a. Health care professionals and the public have an obligation to limit their prescription and demand for antimicrobials respectively

b. Prescribers should prescribe an agent with the broadest available spectrum to ensure coverage of all possible pathogens

c. Prescribers should audit their prescribing patterns against available guidelines

d. Prescribing policies should ensure the restricted use of broad spectrum agents

Oral microbiota and systemic disease

Our knowledge of the interactions between the oral microbiota and the other systems of the human body is constantly evolving. The associations appear to work in both directions; underlying systemic disease may predispose an individual to certain infections or the oral microbiota may initiate or play a role in the progression of systemic disease. An immunocompromised individual is one where there is a congenital or acquired alteration of the immune system. This could be caused by disease such as acquired immune deficiency syndrome (AIDS) or by medical intervention. There are many drugs now used to modify the immune system, for example, during and following solid organ transplant. The oral microbiota in immunocompromised patients is changed either by colonisation with exogenous microorganisms, which are not usually found in the mouth, or by the occurrence of opportunistic infections.

There may be a link in the opposite direction so the presence of a particular microorganism may be associated with or even directly cause a specific systemic disease pathology. An example is the reported association between periodontal disease and atherosclerotic cardiovascular disease. This and other similar associations that are being studied are discussed further in a later section of this chapter.

The status of the teeth and oral soft tissues is often a reflection of systemic health. Oral manifestations of systemic infection and the relevance of the presenting features are therefore important.

SYSTEMIC EFFECTS ON ORAL MICROBIOTA

IMMUNE SYSTEM

An impaired immune system as a result of a genetic cause or acquired disease may result in opportunistic infections, autoimmune disease or malignancy. The resulting opportunistic infections could include fungal and bacterial oral manifestations. An example of this is chronic mucocutaneous candidosis (CMC), which is a collection of syndromes characterised by recurrent, persistent infections of the skin, nails and mucous membranes with the opportunistic yeast *Candida* (see Chapter 8). Patients with CMC are thought to have an immunological abnormality resulting in failure of their T lymphocytes to produce cytokines required for control of candidal infection. In addition, these patients are more prone to both viral and fungal types of pneumonia.

Treatment of underlying disease such as leukaemia with bone stem transplants can result in graft versus host disease. This condition is a complication of allogeneic haematopoietic stem cell transplants and can result in mucositis, lichenoid lesions and xerostomia, leading to a change in the oral microbiota. Patients with rare infections may present primarily to a dental setting before an underlying immunodeficiency disorder is diagnosed.

Individuals with autoimmune conditions such as rheumatoid arthritis may be taking immunosuppressant medication, placing them at higher risk of opportunistic fungal, viral and bacterial infections, for example, acute pseudomembranous candidosis or recurrent herpes labialis.

Following organ transplantation, it is necessary to prescribe immunosuppressive agents to prevent rejection of the transplant. One of the curious consequences of taking these antirejection agents is gingival enlargement caused by overgrowth of fibrous tissue (Fig. 11.1). The gingival overgrowth is more pronounced if the oral hygiene is poor. No specific plaque bacteria have been associated with this condition, which was thought to be directly caused by the systemic action of the immunosuppressive agents. If the patient is treated with low doses of macrolide antimicrobials (e.g., azithromycin), then the overgrowth can be prevented or reduced. This evidence supports the contention that gingival hyperplasia is an infective inflammatory process, but the infecting bacteria have still to be identified.

GENERAL DEBILITATION

Stroke and Parkinson disease

Loss of control of oral musculature can occur following cerebrovascular accidents (strokes) and in conditions such as Parkinson disease. Loss of the oral musculature can result in changes in the oral microbiota, but the reasons for this are not clear. The microbiota becomes predominantly Gram-negative, with *Enterobacter* spp. and *Acinetobacter* spp. frequently isolated. This change in the oral microbiota is clinically significant, as often the patient cannot swallow properly and oral microorganisms, including the Gram-negative colonisers, may be aspirated into the lungs and cause pneumonia. Poor oral and denture hygiene in these vulnerable patient groups has been shown to be a risk factor for the development of pneumonia, and this is discussed further in this chapter.

Staphylococcal mucositis

There is a debate as to how frequently staphylococci infect or colonise the mouth and there would appear to be marked geographic variation. Recently, it has been proposed that there is a discrete condition called staphylococcal mucositis, which occurs in debilitated individuals.

Mucositis is an inflammation of the oral mucosa. The predominant species isolated from this condition is *Staphylococcus aureus* with a minority of these being meticillin-resistant *Staphylococcus aureus* (MRSA). The condition generally affects patients who are debilitated by other systemic conditions or who are terminally ill. In addition, staphylococci have been isolated from orofacial granulomatosis, in particular within fissures of swollen lips (Fig. 11.2). The presenting features of orofacial granulomatosis are identical to those of Crohn's disease, which is a chronic inflammatory condition of the gut.

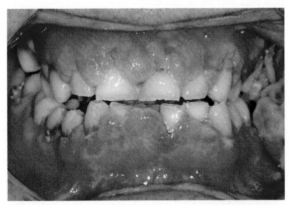

FIGURE 11.1 Hyperplastic gingivae induced by cyclosporine therapy.

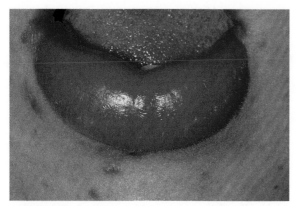

FIGURE 11.2 Lip swelling in orofacial granulomatosis with midline split secondarily infected with *Staphylococcus aureus*.

NUTRITION

The components of an individual's diet will have an influence on the composition and metabolism of the oral microbiota (see Chapter 2). A diet rich in carbohydrates may be associated with a shift in the microbiota and is a risk factor in oral candidosis, in addition to dental caries (see Chapter 6). Diets and nutrition will differ between countries and cultures and this in turn may affect the resident microbiota and subsequent oral disease. Malnutrition, in particular, may affect the susceptibility to and progression of periodontal and infectious disease. A diet deficient in iron, folic acid and vitamins has been linked to an increase in oral candidosis. The mechanism by which dietary factors can affect the pathogenesis of oral candidosis is thought to be both local and systemic.

Cancrum oris (noma, gangrenous stomatitis) is a severe form of necrotising periodontal disease, and is seen occasionally in developing countries, in particular, sub-Saharan Africa (see Chapter 6). The sufferer is characteristically less than 10 years of age, malnourished and has a history of a recent viral infection, such as measles (see Chapter 9). The initial lesion spreads into the cheek, face and neck causing extensive tissue loss. Treatment is with a combination of antibiotics, such as benzylpenicillin with metronidazole, but the combination should include agents active against both Gram-negative and Gram-positive bacteria.

ANAEMIA

Anaemia can be defined as a reduction in the haemoglobin level (below 135 g/L for men and below 115 g/L for women). Anaemia can be categorised as macrocytic or microcytic depending on the mean cell volume (MCV), and both types can lead to oral signs. The orofacial manifestations of anaemia can result in oral ulceration, angular cheilitis, oral candidosis, mucositis and glossitis. In the management of these conditions, it is important to consider an underlying systemic cause, such as anaemia, and particularly if they fail to respond to antimicrobial agents.

MALIGNANCY

Osteoradionecrosis

Cancer in the oral region is usually treated by surgery, radiotherapy, chemotherapy or a combination of all three. Radiotherapy destroys the rapidly dividing cancer cells, but it also destroys surrounding bone. This bone is highly susceptible to secondary radiation as it absorbs a great deal of energy. Bone is affected by radiation in three ways: there is a decrease in the number of cells (hypocellularity) and reduction in blood vessels (hypovascularity) and as a consequence, less oxygen in the tissue (hypoxia). As the bone heals after irradiation, fibrous tissue is generated instead of bone, especially in the mandible. The effects of radiation therapy are not transitory and the hypovascularity increases with time. A simple operation on tissues, which have been irradiated, such as a tooth extraction, can result in spontaneous death of the surrounding bone (necrosis). Death of the bone after irradiation can be progressive and is called osteoradionecrosis and has been associated with oral ulceration caused by ill-fitting dentures, scaling of the teeth, facial bone fractures and root canal therapy. In the past, radiation therapy was not so highly focused (collimated) on the malignant tissue, and the surrounding normal structures were also often affected. In these conditions, the incidence of osteoradionecrosis in oral bone varied from 17% to 37%. With careful collimation, shielding of surrounding tissues, use of small but effective repeated radiation doses (fractionation), the incidence of osteoradionecrosis has been reduced to 2% to 5%.

Osteoradionecrosis is likely to arise because of a combination of radiation, trauma and infection. However, extensive animal studies support a view that the microorganisms are contaminants and cause secondary infection of preexisting necrosis. Interestingly, both cultural and molecular studies of necrotic tissue obtained from cases of osteoradionecrosis have detected a predominantly anaerobic microbiota, including *Porphyromonas* spp. and *Prevotella* spp. Osteoradionecrosis is difficult to manage and treatment failures have been reported despite the provision of appropriate antibacterial agents, such as metronidazole or clindamycin and optimal surgical debridement. Bacterial isolates frequently develop increased antimicrobial resistance during the course of treatment.

Postirradiation mucositis

Another consequence of irradiation of the oral region is non-specific inflammation of the oral mucosa, often called mucositis (Fig. 11.3). This can be extensive and cause considerable pain with difficulties in feeding. Symptoms may be severe enough to influence the patient to abandon the radiation treatment. At first it was thought that radiation mucositis was caused by infection by *Candida* spp., and other yeasts. However, provision of antifungal therapy has no effect, suggesting that yeasts are not causing the condition. More extensive sampling of the mucosa has shown that the microbiota associated with mucositis is mainly composed of Gram-negative aerobic and facultatively anaerobic bacteria such as *Escherichia coli*, pseudomonads, *Klebsiella* spp, and *Acinetobacter* spp. Irradiation mucositis can be largely alleviated by selective decontamination of the oral cavity before and during irradiation therapy by topically applying a combination of non-absorbable antimicrobials onto the tissues to be protected. The usual combinations of antimicrobials are polymyxin and tobramycin, and an antifungal is added to prevent yeast overgrowth. Two antimicrobials are used to prevent the selection of resistance in Gram-negative bacteria. This combination can be used to ameliorate the effects of the mucositis.

XEROSTOMIA

Xerostomia literally means dry mouth and can be caused by a variety of conditions or treatments (Table 11.1). One of the consequences of xerostomia is overgrowth of dental plaque, with acidogenic oral streptococci and lactobacilli predominating within the biofilm. This can induce a dramatic increase in dental caries in dentate individuals. Xerostomia predisposes to the development of mucositis and opportunistic *Candida*

TABLE 11.1 **Causes of xerostomia**
Drug therapy (in particular antidepressants)
Sjögren's syndrome (immunological destruction of salivary tissues)
Damage to salivary glands following radiotherapy
Undiagnosed or poorly controlled diabetes
Dehydration
Congenital absence of salivary glands

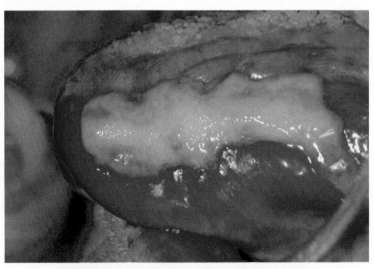

FIGURE 11.3 Postirradiation mucositis on the lingual mucosa.

infections of the oral mucosa in addition to an increased risk of periodontal disease.

MEDICATIONS

Medication-related osteonecrosis of the jaw

Osteonecrosis of the jaw (ONJ) is caused by the use of antiresorptive therapy used mainly in the treatment of osteoporosis, bone metastasis and other malignancies. These medications include bisphosphonates, denosumab and antiangiogenics. Osteoporosis is a serious condition in which there can be spinal compression, long bone fracture and bone pain. The bisphosphonates are pyrophosphate analogues that can prevent osteoporosis by inhibiting osteoclast activity. Unfortunately, some patients who take bisphosphonates can suffer from a failure of bone to heal especially after extractions. The bone around the socket dies and may remain exposed to the oral cavity and get secondarily infected, particularly with obligatory anaerobic bacteria. The exact cause of this condition is not known, but it is likely that this may be similar to the hypovascularity seen in osteoradionecrosis. One other suggestion is that medication-related osteonecrosis is because of an anaerobic infection of the bone, but this is unlikely to be the primary cause as it is not cured by antimicrobials or surgery. The risk of this condition developing is small overall and the greatest incidence reported is 1% to 15% in the oncology patient population where medications are used at high doses. In the osteoporosis patient population, the incidence of ONJ is estimated at 0.001% to 0.01%, with higher incidences reported in the population taking intravenous bisphosphonates compared with an oral preparation. However, the risk of the condition developing increases with age, duration of medication use, concomitant oral disease and underlying systemic disease such as diabetes.

KEY POINTS

Many systemic disorders may affect the oral microbiota and predispose to opportunistic infections. These are summarised in Table 11.2. In addition, there are many situations where the host defence is altered as a result of underlying illness or medication used for treatment, predisposing the individual to oral infections. Optimal oral hygiene may improve the circumstances of patients with general debilitation and in the prevention of systemic respiratory disease. It is also important to consider and rule out systemic disease in patients presenting with oral opportunistic infections.

TABLE 11.2 Orofacial infections that may occur in medically compromised patients

Disorder	Example	Orofacial infection
Endocrine disorders	Diabetes mellitus	Oral fungal infections
Respiratory disorders	Asthma	Oral fungal infections
Neurological disorders	Epilepsy	Gingival hyperplasia and periodontal disease
Neoplastic disease	Oral carcinoma	Dental caries and mucositis following radiotherapy
Chronic infection	Tuberculosis	Oral tuberculosis
Immunological disorders	HIV and AIDS	Oral viral and fungal infections
Haematinic deficiencies	Anaemia	Angular cheilitis and oral fungal infections

AIDS, Acquired immune deficiency syndrome; *HIV*, human immunodeficiency virus.

INFLUENCE OF ORAL MICROBIOTA ON SYSTEMIC DISEASE

It is well established that a healthy oral environment is closely associated with general well-being and self-esteem. A functioning dentition and comfortable, disease-free oral cavity facilitate optimal nutrition and promote normal social interactions. In addition, evidence is emerging that the oral microbiota may have an impact on our general systemic health (Fig. 11.4), and associations are being made between disruptions to the oral microbiota, for example, periodontal disease and conditions such as atherosclerosis and low birth weight infants. This is perhaps not surprising given our growing understanding of the role of the gut microbiota in a number of conditions such as diabetes, obesity and even cognitive ability and mental health. Although there is a lack of consensus on the clinical relevance of some of the associations between the oral environment and systemic disease and a lack of complete understanding of the mechanisms underlying the disease processes, a number of interesting areas for ongoing research have been highlighted.

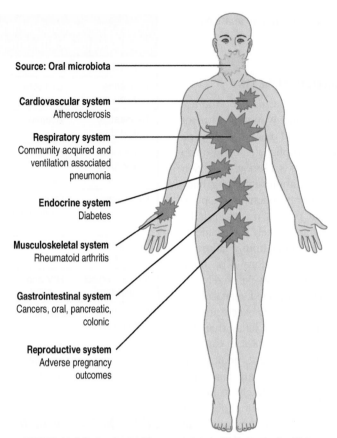

Source: Oral microbiota

Cardiovascular system
Atherosclerosis

Respiratory system
Community acquired and
ventilation associated
pneumonia

Endocrine system
Diabetes

Musculoskeletal system
Rheumatoid arthritis

Gastrointestinal system
Cancers, oral, pancreatic,
colonic

Reproductive system
Adverse pregnancy
outcomes

FIGURE 11.4 Systemic conditions associated with the oral microbiota.

CARDIOVASCULAR DISEASE

Infective endocarditis

Infective endocarditis is an infection of the endothelium (lining) of the heart and is an example of a systemic infection for which there is little doubt that the oral microbiota acts as a source of infection in many patients. If the blood flow through the heart is disrupted either by congenital or acquired disease then it can clot. This is because of the flow being slowed where there is an eddy or whirling of the flow. One common cause of slowing of blood flow is narrowing of the valve exits, where the blood is pumped from a narrow area into a larger area (the so-called Venturi effect). Again the blood is slowed and clots form deposits on the undersides of the valves. These clots are often called vegetations because they resemble vegetationous growths. If bacteria enter the bloodstream (bacteraemia) and enter the heart, they can attach to

these vegetations and start to grow. They grow extremely slowly, often taking between 12 and 18 hours to double in number and form biofilms (Fig. 11.5; see Chapter 5). Eventually they can cause inflammation of the heart lining (called the endothelium) and infective endocarditis can ensue. One source of the infective agents has been postulated to be streptococci from the mouth which are released into the bloodstream during dental procedures.

Infective endocarditis is an extremely dangerous, but fortunately rare condition. Even when prolonged intravenous antibiotics are given promptly to kill the infecting agent, endocarditis still has a high mortality rate of between 25% and 40%. The disease is difficult to diagnose from its initial signs and symptoms which are influenza-like symptoms, night sweats and lassitude which gradually progress. The diagnosis is usually made on the basis of a culture of blood which yields

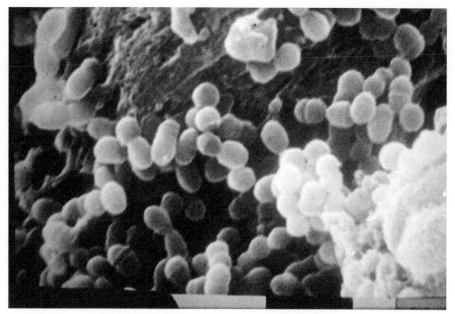

FIGURE 11.5 Scanning electron microscopy showing streptococci colonising a heart valve from a case of fatal endocarditis.

the infective agents. If the patient recovers, the heart valves may need replacement and the vegetations will need removal. This requires open-heart surgery which carries a significant mortality risk. Replacement of the heart valves unfortunately means that the patient may have a 25% chance of getting infective endocarditis again. During the period when the patient has infective endocarditis, small portions of the vegetations may break off and block peripheral blood vessels; this is particularly serious if it is in the brain.

The microorganisms which cause infective endocarditis are listed in Table 11.3. The principal bacteria that cause this disease are now staphylococci (probably derived from the skin), but until recently oral streptococci were the main cause. The rise in the number of people developing infective endocarditis caused by staphylococci is probably because of the use of unsterile needles by intravenous drug addicts.

Oral streptococci have long been associated with the development of infective endocarditis. This is because many dental procedures such as scaling, extractions and gingival manipulations have been shown to release oral bacteria, and in particular streptococci, into the bloodstream (that is, cause a bacteraemia). The principal

TABLE 11.3 Microorganisms isolated from cases of human infective endocarditis	
Microorganism	**% Isolation frequency**
Staphylococci	44
Oral streptococci*	36
Enterococci	12
Aggregatibacter actinomycetemcomitans	3
Coxiella burnetii	2
Candida species	1
Other microorganisms including viruses	2

*Most common species isolated are *S. sanguinis* and *S. oralis*

oral streptococci associated with infective endocarditis are *Streptococcus sanguinis*, but *S. gordonii* and *S. oralis* are also frequently isolated. Although these bacteria are readily found in the mouths of patients with infective endocarditis, they can also be recovered from elsewhere in the body, for example, on the genitalia and in the upper respiratory tract. It is, therefore, by no means certain that the mouth is always the portal of entry for these bacteria on their way to the heart.

The exact mechanism by which oral streptococci cause infective endocarditis is still a matter of debate. Undoubtedly oral streptococci enter the bloodstream and circulate to the heart and attach to the vegetations. Streptococci produce surface glucans and extracellular matrix adhesins (fibronectin binding proteins, FimA) in addition to platelet activating factors which may be involved in the pathogenesis of infective endocarditis. The interaction of bacteria with platelets would appear to be of particular significance and in animal models the ability of *S. sanguinis* to adhere to and activate platelets correlates with increased severity of disease. It has been shown that when platelets are passed over immobilised *S. sanguinis* during conditions of high shear, the platelets roll and then adhere to the bacteria, creating a thrombus. Platelets would appear to bind either via streptococcal surface proteins (platelet aggregation associated proteins PAAPs, SrpA, PblA and PblB) or via indirect bridging molecules such as fibrinogen. Following adhesion, some species seem to be capable of promoting aggregation and activation of the platelets and this ability appears to be distinct from adhesion and is mediated by different protein receptors. For example, *S. mitis*, binds to the platelets via PblA and PblB but does not activate them. The second stage in the pathogenesis of infective endocarditis is thought to involve lipoproteins such as FimA (*S. parasanguinis*) and SloC (*S. mutans*), LPxTz anchored protein and polysaccharides, each of which have been associated with colonisation of the host tissue.

Atherosclerotic cardiovascular disease

The ability of bacteria from the oral cavity to cause infection of a heart valve (infective endocarditis) has been discussed above. More recently, associations between oral microorganisms and other forms of cardiovascular disease, particularly atherosclerosis, have been documented. There appears to be a consistent association between atherosclerotic disease and periodontitis which cannot be explained completely by common risk factors such as diabetes, smoking and hereditary influences. Longitudinal studies have provided evidence that there is an excess risk of cardiovascular events in individuals with periodontal disease. There are a number of proposed mechanisms which include the circulation of inflammatory mediators in response to periodontal disease which contribute to atheroma formation. Furthermore, a range of periodontal pathogens, including *Porphyromonas gingivalis, Fusobacterium nucleatum* and *Aggregatibacter actinomycetemcomitans,* have been detected within atheromatous plaques and been shown to induce inflammatory, immune and procoagulant responses. Some of these bacteria are known to invade endothelial cells, and it has been proposed that endothelial cell dysfunction is an early manifestation of atherosclerotic vascular disease. There is evidence that *P. gingivalis* is able to induce and maintain a chronic state of inflammation at distant sites, including atheromatous plaques, and this species has been shown to accelerate atherosclerosis in animal models. Other potential mechanisms include cross-reactive systemic antibodies that promote inflammation and interact with atheroma components, and the promotion of lipidaemia. Given the prevalence of cardiovascular disease and the associated mortality and morbidity, further research is needed in the form of longitudinal clinical studies involving both physicians and oral health professionals to firmly establish the role of oral bacteria in cardiovascular disease.

RESPIRATORY DISEASE

As there is contiguity between the respiratory tract and the oral cavity, it is perhaps not surprising that the oral microbiota has been associated with the development of respiratory infection. Oral bacteria have frequently been linked to the onset of pneumonia in individuals residing in nursing care homes, hospitals and critical care settings (aspiration pneumonia; Fig. 11.6). Furthermore, studies have shown that dental pain and/or the wearing of dentures are risk factors in the development of community-acquired pneumonia. Periodontal disease has been shown to be a risk factor for hospital-acquired pneumonia with a threefold increased incidence in pneumonia occurring in patients with existing periodontitis. Interestingly, it has been reported that patients who have recently visited the dentist, and who, by implication, may have better oral health, are at lower risk of developing pneumonia. Furthermore, an increasing number of studies are examining the associations between poor oral hygiene and acute exacerbations of chronic obstructive pulmonary disease.

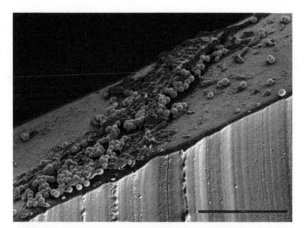

FIGURE 11.6 Scanning electron microscope image of a mixed species biofilm forming on the interior lumen of an endotracheal tube used for mechanical ventilation of critically ill patients. Biofilms at such sites have been shown to contain both oral bacteria and potential respiratory pathogens. (This figure was provided courtesy of Dr Kirsty Wade and Mrs Wendy Rowe (Cardiff University)).

There are several potential mechanisms involved in the promotion of respiratory infections by oral microorganisms. Firstly, members of the normal oral microbiota may cause infection following aspiration into the lower airway. Such aspiration has been documented using molecular and culture approaches in elderly patients with impaired cough reflexes. Furthermore, molecular analysis of bronchoalveolar lavages of patients with community acquired pneumonia demonstrate that oral species such as *Prevotella*, *Fusobacterium* and streptococci are often the predominant bacteria detected.

The oral cavity can harbour pathogenic bacteria capable of causing respiratory infection following aspiration of the microbes or their toxins into the lower respiratory tract. The oral microbiota is dynamic and changes in composition can occur in relation to both local and systemic factors, such as underlying disease, effect of medications including antimicrobials, impairment of salivary flow, changes in diet or reduced oral hygiene practices. These situations can manifest in a number of patient groups including the elderly and those who are critically ill. Indeed, amongst these groups, microbial alteration of dental plaque to involve colonisation by potential respiratory pathogens has been reported. These bacteria include species such as *Pseudomonas aeruginosa* and *Staphylococcus aureus*

(including MRSA), which are detected only infrequently in the dental plaque of healthy patients. Clearly, aspiration of pathogens from the mouth to the lungs could potentiate infection in vulnerable patients.

Another potential means by which members of the oral microbiota can facilitate respiratory infection is by their influence on the oral mucosa. It has been suggested that the inflammatory responses of the oral mucosa may be mirrored at the mucosal surfaces of the lungs thereby facilitating infiltration of this epithelium by respiratory pathogens.

Given the current evidence implicating oral bacteria in respiratory infection, improved oral hygiene in patients' groups susceptible to pneumonia or other respiratory disease would seem to be important. Indeed, improved oral hygiene has been shown to reduce the incidence of pneumonia in a number of studies of ventilated patients and also non-ventilated nursing home residents. Further research is required to better understand the mechanisms underlying these associations, and to determine the most effective oral interventions.

ADVERSE PREGNANCY OUTCOMES

The evidence for a correlation between periodontal disease and an increase in the relative risk of adverse pregnancy outcomes (APO) in some human populations, including preterm and low birth weight babies, is becoming more widely accepted. More than 10 oral bacterial species have been studied in association with APO including *Fusobacterium nucleatum*, *Eikenella corrodens*, *P. gingivalis* and the novel, as yet uncultivated, *Bergeyella* species. *Bergeyella* spp. have been detected in a range of specimens associated with neonatal sepsis including amniotic fluid and cord blood. In addition, there is evidence that the source of these bacteria is the mothers' oral cavity because the phylotypes detected have been matched to those found in plaque and not elsewhere including the mother's vaginal microbiota. This translocation of oral species to the placenta has been supported by animal studies. *Fusobacterium nucleatum* has been extensively investigated in the context of APO and has been documented as the most prevalent species in amniotic fluid from pregnancies complicated by preterm birth and an oral origin of the species has been confirmed in many cases. *Fusobacterium nucleatum* possesses many well-characterised virulence factors which are consistent with the concept of translocation and the propensity to cause infection at sites distant to the oral cavity. These include the ability to adhere to epithelial and endothelial cells and to invade, via both an intracellular and intercellular route. The microorganism can stimulate Toll-like receptor 4 (TLR4) mediated inflammatory responses in placental tissue, a mechanism which has been shown to be the main cause of foetal death in animal models. Other relevant virulence factors are the ability to induce apoptosis of lymphocytes and mediate coaggregation of other oral pathogens.

Despite the plausible pathogenic mechanisms that have been outlined earlier, interventional studies, in which the maternal periodontal condition is treated in an attempt to reduce the risk to the baby, have not consistently shown an effect on birth outcome. Preterm birth is the most common cause of infant morbidity and mortality in developed countries and therefore this area warrants further investigation.

DIABETES

It has been established that diabetes is a risk factor for periodontal disease. Conversely, there is mounting evidence that the presence of periodontal disease may adversely affect diabetes. Although the findings are equivocal, there is some evidence that the severity of periodontal disease may influence glycaemic control. The mechanisms are unclear but chronic periodontal disease is known to result in a continual release of inflammatory mediators into the circulation which is a sustained challenge to the diabetic patient and is known to increase insulin resistance. Intervention studies have reported equivocal results. A review of five clinical studies reported a mean reduction in glycated haemoglobin (a marker of glycaemic control) of 0.4%. It is unclear whether the magnitude of this reduction is clinically significant. However, this area is worthy of further study because it is well established that a decrease in glycated haemoglobin correlates with reduced complications and mortality in diabetic patients.

RHEUMATOID ARTHRITIS

Associations between rheumatoid arthritis (RA) and periodontal disease have been studied for many decades. Individuals newly diagnosed with RA have been shown to have an incidence of periodontal disease higher than would be expected for their age. Subjects with periodontal disease have an increased risk of developing RA and conversely the prevalence of periodontal disease is at least twofold greater in patients with RA. Although this relationship may be the result of shared environmental and hereditary factors, there is some evidence that supports a causal connection. The two conditions show some similarities in that they are associated with a similar host-mediated chronic inflammatory response, have elements of autoimmunity and can be episodic in nature and the activation of underlying and overlapping inflammatory pathways has been proposed as a mechanism to explain the association between these two conditions. Antibodies to Gram-negative pathogens including *Prevotella intermedia*, *Porphyromonas gingivalis* and *Tannerella forsythia* have been detected in the serum and synovial fluid of patients with active RA. Antibodies to *P. gingivalis* have been shown to be significantly associated with the presence of RA-related autoantibodies in individuals at risk for RA. Of particular interest is the demonstration of the ability of *P. gingivalis* to citrullinate proteins by means of peptidylarginine deiminase (PPAD). This enzyme is present in outer membranes or is secreted, and deiminates arginine to citrulline, generating ammonia and leading to a rise in the local pH, which favours the growth of this periodontal pathogen. This property appears to be unique amongst oral pathogens and has been proposed as a potential mechanism for generating antigens that may drive the autoimmune response in RA.

Although these findings are interesting, there is no convincing evidence as yet to suggest that management of periodontal disease leads to improved control of RA. Larger scale studies are required to further examine the relationship between these two diseases and the effects of interventional studies.

CANCER

The role of bacteria in oral and other cancers is currently an active area of research and potential mechanisms include the metabolism and production of carcinogenic products, such as acetaldehyde, the induction of chronic inflammation and direct interference with eukaryotic cell cycle and signalling pathways. Bacteria have been detected within a range of tumour types including oral cancers. Significantly higher levels of *Porphyromonas* and *Fusobacterium* species have been isolated from the surface of oral squamous cell carcinomas compared with adjacent tissue. A diverse range of oral pathogens, including novel phylotypes, has been detected by molecular methods within the tissues of oral carcinoma. With respect to extraoral cancers, a twofold increase in the risk of pancreatic cancer has been documented for those individuals with high levels of antibodies to *P. gingivalis*, independent of known shared risk factors. Large-scale epidemiological studies in the USA have demonstrated an association between orodigestive cancer mortality and levels of *P. gingivalis* antibodies, independent of periodontitis. In relation to colorectal cancer, high levels of *F. nucleatum* have been shown to be present within tumour tissue and levels of antibody to this bacterium were correlated with metastases to lymph nodes. *Fusobacterium nucleatum* expresses a unique adhesin (*Fusobacterium* adhesin A; FadA) that enables the organism to bind to endothelial and epithelial cells. FadA is also classed as an invasin and is involved in the invasion of normal and cancerous cells. *Fusobacterium nucleatum* has been shown to be capable of stimulating the growth of colorectal cancer cells. Both *F. nucleatum* and *P. gingivalis* have been strongly associated with chronic inflammation, often demonstrating intracellular invasion and persistence in epithelial cells and the propensity to translocate to other sites. In addition, their ability to dysregulate the immune system and their effects on apoptotic events are well-documented. The precise role of these microbes in carcinogenesis and the reasons why cancer develops in a relatively limited number of individuals despite the widespread colonisation of the population with these two species remain unclear and require further investigation.

In addition to the diseases outlined earlier, there is a growing body of literature highlighting associations between the oral microbiota and other conditions such as obesity, kidney disease, metabolic syndrome, osteoporosis and cognitive impairment which will require further investigation.

Most of the associations discussed in this section have been in relation to periodontal disease, a term which encompasses a number of heterogeneous conditions. Future epidemiological and interventional studies should ensure robust definitions of the type of periodontal disease under study and accurately record disease outcomes. In addition, given the bias of most studies towards cultured microorganisms and the growing evidence to support pathogenic roles for uncultivated organisms, molecular approaches should be used in the comprehensive analysis of the microbiota. Moreover, because there is evidence that only selected subtypes of a given species may be associated with systemic disease or liable to extraoral translocation (for example *F. nucleatum* subspecies *animalis* with intrauterine infection and *S. mutans* non c serotypes with atherosclerotic disease), any studies of disease associations should include discriminatory subtyping of putative pathogens. Additional, appropriately designed research in these areas will hopefully elucidate the mechanisms underlying any confirmed associations and may help determine the most appropriate strategies for modulation of the oral microbiota in the management of these systemic conditions.

KEY POINTS

In addition to the well-established relationship between oral microorganisms and infective endocarditis, a growing list of systemic conditions is being associated with specific oral bacteria or the chronic inflammatory disease of periodontitis; these include cardiovascular disease, respiratory infection and adverse pregnancy outcomes. Other weaker associations are being explored for rheumatoid arthritis, diabetes and cancer. Although biologically plausible mechanisms have been proposed, the results of intervention studies have been inconsistent and further work is required in this area to confirm associations and better understand the pathogenesis.

ORAL MANIFESTATIONS OF SYSTEMIC INFECTION

TUBERCULOSIS

Tuberculosis (TB) is one of the most prevalent infectious diseases in the world. Globally, there are about 1.5 million deaths and nine million new cases of TB each year. It has been estimated that one third of the world's population is latently infected with TB, and this can reactivate in later years or following immunosuppression (e.g., following human immunodeficiency virus [HIV] infection). Although the incidence of tuberculosis declined during the twentieth century in Western countries, it has increased in recent years because of changing migration patterns from the developing to the developed world, and coinfection with HIV. Every year about 9000 new cases of TB are diagnosed in the United Kingdom. Although nearly 75% of these are caused by the acid-fast bacillus, *Mycobacterium tuberculosis*, other species such as *M. bovis, M. africanum, M. microti* and *M. kansasii* can also cause disease. Infection is spread in droplets of sputum from patients with active pulmonary tuberculosis. In some patients, infection also produces lesions within the oral cavity. The classical intraoral presentation is of a single chronic ulcer on the dorsal surface of the tongue, but lesions may affect any site. The ulcers are irregular with raised borders and may resemble deep fungal infection or squamous cell carcinoma.

Diagnosis of TB may include a mucosal biopsy, sputum culture, tuberculin testing and a chest radiograph. The mucosal biopsy should demonstrate the characteristic granulomatous inflammation with well-formed granulomata, Langhans giant cells and necrosis. Ziehl-Neelsen stain may be used to detect tubercle bacilli. Microbiological culture of suspected clinical material may also be useful to establish the diagnosis of tuberculosis. It is important to inform the microbiologist that tuberculosis is suspected because specialised media (Löwenstein–Jensen) and prolonged incubation (2 to 3 weeks) is required for recovery of the organism. Molecular microbiologic methods are being used increasingly to establish the diagnosis and indicate drug sensitivity profiles. A Mantoux (tuberculin) skin test can be used to screen patients at high risk. It can however show false positive reactions with prior Bacillus Calmette–Guérin (BCG) immunisation and false negative reactions in sarcoidosis and with patients with active TB. Previous infection may occasionally be seen as incidental radio-opacities on radiographs because of calcification within lymph nodes.

Oral lesions will resolve when systemic chemotherapy consisting of rifampicin, isoniazid, pyrazinamide and ethambutol is administered. Typically, combinations of these drugs are given initially for 2 months after which time the therapy is reduced to isoniazid and rifampicin for a further 4 months. There are unpleasant side effects associated with these drug regimens, so that patients may fail to complete the full course of therapy, possibly leading to the emergence of drug-resistant strains. Longer and different regimens are required for the management of patients found to have resistant strains of *M. tuberculosis*. Strains of *M. tuberculosis* that are resistant to the majority of the drugs used to treat this infection are referred to as multidrug (MDR) or extensive (or extreme) drug resistant (XDR) strains. Currently the only vaccine available is live attenuated BCG which has a variable efficacy globally of between 0% and 80%. There has been a lull in new drug development and in the future, difficulties may be encountered in treating this condition.

GONORRHOEA

Gonorrhoea is caused by *Neisseria gonorrhoeae* and is a sexually transmitted disease that principally affects the genital mucosa, although it may also produce pharyngitis and a range of non-specific oral changes including erythema, vesicle formation and pseudomembrane development, as a result of orogenital contact. These symptoms are usually preceded by generalised oral burning or itching and submandibular lymphadenopathy, which make speaking and swallowing difficult. In view of the vague symptoms, diagnosis can only be made by examination of a smear of a lesion, which will show Gram-negative pairs of cocci (diplococci) within neutrophils. Culture of a swab on chocolate agar or Thayer–Martin agar will yield typical translucent oxidase-positive colonies. Identification of *N. gonorrhoeae* can be confirmed by carbohydrate utilisation profiles or fluorescent antibody tests. Treatment has historically involved a single dose of intramuscular penicillin or high-dose oral amoxicillin. The 3 g sachet of amoxicillin was originally developed for the treatment of gonorrhoea. However, the emergence of resistance to amoxicillin has resulted in the need to use alternative antibiotics, such as ceftriaxone or ciprofloxacin. Ceftriaxone 500 mg intramuscularly as a single dose with azithromycin 1 g oral as a single dose are often recommended for management.

SYPHILIS

Recently there has been an increase in the number of new cases of syphilis in the UK. The majority of these cases is in men and can occur with HIV coinfection.

Syphilis, which is caused by the spirochaete *Treponema pallidum*, has four distinct stages, the first three of which (primary, secondary and tertiary) can affect the orofacial tissues. In addition, because *T. pallidum* is one of the few microorganisms that can cross the placenta, this condition may manifest as a congenital disease in childhood. Primary syphilis characteristically develops on the genitalia but can also present initially as a highly infectious indurated red painless ulcer (chancre) on the lip or oral mucosa. Secondary syphilis appears approximately six weeks after the primary infection and, in addition to generalised symptoms, may produce oral lesions described as mucous patches and snail track ulcers. Finally, if unsuccessfully treated, syphilis can become latent and produce tertiary lesions many years after initial infection that manifest as an area of ulceration (gumma) in the palate that may involve bone or leukoplakia affecting the dorsal surface of the tongue which may be potentially malignant.

A provisional diagnosis of syphilis may be made by use of dark-field microscopy to demonstrate numerous structures consistent in size and form with *T. pallidum* in a smear taken from either primary or secondary lesions. The causative spirochaetes cannot be cultured routinely in vitro and therefore serological investigations are used to diagnose syphilis from the late stage of primary infection onwards. *Treponema pallidum* haemagglutination (TPHA) and fluorescent *Treponema* antibody absorbed (FTAabs) tests should be undertaken. A biopsy may be helpful and the spirochaetes may be detected in the tissue section using a silver stain and immunohistochemistry can be performed. The most effective treatment of syphilis is intramuscular benzathine penicillin. However, patients should be followed up for at least 2 years and serological examination repeated during this time.

KEY POINTS

> A range of human systemic infections can on rare occasions primarily infect the orofacial tissues or have secondary manifestations of infection at these sites. Examples of these are tuberculosis, gonorrhoea and syphilis. Appropriate diagnostic tests should be arranged in a patient with orofacial signs and symptoms of such infectious diseases.

HUMAN IMMUNODEFICIENCY VIRUS AND ACQUIRED IMMUNE DEFICIENCY SYNDROME

HIV is the causative agent of acquired immune deficiency syndrome. The infection is thought to affect at least 35 million people worldwide and it has been calculated that HIV infects a new person every 5 minutes. AIDS accounts for 1.5 million deaths each year, the majority being within African countries.

AIDS results from a depletion of CD4$^+$ lymphocytes (T-helper cells) so there is no functional immunity, particularly to infection. T-helper cells mediate both humoral and cellular immunity, and are able to direct the host response to different infectious agents to give predominantly either humoral or cell-mediated immunity. The loss of CD4$^+$ lymphocytes results in an inadequate host response to a range of frank or opportunistic pathogens.

A huge variety of infections, lesions, signs and symptoms are associated with HIV infection and some of the oral manifestations are listed in Table 11.4. Note that AIDS is a syndrome, which is a collection of potential signs and symptoms which may occur, in contrast to a disease, which is a collection of signs and symptoms that always go together.

HIV can easily penetrate the blood-brain barrier and one of the early signs of AIDS may be mental deterioration of the patient because of infection of the brain. Such neurological deterioration can be misdiagnosed as dementia.

HIV can be found in a wide range of body fluids including blood, saliva, sputum, semen, vaginal secretion, perianal secretion and breast milk. The main test used for detection of HIV uses the antibody produced in response to infection by the virus. The HIV antibody test is relatively simple, using an enzyme linked immunosorbent assay (ELISA). The detection of this virus relies on the virus stimulating an antibody response and this can take between 22 days and 11 months. There are periods, therefore, when the virus has infected lymphocytes and macrophages but is not being released into the bloodstream and has not stimulated an antibody response. In this time period the person infected would give a negative antibody test, but would still be infectious.

In the early stages of infection, HIV releases a protein, present in its core, called p24. This protein can sometimes be detected within one week of infection,

TABLE 11.4   Lesions associated with human immunodeficiency virus infection

Group 1	Group 2	Group 3
Lesions strongly associated with HIV	Lesions less commonly associated with HIV	Lesions sometimes associated with HIV
Candidosis: Erythematous Pseudomembranous	Bacterial infections: *Mycobacterium tuberculosis* *Mycobacterium avium-intracellulare*	Bacterial infections: *Actinomyces israelii* *Escherichia coli* *Klebsiella pneumoniae*
Hairy leukoplakia Periodontal disease Linear gingival erythema Necrotising periodontal diseases Kaposi's sarcoma	Melanotic hyperpigmentation Necrotising stomatitis Non-specific ulceration	Cat scratch disease Drug reactions Fungal infections: *Cryptococcus, Geotrichum, Mucor,* *Aspergillus*
Non-Hodgkin lymphoma	Salivary gland disease Thrombocytopenic purpura	
	Viral infections: Herpes simplex type 1, Human papilloma virus, Varicella zoster virus	

HIV, Human immunodeficiency virus.

but always within one month. This is a direct test, which confirms the presence or absence of the virus, but it is more complex and expensive than the detection of antibody.

The screening of individuals for HIV is subject to varying legislation in different countries and involves consideration of civil liberties. In some countries, including the UK, screening is carried out as part of healthcare worker occupational checks and antenatal screening tests. In some countries, no precise records are kept of HIV infection rates and the prevalence of the disease can only be estimated from the number of those who seek treatment, develop AIDS, or indirectly by the screening of blood donations. Testing for HIV infection is a highly emotive issue, which, because of the serious social and medical consequences, has to be undertaken carefully and sensitively. Individuals should be encouraged to undergo testing as soon as a diagnosis is suspected, and be reassured that in most countries they no longer need to tell life insurance companies about testing, but only in the event of a positive result. One of the most difficult situations is the testing of patients who have been treated by HIV-infected healthcare workers, where there could have been blood contamination; these are often called

exposure prone procedures. To assess whether HIV or other infection has been transmitted, all the patients who have been treated by the healthcare worker are contacted and offered counselling, or HIV tests. The value of such retrospective surveys has been questioned, as the risk of transmission is low and not worth the anxiety generated in the population who are offered the counselling or the tests. There have been very few proven transmissions of HIV by healthcare workers to patients. However, a small number of cases involving, for example, an orthopaedic surgeon and a dentist have been documented.

The value of such retrospective surveys is also scientifically questionable as the test may be taken when no HIV markers are detectable and false negative results will be obtained. The risk of transmission of HIV by healthcare workers is very low, unless a significant amount of blood is transferred directly into the recipient's bloodstream. Even if this occurs the risk of transmission is thought to be only 0.4%.

One of the most significant advances in the treatment of HIV is the use of highly active antiretroviral therapy (often given the acronym HAART or ART). The use of a combination of a deoxyribonucleic acid (DNA) analogue and two protease inhibitors has been found to stop HIV replication. The agents penetrate the HIV infected cell and the DNA analogue integrates into the elongating DNA chain stopping further replication. It is important to stress that this is not a cure for HIV infection; the person remains infected but does not progress to develop AIDS.

The use of HAART therapy is not without its problems. Such anti-HIV therapy has significant side effects and must be continued for the life of the infected person without any interruption. If interruption of the drug does occur the individual is at risk of rebound infection. Treating the disease early in the primary seroconversion phase has been shown to have a better prognosis than late treatment. Treatment is usually only started when the CD4 count falls below 350 because above this the level of the disease and symptoms are monitored rather than initiating treatment. The long-term prognosis of patients with HIV is now much better with HAART and patients generally live longer than those with other long-term systemic conditions such as diabetes. However, such treatment regimens present an enormous economic problem, which can be an insuperable barrier to appropriate management in poorer countries of the world.

Anti-HIV therapy can also be used to prevent the transmission of HIV. If a healthcare worker suffers a significant injury and exposure to HIV-infected blood, then the prompt use of anti-HIV therapy can prevent infection. The therapy has to be instituted as soon as possible; preferably within 24 hours and continued for 28 days. This use of anti-HIV therapy is often described as post-exposure prophylaxis (PEP).

The dental management of HIV-infected individuals is no different to any non-infected person and universal or standard precautions are applied to all patients (see Chapter 12). The aim is to get rid of any incipient sepsis and to ensure good periodontal health. Patients on HAART can be managed in general dental practice, and consideration given to the large number of other medications that they may be taking.

MICROORGANISMS OF RELEVANCE TO INFECTION CONTROL IN DENTISTRY

HEPATITIS B

The outcome of infection with hepatitis B virus includes recovery and the development of immunity,

KEY POINTS

Acquired immune deficiency syndrome (AIDS) represents a cell-mediated immunodeficiency, principally T lymphocytes, because of infection by an RNA retrovirus known as the human immunodeficiency virus (HIV). Once infected, an individual may remain HIV positive for many years, particularly since the development of antiretroviral drugs, before progressing to AIDS. The conditions that define AIDS include a reduced CD4$^+$ lymphocyte count accompanied by a number of orofacial signs and symptoms, including candidosis, hairy leukoplakia, Kaposi sarcoma and herpetic ulceration. Because oral manifestations of HIV infection are relatively common, changes in the mouth may be the first indication of infection. Although it is unlikely that HIV is spread in saliva, it is relevant to dentistry because of the potential for contact with blood during the provision of dental treatment. Standard infection control procedures must be applied and a high standard of instrument decontamination practiced (see Chapter 12). In many countries, some HIV positive healthcare workers including dentists can undertake exposure prone procedures as long as they are receiving appropriate antiretroviral treatment and have regular testing to safeguard patients. Dental school applicants are often required to show evidence of HIV negativity as part of a health clearance screen before admission.

death from fulminant acute hepatitis or the development of chronic infection and associated complications such as cirrhosis and hepatocellular carcinoma. Chronic infection with hepatitis B has a varied geographical distribution with the highest prevalence being in sub-Saharan Africa and East Asia, where between 5% and 10% of the adult population is infected. Less than 1% of the population in Western Europe and North America are chronic carriers of the disease. The primary route of transmission of hepatitis B is sexual, but blood to blood transmission in unvaccinated persons has a 40% transmission rate. Patients who have active acute hepatitis or who are chronic carriers will have many infectious viral particles present in their blood and can release intact hepatitis B into saliva where it could potentially be a source of infection for other patients. It has been estimated that as little as 0.0001 ml of blood could transmit the disease. The virus consists of a double-layered coat which contains an important glycoprotein called hepatitis B surface antigen (HBsAg). The production of antibodies to HBsAg is a significant event in clearing infection. Two further internal antigens are of relevance, the hepatitis core antigen (HBcAg) and hepatitis B e antigen (HBeAg). The presence of these antigens and antibodies to them is used to determine the status of an individual with hepatitis B, for example whether a patient has experienced previous infection, is immune to infection or has active disease. The period taken from exposure to this virus to the development of symptoms can be up to 8 weeks. An effective vaccine against hepatitis B is available and in many countries satisfactory levels of protective antibodies are a prerequisite to patient treatment by healthcare workers.

HEPATITIS C

Hepatitis C is an enveloped ribonucleic acid (RNA) virus which although transmitted primarily by the sexual route, can also be transmitted by other routes including unsafe injection techniques, inadequate sterilisation of medical equipment and unscreened blood products. The virus can cause mild asymptomatic illness, or chronic disease, often progressing to liver cirrhosis or cancer. There is some controversy as to whether or not dental procedures are a frequent mode of transmission of this virus. Members of the dental team demonstrate a prevalence of antibodies to the virus which is similar to that of the general population (0.1% to 5%), suggesting that it is not a significant occupational hazard. However, a case of transmission of hepatitis C within a dental practice has been reported and suboptimal infection control practices may have facilitated transmission. Infection is detected serologically by the detection of antibodies to the virus (HCV antibodies) and confirmed by direct detection of the virus using the polymerase chain reaction (see Chapter 9). No completely effective vaccine against this disease has been developed. New direct antiviral agents are becoming available, which can cure a high percentage of those infected with Hepatitis C.

Analysis of a large number of percutaneous injuries of individuals who may have been exposed to the hepatitis C virus has shown that the risk of transmission is approximately 3%.

KEY POINTS

Hepatitis B virus (HBV) is a double-shelled DNA virus that can be spread by extremely small volumes of blood and, as such, is a potential risk during the provision of dental treatment. Markers of infection include surface antigen (HBsAg) and a breakdown product of core antigen termed e antigen (HBeAg). An effective vaccine against HBV is available and members of the dental team including dental undergraduates must show evidence of protection by adequate antibody titres and absence of active infection with hepatitis B. Hepatitis C virus (HCV) is an enveloped RNA virus that is spread mainly via blood. The risk of transmission of HCV during dental treatment is low but has been documented. Active infection with HCV is confirmed serologically and by molecular detection of viral nucleic acid. An effective vaccine is not available at the present time. Potential dental students may be required to demonstrate the absence of HCV infection before entry to studies. Dental healthcare workers who become infected with HCV must not treat patients until their viral load is reduced below an infectious threshold.

TRANSMISSIBLE SPONGIFORM ENCEPHALOPATHIES

Prions are the agents thought to be responsible for the transmissible spongiform encephalopathies (TSE) leading to a variety of unusual, lethal, neurological conditions, which are listed in Table 11.5. All of the TSE produce the same range of pathological changes, which include progressive and often rapid loss of voluntary and autonomic function (non-voluntary), resulting in loss of vital processes (e.g., breathing) and eventual death. The signs and symptoms may vary, as does the rapidity of the degeneration, but the result is always death. The most common forms of TSE are those called Creutzfeldt–Jakob disease (CJD).

TABLE 11.5 **Prion–induced diseases**
Kuru
Creutzfeldt–Jakob disease (CJD)
Variant Creutzfeldt–Jakob disease (vCJD)
Fatal familial insomnia
Gertmann–Straussler–Scheinker syndrome
Protease sensitive prionopathy

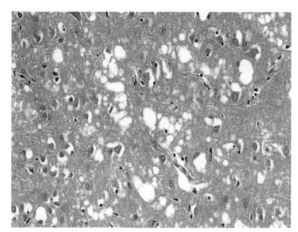

FIGURE 11.7 Section of human brain showing typical degeneration caused by prion disease.

Prions can enter the body through contaminated surgical instruments, surgical grafts, hormones, blood or through the food chain. The mechanism and exact site of entry of prions through the food chain is not precisely known, but is thought to be in the first part of the small intestine. Once in the body, the prions migrate to the brain either through the lymphoid system, or by passage along nerves. Once in the brain, the prions can trigger gross destruction of brain tissue and can lead to vacuolation (holes in the brain, hence spongiform neuropathies; Fig. 11.7).

There are four forms of CJD – sporadic, variant, genetic and iatrogenic. The most common form of CJD is the sporadic form and, fortunately, this is rare. Sporadic CJD has been found in every country in the world where it has been sought. CJD occurs worldwide at a rate of about one case per million population per year. This form of CJD also occurs in vegans and people who have not been exposed to meat. It is thought to be caused by a spontaneous change in a protein in the brain which initiates CJD onset but this is theoretical and as yet unproven.

A new variant of CJD was identified during the UK epidemic of Bovine Spongiform Encephalopathy (BSE; mad cow disease) in the 1990s. Sporadic CJD tends to affect people in their sixth and seventh decades of life and takes a few months to be fatal. In mid-1995, a new variant of CJD that affected people in their twenties was recognised in the UK. This was initially called new variant CJD, but later shortened to variant CJD with the acronym vCJD. Not only did this new clinical type of CJD affect younger individuals than previous forms of CJD but it also had a longer clinical course, with affected persons taking about a year to die. After extensive research, it was concluded that vCJD arose as a result of the consumption of prion-infected beef products.

Genetic forms of CJD are very rare and are due to an abnormal gene; it is not transmitted but tends to affect families. This form of CJD can be found in families which have not been affected before.

Iatrogenic CJD is the transmission of CJD by an intervention, usually a medical or surgical procedure. It was first reported following neurosurgery to remove a central brain tumour in a patient subsequently found to be also suffering from CJD. The instruments used in the operation were sent to the central sterile services in the hospital where they were decontaminated by the usual processes for reuse. Four patients on whom the instruments were subsequently used developed CJD. There have been small number of other cases in which CJD has been transmitted by the administration of contaminated human derived growth hormone and dura mater grafts.

There are no simple diagnostic tests for the identification of prion disease and often the diagnosis is made on typical clinical symptoms and signs. There is currently no treatment for prion disease but there is continued research is this area.

Prions are resistant to normal methods of deactivation, including strong disinfectants, heat, autoclaving and enzyme activity and, currently, we rely on effective cleaning in the decontamination process to reduce the likelihood of onward transmission. Although the numbers of individuals presenting with variant CJD (directly related to the eating of contaminated beef in the UK) is falling, there is evidence from anonymised studies of appendix tissues that approximately 1 in 2000 individuals in the UK is infected with abnormal prions. The concern is that these individuals may pass on infection via inadequately decontaminated instruments and that this form of the disease has longer incubation periods with symptoms presenting perhaps decades after exposure. The tissues encountered in routine dentistry are considered to be low risk, and instruments used, even for individuals with confirmed CJD, may be reprocessed provided there are optimal decontamination processes in place. In this context, the emphasis is on the cleaning stage in the decontamination cycle, because prion agents are unreliably destroyed by the standard sterilisation parameters. Instruments that cannot be cleaned adequately, such as endodontic files and matrix bands, must be regarded as single use.

KEY POINTS

Prions are self-replicating low molecular weight proteins (PrP) that are the cause of rare and fatal transmissible spongiform encephalopathies (TSE), the most important being variant Creutzfeldt–Jacob disease (vCJD). The relevance of the possible presence of prions in dental tissues and provision of dental healthcare is uncertain. However, in view of the difficulty in inactivating and removing prions from equipment, there have been recommendations for single usage of some types of dental instruments and a renewed focus on the cleaning stages of the decontamination cycle.

OTHER MICROORGANISMS OF SIGNIFICANCE

The microbes causing the most serious infections which may be transmitted in the dental surgery have been outlined earlier. A summary of proven cases of infection transmitted by dentistry is shown in Table 11.6. Because patients and staff may be colonised by numerous potential pathogens, it is possible to transmit a wide range of other infections in the dental care environment. These include bacterial pathogens such as MRSA, and other multiresistant bacteria that may have colonised patients and be present on the skin or in the oral cavity. *Clostridium difficile* is an endogenous gut pathogen and is the cause of *C. difficile*-associated diarrhoea. The role of the dental surgery in the transmission of this pathogen is unknown but merits further study because the spores of these bacteria contaminate the environment and are more resistant to cleaning by standard procedures. It is established that direct and indirect contact with nasal secretions is an efficient route of transmission of the respiratory viruses including influenza and parainfluenza. The fundamental processes of infection control to break the chain of infection including hand hygiene and appropriate environmental cleaning must be practised to avoid transmission of these and similar pathogens (see Chapter 12).

TABLE 11.6 Proven cases of infection transmitted by dentistry

Infectious agent	Route of infection
HIV	Use of infected instruments or direct injection of blood
Hepatitis B virus	Sharps injury
Hepatitis C virus	Suboptimal infection control practices including reuse of needles
Herpes simplex type 1 virus	Contact of infected material with skin or eyes
Coxsackie viruses	Contact with skin
Legionella spp	Inhalation of contaminated dental unit water supplies
Pseudomonads (e.g., *Pseudomonas aeruginosa*)	Contact with contaminated dental unit water supplies
MRSA (Methicillin-resistant *Staphylococcus aureus*)	Contact with skin
Mycobacterium tuberculosis	Inhalation of infected droplets

CHAPTER SUMMARY

The systemic status of an individual and the medications taken will impact on the oral microbiota and manifestations of oral disease and infection. A good example of this is the treatment of head and neck cancer, which can lead to Gram-negative enteropathogens colonising the mouth, and cause destructive changes in bone following extractions. A further example of the effect of general health changes on the oral microbiota is when there is impairment of the immune system, which can result in chronic mucocutaneous candidosis. Changes may also be related to the individual's nutrition leading to anaemia and increased risk of, in particular, opportunistic infections. The oral tissues can be directly impacted by the medication taken by the patient for prevention of conditions as evident following receipt of bisphosphonates taken for osteoporosis. A number of systemic infections may be transmitted in the dental care environment, the most significant of which are tuberculosis, HIV, hepatitis B and C and prion disease. The conditions discussed in this chapter indicate the importance of obtaining a thorough medical and drug history for any patient that presents with an oral infection, as there may be implications for diagnosis and management.

In addition, there is growing evidence that the oral microbiota may have an effect on the rest of the body and be important in a number of conditions including cardiovascular and respiratory disease and pregnancy outcomes. More research is required in these areas to establish the nature of the associations and whether modulation of the oral microbiota could play a role in management of these systemic conditions

FURTHER READING

Gibson J, Wray D, Bagg J. Oral staphylococcal mucositis: a new entity in orofacial granulomatosis and Crohn's disease. *Oral Surg Oral Med Oral Pathol Oral Radiol Endod.* 2000;89:171-176.

Guidance for clinical health care workers: Protection against infection with blood-borne viruses. Recommendations of the Expert Advisory Group on AIDS and the Advisory Group on Hepatitis. <www.open.gov.uk/doh/chcguid1.htm>.

Han YW, Wang X. Mobile Microbiome: Oral bacteria in extra-oral infections and inflammation. *J Dent Res.* 2013;92:485-491.

Hooper SJ, Wilson MJ, Crean SJ. Exploring the link between microorganisms and oral cancer: a systematic review of the literature. *Head Neck.* 2009;31:1228-1239.

Khan AA, et al. Diagnosis and Management of Osteonecrosis of the Jaw: A systematic review and international consensus. *J Bone Miner Res.* 2015;30:3-23.

Kholy KE, Genco RJ, Van Dyke TE. Oral infections and cardiovascular disease. *Trends Endocrinol Metab.* 2015;26:315-321.

Lewis MAO, Jordan RCK. *A colour handbook of oral medicine.* 2nd ed. London: Manson publishing; 2012.

Lyons A, Ghazali N. Osteoradionecrosis of the jaws: current understanding of its pathophysiology and treatment. *Br J Oral Maxillofac Surg.* 2008;46:653-660.

Nobb AH, Lamont RJ, Jenkinson HF. *Streptococcus* adherence and colonization. *Microbiol Mol Biol Rev.* 2009;73:407-450.

Ramalho VL, Ramalho HJ, Cipullo JP, et al. Comparison of azithromycin and oral hygiene programs in the treatment of cyclosporine-induced gingival hyperplasia. *Ren Fail.* 2007;29: 265-270.

Roy A, Eisenhut M, Harris RJ, et al. Effect of BCG vaccination against *Mycobacterium tuberculosis* infection in children: systematic review and meta-analysis. *BMJ.* 2014;349:g4643.

Ruggiero SL, Dodson TB, Fantasia J, et al. American Association of Oral and Maxillofacial Surgeons Position Paper on Medication-Related Osteonecrosis of the Jaw-2014 update. *J Oral Maxillofac Surg.* 2014;72:1938-1956.

Shi Z, Xie H, Wang P, et al. Oral hygiene care for critically ill patients to prevent ventilator-associated pneumonia. *Cochrane Database Syst Rev.* 2013;13(8):CD008367.

Walker JT, Dickinson J, Sutton JM, et al. Implications for Creutzfeldt-Jakob disease in dentistry: a review of current knowledge. *J Dent Res.* 2008;87:511-519.

<www.who.int/mediacentre/factsheets/fs204/en/> (Hepatitis B Fact sheet Accessed 06.08.15).

<www.who.int/mediacentre/factsheets/fs164/en/> (Hepatitis C Fact sheet Accessed 06.08.15).

MULTIPLE CHOICE QUESTIONS

Answers on p. 250

1 *Which of the following microorganisms are associated with postirradiation mucositis?*
   a. *Candida albicans*
   b. Non-oral Gram-negative facultatively anaerobic bacteria
   c. Oral Gram-negative obligate anaerobes
   d. Staphylococci

2 *In patients suffering from loss of oral musculature caused by Parkinson disease or following a stroke, which of the following changes has been observed in the oral microbiota?*
   a. An increase in the prevalence of yeasts
   b. An increase in the prevalence of enterobacteria and *Acinetobacter*
   c. An increase in the prevalence of staphylococci, including methicillin-resistant *Staphylococcus aureus*
   d. An increase in the prevalence of mycoplasmas

3 *Which of the following tests assess the extent of susceptibility to infection of an immunocompromised patient?*
   a. Proportion of white blood cells
   b. High-density lipoprotein (HDL)
   c. Liver biopsy
   d. Alanine aminotransferase (ALT)

4 *Radiation affects bone in which of the following ways?*
   a. Hypercellularity
   b. Increases risk for fracture (osteoporotic)
   c. Hypervascularity
   d. Tissue hypoxia

5 *A simple operation on irradiated tissues, such as a tooth extraction, can result in which of the following?*
a. Scar tissue formation
b. Spontaneous death of the surrounding bone (necrosis)
c. Very sensitive tissue
d. Contact dermatitis

6 *The non-specific inflammation of the oral mucosa resulting from irradiation is called which of the following?*
a. Aphthous stomatitis
b. Mucositis
c. Gingivostomatitis
d. Candidiasis

7 *Xerostomia has several causes including which of the following?*
a. Coxsackie virus infection
b. Antimicrobial rinses
c. Pharmaceutical and over-the-counter (OTC) drugs
d. Excess of Vitamin D

8 *Transmissible spongiform encephalopathies (TSEs) are caused by which of the following infectious agents?*
a. Virion
b. Prion
c. Unculturable bacteria
d. HBsAg

9 *Which of the following lesions is strongly associated with human immunodeficiency virus (HIV)?*
a. Necrotising stomatitis
b. Thrombocytopenic purpura
c. Candidosis
d. Hand, foot and mouth disease

10 *Syphilis can present with oral lesions. Which of the following is the causative bacterium?*
a. *Treponema denticola*
b. *Treponema socranskii*
c. *Treponema pallidum*
d. *Treponema putidum*

11 *The current vaccine for tuberculosis (TB) is known as which of the following?*
a. MDR-TB
b. MMR
c. BCG
d. XDR-TB

12 *Oral bacteria have been associated with which of the following conditions?*
a. Atherosclerosis
b. Congenital heart defects
c. Osteoarthritis
d. Postnatal Group B streptococcal septicaemia

13 *Which of the following oral microbiota have not been associated with carcinogenesis?*
a. *P. gingivalis*
b. *F. nucleatum*
c. *S mutans*
d. *C. albicans*

14 *F.* nucleatum *has been liked to many systemic conditions. Which of the following features has* not *been proposed as possible virulence factors in this context?*
a. Helical morphology
b. FadA adhesin
c. Anaerobic growth
d. Interactions with other bacteria

15 *Hepatitis B can be found in the blood of infected patients. The detection of which of the following can be used to diagnose hepatitis B?*
a. HBsAg
b. HBcAg
c. Genomic viral deoxyribonucleic acid (DNA)
d. Genomic viral ribonucleic acid (RNA)

CHAPTER 12

Infection control

IMPORTANCE OF INFECTION CONTROL IN DENTISTRY

The term infection control is defined as all the processes and precautions that can be taken to control the spread of infection. Members of the dental team operate in a unique environment; the oral cavity contains both a higher microbial load and greater bacterial diversity than the rest of the human body. Saliva or plaque may harbour clinically significant viruses such as human immunodeficiency virus (HIV), hepatitis and herpes, in addition to bacterial pathogens that have been associated with infection. Moreover, the practice of dentistry requires the use of a range of sharp instruments and the generation of microbially contaminated aerosol and splatter, providing routes of transmission for these microorganisms. The small size of the typical surgery environment and the fact that patients undergoing treatment are often anxious increases the risk of incidents which may transmit infection. Indeed, from the perspective of the pathogens, it could be suggested that the dental surgery provides an ideal environment for their requirements, that is, for survival and transmission to other human hosts.

The classification of infection control procedures is based on the risk of transmission of the diseases encountered and the procedures undertaken, and are described as high, medium or low level. High-level infection control is where a patient is isolated from all contact with healthcare professionals or family members and every procedure is done with appropriate barriers in place. High-level disinfection is employed when patients contract highly infectious disease such as the haemorrhagic fevers, which if transmitted are fatal. Medium-level infection control is where barrier protection is used, but the risk of contracting the disease is not high but still possible. Low-level infection control measures are used where the risk of transmission is low and only standard hygiene practices are required.

There are problems in categorising which level of infection control is appropriate for dentistry. Many of the patients who attend dental surgeries may asymptomatically carry potentially infectious diseases, but they do not know they are infected (e.g., hepatitis B or C). The risk of transmission could be high in dentistry if there is blood to blood contact through, for example, an inoculation (sharps) injury. In addition, the major fluids encountered in dentistry are blood and saliva and these could potentially transmit agents of infectious disease. Therefore the risk for most of the surgical procedures undertaken in dentistry is in the medium category. Because most dental patients who asymptomatically carry disease are unaware of their infectious status, it is wise to treat all patients and all potentially infectious bodily fluids with the same precautions; these are often described as Standard or Universal Precautions.

WHICH INFECTIOUS DISEASES ARE TRANSMITTED BY DENTISTRY?

Many communicable diseases can potentially be transmitted in the dental care environment, including a range of infections circulating in the community. However, the number of proven cases of infectious diseases that have been transmitted by dental personnel, treatment or patients is very limited and such diseases are listed in Table 11.5. The pathogens include *Mycobacterium tuberculosis* (the causative organism of the majority of cases of tuberculosis in humans), bloodborne viruses (BBVs) such as HIV, hepatitis B and C, meticillin-resistant *Staphylococcus aureus* (MRSA), *Pseudomonas* species, and the hand, foot and mouth virus (see Chapters 9 and 11).

In parallel with other countries, the number of individuals infected with the BBVs (HIV, hepatitis B and hepatitis C) continues to increase, with thousands of newly diagnosed individuals each year in the UK. It is theoretically possible for BBVs to be transmitted both from a healthcare worker (HCW) to a patient and from a patient to a HCW. The transmission of hepatitis B to the dental team has reduced significantly with the increased uptake of vaccination for HCWs. However, a recent case of transmission of hepatitis B between patients in a dental surgery following multiple extractions highlights the fact that patients may not be protected against this virus. Herpes simplex virus is highly infectious and can be transmitted in the dental surgery by direct contact with either lesions or contaminated aerosols and splatter. It is important to remember that patients without obvious signs of infection, such as cold sores, can still transmit infection, as they may be shedding the virus in their saliva. This virus has been responsible for blindness, usually in dental personnel who do not wear protective spectacles. The recent influenza pandemic and the discovery of new viruses such as the agents associated with severe acute respiratory syndrome (SARS) and Middle East respiratory syndrome (MERS) have highlighted the need for the dental profession to remain vigilant and to be prepared to respond appropriately to the threat of novel pathogens by understanding that additional measures may be required to protect patients and team members.

Tuberculosis (TB) is a global problem. Following an increased incidence in the United Kingdom from 1990 to 2005, rates of newly diagnosed TB have stabilised. However, the incidence in the UK is still higher than most other European countries with over 8000 new cases in 2012. Members of the dental team should be aware of the signs and symptoms of TB in staff and patients, and encourage them to seek early diagnosis and treatment (see Chapter 11). Untreated TB is highly infectious, and patients should not be treated in the primary care environment until two weeks after they have commenced appropriate antibiotic therapy.

Dental unit waterlines are almost universally contaminated with a range of bacteria to levels well above the drinking water recommendations. Pathogens such as *Pseudomonas* and *Legionella* species may be present. Legionnaire's disease is rare in the UK with just over 100 cases on average per year originating in this country, but the infection may be associated with high mortality. *Pseudomonas* infections from infected dental unit waterlines are rare in otherwise healthy individuals. However, it seems reasonable to ensure that the water provided for patients conforms to drinking water guidelines (see later section on dental unit waterline maintenance).

Some authors have reviewed the low number of transmissions of infection in dentistry and have questioned whether many of the precautions used are necessary or justified, based on a risk assessment. Whether or not infection control measures in dentistry are necessary cannot now be answered, as it would be impossible to revert to anything but standard precautions. Public pressure and ethical responsibility would prevent any diminution in the standard of precautions or to test a reduced level of protection. In addition, most regulatory authorities outline requirements for infection control in dentistry and litigate if the standards are not met.

ROUTES OF TRANSMISSION

Bacteria and viruses may be transmitted by direct contact between patients and staff in the dental surgery, and indirect contact via the environment, equipment or instruments. In this way MRSA, coliform bacteria, herpes simplex virus and the influenza virus may be transmitted. Other infections, such as TB, are spread predominantly by the airborne route. The most significant route of transmission in the dental surgery is via inoculation, which includes percutaneous injury via breaches in the skin, as well as splash injuries, whereby pathogens gain access to the body via the mucous membranes of the eye, nasal or oral mucosa. Although the majority of cases of transmission of BBVs have been via a sharps injury penetrating the skin, it is possible for these viruses to cause infection via a splash injury, albeit at a much lower rate. A rare route for the transmission of infection is via human bites. Aerosols are generated on a daily basis in the practice of dentistry, and these may be contaminated with bacteria and BBVs. The smaller particles may remain airborne for several hours and migrate through the local environment, for example, into the waiting room, and although unlikely to transmit BBVs, may be a reservoir of bacterial pathogens. The larger particles, known as splatter, generally settle within 1 metre of the point of origin, that is, the patient's mouth, and these particles may contain both bacterial pathogens and BBVs at levels high enough to transmit infection to subsequent patients or staff by direct contact. A further potential route of infection in the dental surgery environment is via instruments not adequately decontaminated.

KEY POINTS

A large number of microorganisms may be transmitted between patients and staff in the dental surgery environment, including potentially serious infectious agents such as the blood-borne viruses, tuberculosis and prions. The main routes of transmission are via inoculation; percutaneous for sharps injuries; transmucosal for splash injuries. Inoculation of infectious material into patients may occur via instruments that have been inadequately decontaminated. In addition, transmission of communicable diseases and opportunistic pathogens circulating in the community may occur via the aerosol or droplet route and via direct and indirect contact.

BREAKING THE CHAIN OF INFECTION
PERSONAL PROTECTION

Personal protection is an important part of infection control and includes immunisation, protection of hands, eye and face, protective clothing and the avoidance and appropriate management of inoculation (sharps and splash) injuries. Protection of the HCW in this way also protects the transmission of any infections to subsequent patients.

IMMUNISATION

The protection of dental personnel by immunisation before they engage in dental procedures is an important part of infection control. Nowadays, many regulatory authorities require that dentists, nurses, hygienists and therapists are not carrying any potentially infectious disease before they undertake or assist with any dental procedures. Some countries will permit individuals infected with, for example, BBVs to continue to treat patients provided they have received treatment which reduces the level of the virus to below the threshold considered to be capable of transmitting infection. Freedom from infectious disease and satisfactory records of immunisation should be a contractual prerequisite before dental personnel are employed. Although recommendations will vary between countries, examples of recommended vaccinations are listed in Table 12.1 and include those that are part of the routine vaccination schedules of childhood. In most parts of the world, a full course of hepatitis B vaccination needs to be satisfactorily completed before any exposure to clinical procedures or equipment contaminated with oral tissue or fluids.

HAND PROTECTION

Hands of dental personnel are potentially one of the most vulnerable areas of the body to infectious disease and also may be a potential vector for infection. The maintenance of an intact layer of epithelium is an important part of protection. The problem is that procedures such as handwashing in soap and water, and covering hands with gloves, can have a serious and deleterious effect on the integrity and pliability of the skin. Both glove wearing and handwashing can have a hyperosmotic effect on the hands and cause the skin to crack and lose its pliability, thereby rendering it

TABLE 12.1 Recommended vaccinations for all dental personnel

Vaccine	Length of protection
Diphtheria	Probably lifelong
Tetanus	At least 10 years but probably lifelong
Pertussis (Whooping Cough)	Probably lifelong
Poliomyelitis	Probably lifelong
Measles, Mumps, Rubella	Probably lifelong
Varicella-zoster virus (chickenpox)	Varies, but on average at least 10 years.
Influenza	Annual vaccinations required
Tuberculosis (BCG)	Probably less than lifelong in most recipients
Hepatitis B	At least 5 years but probably lifelong

susceptible to microbial ingression. Hand creams used after every session restore essential oils to the skin and help retain pliability.

Handwashing should be performed by a systematic method, such as the technique devised by Ayliffe (Fig. 12.1) to ensure all surfaces are washed and rinsed. If the hands are not visibly contaminated, then combined alcohol and disinfectant hand rubs may be used. One advantage of hand rubs is that they are less injurious to the integrity of hand skin and many contain emollients that help protect the skin from drying.

GLOVES

Gloves are an essential part of infection control in dentistry. They provide a physical barrier which protects the hands from the ingress of microorganisms and should be worn for all dental procedures. They are a single-use item, a new pair should be used for each patient and they should be changed when torn. Most gloves are made out of natural latex rubber and

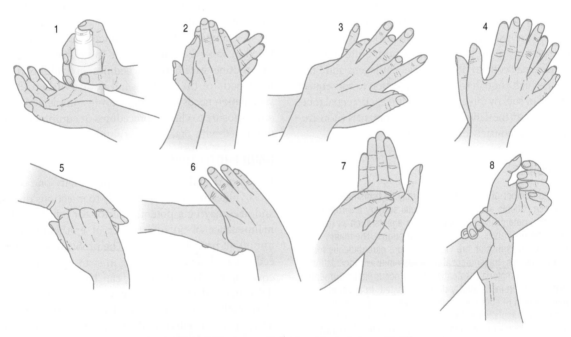

FIGURE 12.1 The systematic handwashing technique of Ayliffe.

contain low-molecular-weight proteins that can be immunologically active. These low-molecular-weight proteins can penetrate the skin and induce inflammation; this condition is called irritant contact dermatitis. All rings and watches should be removed before handwashing or donning gloves, otherwise irritant contact dermatitis can ensue. Poor handwashing technique with soap and water can also cause irritant contact dermatitis, and this condition can be cured by changing the make of gloves and careful attention to handwashing. Topical steroids may help alleviate the condition in more severe cases of irritant contact dermatitis. In one major survey of hand problems in dental personnel, approximately 20% were shown to suffer intermittently from irritant contact dermatitis.

Immunological reactions to latex proteins are more serious and can be life-threatening if they progress to anaphylaxis. Sensitivity to latex proteins is fortunately still rare, but in the USA it has been estimated that 40% of medical personnel have detectable antibodies to latex proteins. Immunological contact dermatitis is immediate and the inflammation spreads well beyond the glove-wearing area (Fig. 12.2); it is not controlled by handwashing and always requires steroid or other systemic therapy. Concern about latex proteins is now so serious that latex-free gloves are increasingly being used as a matter of routine in many healthcare facilities.

Some gloves contain donning agents which help them to be put on dry hands. One agent that has been extensively used as a donning agent is starch, but it should be avoided because it causes latex allergens to be dispersed in the atmosphere. If allowed to contaminate wounds, starch can cause granulomas (excessive fibrous tissue) to form and it can prevent restorations such as veneers from adhering properly to teeth.

EYE AND FACE PROTECTION

Eye protection is mandatory for all dental operators. The eye can be contaminated by patients who cough pooled saliva and blood from the floor of the mouth into the face of the operators (this is called 'splatter'). Eyes can also be contaminated from aerosols generated from the mouth when high-speed instruments are used with coolants (Fig. 12.3). Because 30% of patients will have significant numbers of herpes simplex type 1 virus in the mouth, even in the absence of obvious herpetic lesions, the risk of infection is high. Herpetic infections of the eye have a significant chance of causing blindness, and this has been documented in a number of dental personnel in the UK. Protective or

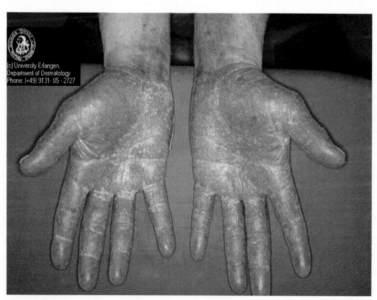

FIGURE 12.2 Immunological contact dermatitis caused by glove wearing. Note the inflammation spreads beyond the glove wearing area (courtesy of the University of Ehlingham).

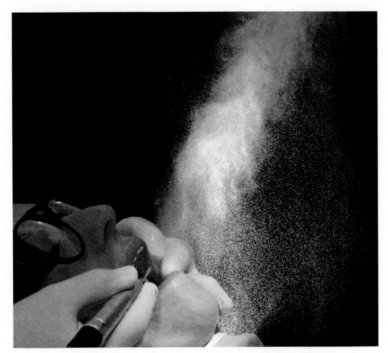

FIGURE 12.3 Aerosol generated by high-speed dental handpiece.

prescription glasses with appropriate side protection should be worn during treatment; these require washing and drying after use. An alternative form of eye protection is a visor, and some designs incorporate a mask.

The basic surgical type of mask worn in dentistry does not provide full microbiologic protection; they provide protection against splatter but not against aerosols. They are a single-use item and should be thrown away after use. The best protection against aerosols is high-vacuum suction which should be switched on before any coolants are used. The role of aerosols in the transmission of infection in dentistry is still unproven, but it is well-established that many diseases such as TB, Legionnaires' disease and infectious mononucleosis are spread by this route.

SURGERY CLOTHING

There is a wide variety of surgery clothing available, and it is clear that these items become contaminated by aerosol and splatter during operative procedures. Surgery clothing should be capable of being washed at temperatures greater than 60°C as this kills many potentially pathogenic microorganisms. The debate

about whether surgery clothing should have long or short sleeves is still unresolved. Many argue that long sleeves protect the arms from microorganisms. However, there is a potential to transmit the microbes present on the sleeves to subsequent patients. Disposable long-sleeved gowns are an option, but come with a considerable economic and environmental burden. Others argue that bare arms can be easily washed and facilitate optimal hand hygiene. Consequently, many healthcare facilities have adopted a 'bare below the elbows' policy.

INOCULATION INJURIES

Inoculation injuries have a high potential for the transmission of serious infection as they can involve blood-to-blood contact. Injuries may be sustained via a percutaneous or mucosal route. Percutaneous injuries are caused by needles or other sharp instruments piercing the skin or, less commonly in dentistry, following human bites. Mucosal injuries include splashes or other contact with the mucosa of the mouth, nose or eye. Injury rates can be reduced in a number of ways including the use of safety local anaesthetic

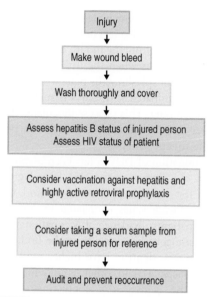

Injury

↓

Make wound bleed

↓

Wash thoroughly and cover

↓

Assess hepatitis B status of injured person
Assess HIV status of patient

↓

Consider vaccination against hepatitis and
highly active retroviral prophylaxis

↓

Consider taking a serum sample from
injured person for reference

↓

Audit and prevent reoccurrence

FIGURE 12.4 Management of an inoculation injury.

syringes, extra care when handling sharp instruments, and policies that restrict resheathing of needles or that encourage the use of needle-resheathing devices. A schema for dealing with sharps injuries is shown in Fig. 12.4. After immediate first aid, a risk assessment as to the likelihood of transmission of any infectious agents should be undertaken and the need for prophylaxis for hepatitis B and/or HIV determined. In most cases, baseline blood will be taken from the injured party and tested for the presence of BBVs. An audit of the reasons for the sharps injury should take place and action taken to prevent reoccurrence.

KEY POINTS

> Breaking the chain of infection involves a number of strategies including bolstering the immunity of staff (and the public), the use of protective clothing, face and eye wear, and optimal hand hygiene. Staff must take steps to avoid inoculation injuries and know how to manage them when they occur.

DECONTAMINATION OF SURGERY ENVIRONMENT AND EQUIPMENT

Decontamination is a term used to define a number of processes generally involving cleaning, disinfection and in some cases sterilisation of an object to remove contaminants, including microorganisms to make that object safe, in that it no longer poses a risk. The term can be used in the context of the surgery environment, equipment, appliances or dental instruments. The two main stages in the decontamination process are cleaning followed by either disinfection or sterilisation. Disinfection eliminates nearly all recognised pathogenic microorganisms but not necessarily all microbial forms (for example bacterial spores) on inanimate objects. Sterilisation is the removal of all viable infectious agents.

SURGERY DESIGN

To reduce the risk of cross infection, most surgeries incorporate three distinct areas or zones: an operator's zone, an assistant zone and a separate room for the decontamination of instruments. The first two zones should have hand-hygiene basins and should not be used for any decontamination processes. Surgeries should be tidy and uncluttered and designed to allow optimal disinfection.

SURFACE DECONTAMINATION

The most important element of surface disinfection is cleaning. Surfaces should be thoroughly cleaned, ideally with a detergent initially and then disinfected with an appropriate agent. Cleaning is a vital stage because disinfectants will not act effectively in the presence of organic matter. Although a large number of types of surface disinfectant are available, it is how they are used that is probably more important than their disinfectant action. The aim of surface cleaning is to remove the maximum number of microorganisms by dilution and cleaning; when this is complete then the disinfectant will kill the remainder. Disinfectant should be applied to surfaces, wiped off using a lot of energy and the process repeated. This is a progressive dilution technique with each application of disinfectant further reducing the number of microorganisms present.

DRAINS AND SPITTOONS

Drains and spittoons are heavily contaminated areas as they collect saliva, blood and other material. These areas are prone to the formation of tenacious biofilms on the surfaces of their tubes. Biofilms are formed on the inner surfaces of tubing and are held together by extracellular slime-like materials secreted by the constituent micro-organisms (see Chapter 5). Microorganisms in biofilms are highly tolerant of disinfectants and very difficult to remove. A combination of a bactericidal disinfectant and a detergent should be used on drains and spittoons, and this should be done after every session to prevent biofilm accumulation.

DENTAL UNIT WATER SYSTEMS

Water delivered from dental unit water systems (DUWS) is not sterile and can contain high numbers of bacteria (sometimes exceeding one million colony forming units (CFU)/ml), including opportunistic pathogens such as *Legionella pneumophila, Mycobacterium* species, *Pseudomonas aeruginosa* and *Candida* species. The source water is often tap or deionised water, and this should have low microbial counts. The high microbial load in the outflowing water is because of the rapid development of biofilms (see Chapter 5) on the inner surfaces of tubing in DUWS (Fig. 12.5), from which large numbers of microorganisms are shed into the water. The water in DUWS is static for long periods of time and is constantly heated to a temperature of between 22°C (room temperature) and 37°C (body temperature), which also encourages microbial growth. DUWS can also be contaminated with microorganisms derived from the mouth by back-siphonage. The latter occurs as when the turbine drill is deactivated, to prevent splashing the patient, a small amount of water contaminated with saliva is sucked back into the turbine tubing. This process inoculates the dental unit water with oral microbes, which can be passed on to subsequent patients.

Contamination of DUWS has been responsible for the death of a dentist in the USA from legionellosis, and also for amoebic eye infections and infections caused by *Pseudomonas aeruginosa* in immunocompromised patients. Evidence of occupational exposure to such pathogens has come from the finding that in some countries, dentists have higher antibody titres to *L. pneumophila* than other employment groups. Although the evidence is conflicting, contamination has also been implicated as a cause of late onset asthma in dental personnel from endotoxins released from the Gram-negative bacteria present in aerosols from DUWS (see Fig. 12.3). Guidelines have been introduced to set standards for the maximum microbial load delivered by water from dental units. In the USA, this is 200 CFU/ml, and other countries are setting equivalent standards. To achieve these levels, DUWS need purging with disinfectants that are effective not only against microorganisms in the liquid phase, but which are also active against established biofilms, as these are inherently more tolerant of antimicrobial agents (see Chapter 5). Products containing hydrogen peroxide and silver ions have been found to be particularly effective. Care has to be taken to ensure that any disinfectant is used according to the manufacturer's instructions (e.g., frequency of application and concentration), and is compatible with the materials used in the construction of the particular dental unit.

DECONTAMINATION OF APPLIANCES AND IMPRESSIONS

Before leaving the surgery, appliances and impressions should be washed to remove debris and then disinfected by immersion. Spraying of disinfectants onto the surface is ineffective. A number of immersion disinfectants are now available which minimise distortion of impression materials. Likewise, appropriate

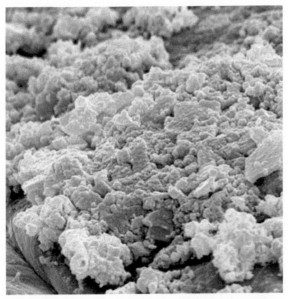

FIGURE 12.5 Scanning electron micrograph of a biofilm formed on the inner surface of tubing in a dental unit.

decontamination of appliances should take place upon receipt from the laboratory, before placement in the patient's mouth.

DECONTAMINATION OF INSTRUMENTS

The term decontamination has been defined in the previous section, and in the context of instrument decontamination, there are many processes that contribute to the decontamination cycle (Fig. 12.6): cleaning, disinfection, sterilisation and safe storage to prevent recontamination.

CRITICAL AND NON-CRITICAL INSTRUMENTS

Critical instruments are those that may come into contact with sterile body sites and will require sterilisation before reuse. When critical instruments are purchased, the manufacturer must provide a statement of how they are to be cleaned and sterilised. Semicritical items are those that may come into contact with intact mucous membranes and require either sterilisation or

high-level disinfection. Often items are difficult if not impossible to sterilise and disposal is the best option; a good example of this is saliva ejectors and other items with lumens that are difficult to clean effectively. Equipment such as patient spectacles and bib chains are not heavily contaminated and so are not critical instruments and are best decontaminated by cleaning and disinfection.

Unless critical instruments are cleaned they cannot be sterilised. This presents a particular problem in dentistry in relation to transmissible spongiform encephalopathies such as Creutzfeldt-Jakob disease (CJD) because none of the currently available methods can be guaranteed to remove prion contamination, but may reduce it to levels below the threshold for transmission (see Chapter 11). All methods used for cleaning must be validated (shown to work), and be regularly checked. The three methods currently used for instrument cleaning in dentistry are manual washing, ultrasonics and washer disinfectors.

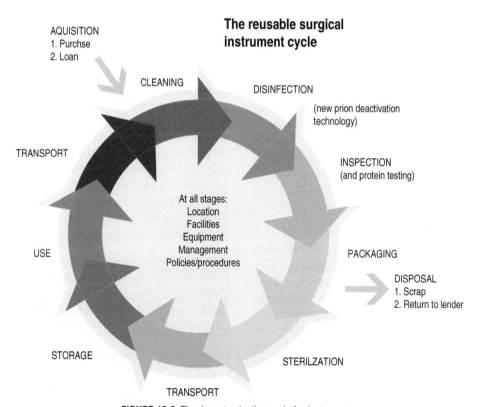

FIGURE 12.6 The decontamination cycle for instruments.

MANUAL CLEANING

This is by far the most common method of cleaning instruments, but it is the least efficient and is difficult to validate reliably. Inherently it is dangerous as it increases the risk of percutaneous sharps injuries and generates contaminated aerosols. Consequently, this method of cleaning is not recommended.

ULTRASONIC CLEANING

Cleaning by the ultrasonic method involves placing the instruments into a bath containing a detergent and applying an ultrasonic generator to create vacuums within the liquid, which collapse on the instrument surface and release energy. The energy dislodges material adherent to the instrument. Ultrasonic baths have to be properly commissioned and periodically validated if they are to be effective. The correct detergent has to be used in the bath and the instruments must be separated so the liquid can flow round them. The instruments must be subjected to the manufacturer's recommended length of time without interruption, that is, instruments may not be added midcycle. Ultrasonic baths need periodic testing, and the easiest test to use is the foil ablation test in which pieces of foil are placed in the bath and are destroyed by the ultrasonics. Another test that is recommended for ultrasonic baths is a residual protein test. This test employs detection of a test soil which is placed on an instrument before decontamination. The reader is recommended to textbooks and guidelines on infection control that are cited in the Further Reading section at the end of this chapter. Ultrasonics are effective cleaning methods if used properly and checked regularly but are not as efficient as the use of a washer disinfector.

WASHER DISINFECTORS

These machines are designed to clean and disinfect instruments to a high and reproducible standard. They first rinse the instruments in cold water which removes most of the debris. The machine then washes the instruments in hot water and detergent, rinses them and then heats the instruments to a temperature between 80°C and 90°C for 1 to 3 minutes. Some washer disinfectors incorporate a subsequent drying cycle. The length of the cycles of these machines is between 20 and 60 minutes. They require a good standard of water which can be produced by cleaning mains supplies with ion exchange resins or by reverse osmosis. Washer disinfectors require daily monitoring to check that the manufacturer's parameters for the machine are met. They need periodic residual protein tests as described for ultrasonic machines.

STERILISATION OF INSTRUMENTS

An instrument has to be clean before sterilisation, otherwise residual material can protect microorganisms in biofilms retained on the surface and they can remain viable. Sterilisation is defined as the complete killing of all forms of life including prions. In practice, sterility is probably never achieved as the type of process used does not kill or inactivate prions (see Chapter 11).

In dentistry, the process used most often for sterilisation is the autoclave which uses the latent heat of steam to achieve its killing of microorganisms. Water is heated under pressure beyond its boiling point and circulates around the instruments in a pressure-resistant chamber. The steam condenses on the instruments until they are heated to the temperature of the steam. This temperature is then held until the instruments are sterile. The temperature-time combinations that are necessary for sterility in autoclaves are shown in Table 12.2. The efficiency of killing in an autoclave is partly dependent on the amount of air that is driven out of the chamber. The more air that is driven out of the autoclave chamber, the more efficient the penetration of steam. The penetration of the steam is important when instruments containing small diameter tubes are being sterilised (e.g., dental handpieces). The most common form of autoclave is called a type N in which the air is pushed out of the chamber by the steam; this type of autoclave is only suitable

TABLE 12.2 Recommended temperature, time and pressure combinations for sterilisation		
Temperature (°C)	Time (min)	Pressure (bar)
134	3	2
115	30	1
121	15	1

for solid instruments. Type S autoclaves pump the air out and a large amount of residual air is removed; these autoclaves are suitable for some instruments with tubes as specified by the manufacturer. Type B autoclaves repeatedly pump out the air from the chamber and the amount of residual air remaining is small; these autoclaves are recommended for any instrument. The autoclaves recommended for dental instruments are type B or S. Autoclaves need periodic testing and this is best done by thermocouples. In some countries the mandatory testing of autoclaves is done by assessing the killing of the heat-resistant bacterium, *Geobacillus stearothermophilus*. The spores are contained on strips in the autoclave for one cycle and then incubated; if the autoclave works then no growth should occur.

STORAGE OF INSTRUMENTS

Once sterilised, instruments are best stored in dry cassettes, bags or pouches. They can remain sterile for considerable periods of time if kept airtight and dry. If stacked and covered, it is considered acceptable to use unwrapped trays of decontaminated instruments within one clinical session as long as there is no recontamination from the surgery environment. The length of storage for wrapped instruments is a cause of much debate and is dependent on the nature of processing including particularly the type of steriliser that is used. However, the guiding principles are the prevention of recontamination and the examination of instruments before use.

WASTE DISPOSAL

Clinical waste is material which has been exposed to blood, saliva, tissue or other bodily fluids. It has to be disposed of separately from other non-clinical waste by incineration or by burial in deep landfill sites. Sharps must be kept in rigid containers until disposal. Different countries have varying regulations for the disposal of this material with the primary aim of protecting the public and the environment.

CHAPTER SUMMARY

Infection control in dentistry is important and standard precautions must be used for all patients. Personal

KEY POINTS

Decontamination is a term used to define a number of processes to remove microorganisms to make objects safe for use. The term can apply to the surgery environment, equipment, appliances or dental instruments. The basic procedure involves two stages: cleaning followed by either disinfection or, in the case of critical instruments, sterilisation. A number of different cleaning methods are available for instruments and include manual processes, the use of ultrasonic equipment or a washer disinfector. The latter cleans most efficiently, can be validated reliably and is, therefore, the preferred approach. The microbial load within dental unit water systems must be managed to ensure that the water is at least of drinking water quality.

protection includes ensuring optimal vaccination against infectious diseases, the wearing of protective equipment (gloves, face and eye protection) and clinical clothing that is capable of being washed above 60°C. Members of the dental team must take care in handling sharps and be aware of how to assess risk and manage injuries should they occur. The surgery, equipment and instruments must be decontaminated appropriately, which usually involves a preliminary cleaning step followed by disinfection or sterilisation. The most effective method for the decontamination of instruments is via a washer disinfector and a steam steriliser. Consideration must be given to instrument storage to prevent recontamination. Clinical waste must be disposed of safely according to local regulations.

FURTHER READING

Gill ON, Spencer Y, Richard-Loendt A, et al. Prevalent abnormal prion protein in human appendixes after bovine spongiform encephalopathy epizootic: large-scale survey. *BMJ.* 2013;15:347.

Martin MV, Fulford MR, Preston AJ. *Infection control for the dental team.* Quintessence Publications, Surrey, UK; 2008.

Oosthuysen J, Potgieter E, Fossey A. Compliance with infection prevention and control in oral health-care facilities: a global perspective. *Int Dent J.* 2014;64:297-311.

Redd JT, Baumach J, Kohn W, et al. Patient to patient transmission of hepatitis B virus associated with oral surgery. *J Infect Dis.* 2007;195:1311-1314.

Walker JT, Dickinson J, Sutton JM, et al. Cleanability of dental instruments-implications of residual protein and risks of Creutzfeldt-Jakob disease. *Br Dent J.* 2007;203:395-401.

Walker JT, Marsh PD. Microbial biofilm formation in DUWS and their control using disinfectants. *J Dent.* 2007;35:721-730.

MULTIPLE CHOICE QUESTIONS

Answers on p. 250

1 *Which of the following diseases may be transmitted in the dental surgery?*
a. Influenza
b. Measles
c. Chicken pox
d. All of the above

2 *Which statement is false regarding hepatitis B?*
a. The vaccine usually provides lifelong protection
b. Dental nurses do not need to receive the vaccine
c. It may be spread via splatter
d. It is more likely to be spread by the percutaneous route than the mucosal route

3 *Select the false answer from these statements regarding gloves.*
a. Gloves must be changed between patients
b. Gloves should be changed when torn
c. Gloves may be decontaminated using alcohol rub
d. The use of latex gloves is being phased out

4 *Which is the true statement concerning facial protection?*
a. Masks provide complete microbiological protection
b. A mask must be worn in addition to a full face visor
c. Masks may be reused for each patient over the course of one clinical session
d. Masks must be changed after every patient use

5 *Which one of the following statements is false?*
a. Long sleeved garments must be worn to protect the forearms from splatter
b. Bare below the elbows facilitates optimal hand hygiene
c. Surgery clothing should be washed at temperatures of greater than 60°C
d. It is considered unacceptable to wear protective clothing outside the surgery

6 *Which of the following is the correct definition of decontamination?*
a. The removal of all microorganisms except spores
b. The killing of all microorganisms including spores
c. The physical removal of organic matter
d. A combination of processes which removes or destroys contamination so that infectious agents or other contaminants cannot reach a susceptible site in sufficient quantities to initiate infection or other harmful response

7 *Choose the false statement from the following relating to dental unit water supplies (DUWS)*
a. Those with an independent reservoir are immune to contamination
b. Microbial contamination must be limited to below approximately 200 bacteria per ml of water
c. Biofilms form inside the waterlines, and these are more tolerant of biocides than the free floating (planktonic) bacteria
d. The bacteria that cause Legionnaire disease may be isolated from some dental unit water supplies

8 *Regarding the cleaning of instruments, which statement is true?*
a. Manual cleaning is better than ultrasonic cleaning
b. Ultrasonic cleaning machines do not need to be tested
c. Washer disinfectors sterilise instruments
d. Manual cleaning is associated with a higher incidence of inoculation injuries

Multiple choice answers

CHAPTER 1

1	b	5	b
2	b	6	d
3	d	7	a
4	d	8	b

CHAPTER 2

1	a	6	b
2	c	7	b
3	a	8	b
4	d	9	a
5	d	10	d

CHAPTER 3

1	a	6	c
2	d	7	b
3	c	8	c
4	a	9	a
5	b	10	b

CHAPTER 4

1	c	7	b
2	b	8	d
3	d	9	c
4	a	10	b
5	b	11	c
6	d	12	c

13	a	15	a
14	b		

CHAPTER 5

1	c	9	c
2	a	10	a
3	d	11	b
4	a	12	d
5	d	13	b
6	c	14	a
7	c	15	c
8	a		

CHAPTER 6

1	c	11	b
2	a	12	a
3	b	13	d
4	b	14	c
5	b	15	d
6	c	16	b
7	b	17	a
8	c	18	b
9	d	19	c
10	a	20	b

CHAPTER 7

1 a	9 a and b
2 c	10 c
3 d	11 b
4 b	12 c
5 b	13 b
6 b	14 a
7 b	15 b
8 c	

CHAPTER 8

1 c	6 d
2 c	7 c
3 d	8 a
4 b	9 a
5 d	10 b

CHAPTER 9

1 d	7 a
2 b	8 b
3 d	9 b
4 c	10 b
5 b	11 d
6 b	12 d

CHAPTER 10

1 d	8 c
2 c	9 b
3 c	10 c
4 b	11 a
5 d	12 b
6 a	13 c
7 d	14 b

CHAPTER 11

1 b	9 c
2 b	10 c
3 a	11 c
4 d	12 a
5 b	13 c
6 b	14 a
7 c	15 a
8 b	

CHAPTER 12

1 d	5 a
2 b	6 d
3 c	7 a
4 d	8 d

Index

Page numbers followed by 'f' indicate figures, 't' indicate tables, and 'b' indicate boxes.